THE ECG HANDBOOK OF CONTEMPORARY CHALLENGES

THE ECG HANDBOOK OF CONTEMPORARY CHALLENGES

EDITORS

Mohammad Shenasa, MD

Mark E. Josephson, MD

N.A. Mark Estes III, MD

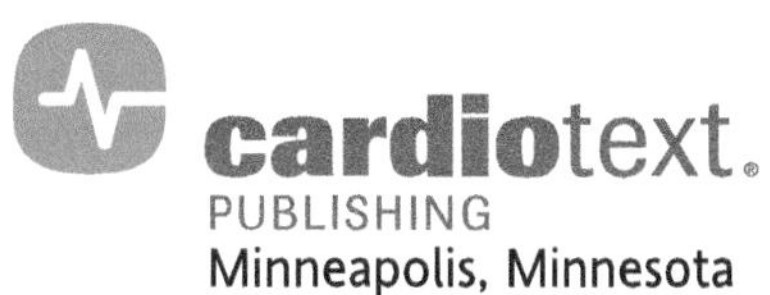

Cardiotext Publishing, LLC
3405 W. 44th Street
Minneapolis, Minnesota 55410
USA

www.cardiotextpublishing.com

Any updates to this book may be found at: www.cardiotextpublishing.com/ecg-handbook-of-contemporary-challenges

Comments, inquiries, and requests for bulk sales can be directed to the publisher at: info@cardiotextpublishing.com.

This book is intended for educational purposes and to further general scientific and medical knowledge, research, and understanding of the conditions and associated treatments discussed herein. This book is not intended to serve as and should not be relied upon as recommending or promoting any specific diagnosis or method of treatment for a particular condition or a particular patient. It is the reader's responsibility to determine the proper steps for diagnosis and the proper course of treatment for any condition or patient, including suitable and appropriate tests, medications or medical devices to be used for or in conjunction with any diagnosis or treatment.

Due to ongoing research, discoveries, modifications to medicines, equipment and devices, and changes in government regulations, the information contained in this book may not reflect the latest standards, developments, guidelines, regulations, products or devices in the field. Readers are responsible for keeping up to date with the latest developments and are urged to review the latest instructions and warnings for any medicine, equipment or medical device. Readers should consult with a specialist or contact the vendor of any medicine or medical device where appropriate.

Except for the publisher's website associated with this work, the publisher is not affiliated with and does not sponsor or endorse any websites, organizations or other sources of information referred to herein.

The publisher and the authors specifically disclaim any damage, liability, or loss incurred, directly or indirectly, from the use or application of any of the contents of this book.

Unless otherwise stated, all figures and tables in this book are used courtesy of the authors.

Library of Congress Control Number: 2015931353

ISBN: 978-1-935395-88-1

Printed in The United States of America

CONTENTS

CONTRIBUTORS

Editors

Mohammad Shenasa, MD, FACC, FHRS, FAHA, FESC
Attending Physician, Department of Cardiovascular Services, O'Conner Hospital; Heart & Rhythm Medical Group, San Jose, California

Mark E. Josephson, MD, FACC, FHRS, FAHA
Chief, Cardiovascular Medicine Division; Director, Harvard-Thorndike Electrophysiology Institute and Arrhythmia Service, Beth Israel Deaconess Medical Center; Herman C. Dana Professor of Medicine, Harvard Medical School, Boston, Massachusetts

N.A. Mark Estes III, MD, FACC, FHRS, FAHA, FESC
Professor of Medicine,
Tufts University School of Medicine;
Director, New England Cardiac Arrhythmia Center,
Tufts Medical Center, Boston, Massachusetts

Contributors

Dominic J. Abrams, MD, MRCP
Assistant Professor of Pediatrics, Harvard Medical School; Director, Inherited Cardiac Arrhythmia Program, Boston Children's Hospital, Boston, Massachusetts

Arnon Adler, MD
Tel Aviv Medical Center, Tel Aviv University, Tel Aviv, Israel

Konstantinos N. Aronis, MD
Senior Resident, Department of Medicine, Boston University Medical Center, Boston, Massachusetts

Yousef Bader, MD
Senior Fellow in Clinical Cardiac Electrophysiology, Tufts Medical Center, Division of Cardiac Electrophysiology; Instructor in Medicine, Tufts University School of Medicine, Boston, Massachusetts

Hiroko Beck, MD
Assistant Professor, Clinical Cardiac Electrophysiology, University of Buffalo, Buffalo, New York

Josep Brugada, MD, PhD
Chairman, Cardiovascular Center; Professor, Fundacio Clinic; Medical Director, Hospital Clinic, Barcelona, Spain

Pedro Brugada, MD, PhD
Heart Rhythm Management Center, Cardiovascular Center, Free University of Brussels, Brussels, Belgium

Ramon Brugada, MD, PhD
Dean of Faculty of Medicine, Reial Academia de Medicinia de Catalunya, Barcelona, Spain

Alan Cheng, MD
Associate Professor of Medicine; Director, Arrhythmia Device Service, John Hopkins Hospital, Baltimore, Maryland

Anne B. Curtis, MD, FACC, FHRS, FACP, FAHA
Charles and Mary Bauer Professor and Chair, UB Distinguished Professor, Department of Medicine, School of Medicine and Biomedical Sciences, University of Buffalo, Buffalo, New York

Victor Froelicher, MD, FACC, FAHA, FACSM
Professor of Medicine,
Department of Cardiovascular Medicine,
Stanford University, Stanford, California

Michel Haïssaguerre, MD
Hôpital Cardiologique du Haut-Lévêque and
the Université Victor Segalen Bordeaux II,
Bordeaux, France

Ofer Havakuk, MD
Tel Aviv Medical Center, Cardiology Department,
Tel Aviv, Israel

Mélèze Hocini, MD
Hôpital Cardiologique du Haut-Lévêque and
the Université Victor Segalen Bordeaux II,
Bordeaux, France

Stefan H. Hohnloser, MD
Professor of Medicine and Cardiology,
J.W. Goethe University,
Department of Cardiology,
Division of Clinical Electrophysiology,
Frankfurt, Germany

Henry D. Huang, MD
Clinical Electrophysiology Fellow,
Harvard-Thorndike Arrhythmia Institute,
Harvard Medical School; Beth Israel Deaconess
Medical Center, Boston, Massachusetts

Rahul Jain, MD, MPH
Assistant Professor, Indiana University School of
Medicine; Cardiac Electrophysiology Service, VA
Hospital, Indianapolis, Indiana

Pierre Jaïs, MD
Department of Rhythmologie,
Hôpital Cardiologique du Haut-Lévêque
and the Université Bordeaux II,
Bordeaux, France

Mohammad-Reza Jazayeri, MD, FACC, FAHA
Director of Electrophysiology,
Laboratory and Arrhythmia Service,
Heart and Vascular Center,
Bellin Health Systems, Inc.,
Green Bay, Wisconsin

Eyad Kanawati, MD
Cardiovascular Disease Fellow,
Department of Cardiology,
Lankenau Medical Center,
Wynnewood, Pennsylvania

Peter Kowey, MD, FACC, FAHA, FHRS
Professor of Medicine and Clinical Pharmacology,
Jefferson Medical College; William Wikoff
Smith Chair in Cardiovascular Research, Lankenau
Institute for Medical Research,
Wynnewood, Pennsylvania

Eric L. Krivitsky, MD
Electrophysiologist, Chattanooga Heart Institute,
Chattanooga, Tennessee

Hervé Le Marec, MD, PhD
Professor of Cardiology, Director of L'institut du
thorax, Nantes University Hospital, Nantes, France

Mark S. Link, MD
Professor of Medicine, Tufts University School of
Medicine; Co-Director, Cardiac Electrophysiology
and Pacemaker Laboratory; Director, Center for the
Evaluation of Heart Disease in Athletes,
Boston, Massachusetts

Jared W. Magnani, MD, MS
Assistant Professor, Department of Medicine,
Boston University School of Medicine,
Boston, Massachusetts

John M. Miller, MD
Professor of Medicine, Indiana University School of
Medicine; Director, Clinical Cardiac
Electrophysiology, Indianapolis, Indiana

Victor Nauffal, MD
Postdoctoral Fellow, Division of Cardiology,
Department of Medicine, Johns Hopkins Hospital,
Baltimore, Maryland

Chinmay Patel, MD, FACC
Clinical Cardiac Electrophysiologist,
Pinnacle Health Cardiovascular Institute,
Harrisburg, Pennsylvania

Vincent Probst, MD, PhD
Professor of Cardiology, Director of the Cardiologic
Department, L'institut du thorax
Nantes University Hospital, Nantes, France

Sergio Richter, MD
Associate Professor of Medicine and Cardiology,
Department of Electrophysiology,
Heart Center – University of Leipzig,
Leipzig, Germany

John Rickard, MD, MPH
Assistant Professor of Medicine Electrophysiology,
John Hopkins University, Baltimore, Maryland

Raphael Rosso, MD
Atrial Fibrillation Service, Director,
Cardiology Department, Tel Aviv Medical Center,
Tel Aviv, Israel

Ashok J. Shah, MD
Hôpital Cardiologique du Haut-Lévêque and
the Université Victor Segalen Bordeaux II,
Bordeaux, France

Hossein Shenasa, MD
Attending Physician, Department of Cardiovascular
Services, O'Conner Hospital;
Heart & Rhythm Medical Group,
San Jose, California

Alexei Shvilkin, MD
Assistant Clinical Professor of Medicine,
Department of Medicine, Beth Israel Deaconess
Medical Center, Boston, Massachusetts

Cory M. Tschabrunn, CEPS
Principal Associate of Medicine,
Harvard Medical School; Technical Director,
Experimental Electrophysiology,
Harvard-Thorndike Electrophysiology Institute,
Beth Israel Deaconess Medical Center,
Boston, Massachusetts

Sami Viskin, MD
Associate Professor of Cardiology,
Sackler School of Medicine, Tel-Aviv University;
Director, Cardiac Hospitalization, Sourasky Tel-Aviv
Medical Center, Tel Aviv, Israel

Galen S. Wagner, MD
Associate Professor of Medicine, Department of
Cardiology, Division of Department of Medicine,
Duke University, Durham, North Carolina

Edward P. Walsh, MD, FHRS
Professor of Pediatrics, Harvard Medical School;
Chief, Cardiac Electrophysiology Service,
Boston Children's Hospital,
Boston, Massachusetts

FOREWORD

The electrocardiogram (ECG), which is now more than 100 years old, is available all over the planet, easy and rapid to make, noninvasive, reproducible, inexpensive, and patient-friendly.

Worldwide, approximately 3 million ECG recordings are made daily. It is an indispensible tool, giving immediate information about the diagnosis, management, and effect of treatment in cases of cardiac ischemia, rhythm- and conduction disturbances, structural changes in the atria and ventricles, changes caused by medication, electrolyte and metabolic disorders, and monogenic rhythm and conduction disturbances.

During those more than 100 years, the value of the ECG continued to improve by reanalyzing the ECG in the light of findings from invasive and non-invasive studies such as coronary angiography, programmed electrical stimulation of the heart, intracardiac mapping, echocardiography, MRI and CT, nuclear studies, and genetic information. Also, by epidemiologic studies with long-term follow-up, we learned about the value of the ECG for risk estimation.

The unraveling of basic mechanisms, the clinical application of new information, and the essential contribution of medical technology are the three overlapping circles leading to these major and always continuing advancements.

Essential for the optimal interpretation of the ECG is the distribution of new information, which is the challenge addressed in this volume.

By selecting authors who made important contributions in their respective areas of interest and knowledge, the editors have succeeded to make a text that will bring the reader up to date about these new developments. As such, this book deserves to be studied carefully by all those who are using the ECG as their daily "work horse"!

Hein J. J. Wellens, MD, PhD, FACC, FAHA, FESC
Professor of Cardiology, Cardiovascular Research Institute,
Maastricht, The Netherlands

PREFACE

It is now over a century (112 years, to be accurate) since Willem Einthoven reported the first use of the electrocardiogram (ECG) to register the electrical activity of the human heart. Since then, the ECG has become part of routine work-ups in clinical practice and is used for the diagnosis and management of a variety of cardiac and non-cardiac disorders. Today, there are no other diagnostic tests in clinical practice that have been used as frequently. ECGs are readily available, noninvasive, and relatively low in cost, yet they are challenging to interpret. The ECG captures the diagnosis immediately and provides a window, not only to cardiac conditions, but also to other pathologies. Amazingly, a century after the discovery of the ECG, new ECG patterns are being discovered. The modern ECG is not only a method to obtain heart rate and rhythm, QRS duration, A-V conduction disease, etc., but it is also implemented into many guidelines and used as a part of screening for many diseases even at a pre-clinical stage.

In the last few decades, several new electrocardiographic phenomenon and markers have emerged that are challenging to physicians who interpret ECGs, such as early repolarization, ECGs of athletes, Brugada Syndrome, short and long QT syndrome, various channelopathies, and cardiomyopathies.

Despite several textbooks on electrocardiography, recent guidelines, and consensus reports from different societies, there is still a definite need to put together a handbook related to these new observations for those involved in the interpretation of ECGs. To date there is no such collective.

The purpose of this handbook is to prepare a state-of-the-art reference on contemporary and challenging issues in electrocardiography. This handbook is not designed as a classic textbook that covers all aspects of the subject, nor is it meant to discuss other cellular and imaging modalities related to this topic.

We are confident that this text will be useful for medical students, physicians who are involved in sports medicine, ECG readers, and pediatric and adult cardiologists/electrophysiologists. We have attempted to make this handbook easy to use and understand; therefore, we believe it should be in the hands of any physician who reads ECGs as their very own "No Fear, Shakespeare."

We are privileged and thankful that a group of experts on the subjects provided the most recent evidence-based information of related-topics.

We wish to thank the Cardiotext staff for their professionalism, namely Mike Crouchet, Caitlin Crouchet Altobell, and Carol Syverson.

Mohammad Shenasa, MD
Mark E. Josephson, MD
N.A. Mark Estes III, MD

ABBREVIATIONS

ACC/AHA	American College of Cardiology and American Heart Association
AF	atrial fibrillation
ALCAPA	Anomalous origin of the left coronary artery from the pulmonary artery
AMI	acute myocardial infarction
AP	accessory pathway
AP	action potential
APD	action potential duration
ARIC	Atherosclerosis Risk in Communities
ART	antidromic reentrant tachycardia
ARVC	arrhythmogenic right ventricular cardiomyopathy
ARVD/C	arrhythmogenic right ventricular dysplasia/cardiomyopathy
ASD	atrial septal defect
AT	atrial tachycardia
AVNRT	AV-node reentrant tachycardia
AVRT	atrioventricular reentrant tachycardia
AWP	alternate-beat Wenckebach periods
BBB	bundle branch block
BBre-VT	bundle branch reentry VT
BBs	bundle branches
BMI	body mass index
bpm	beats per minute
BrS	Brugada syndrome
CABG	coronary artery bypass grafting
CAD	coronary artery disease
CC	concealed conduction
CCB	calcium channel blockers
CHB	complete heart block
CHD	congenital heart disease
CHF	congestive heart failure
CL	cycle length
CM	cardiac memory
CMR	cardiac magnetic resonance
CPVT	catecholaminergic polymorphic ventricular tachycardia
CRT	cardiac resynchronization therapy
CS	coronary sinus
CSE	Computer Society of Electrocardiography
CTA	computed tomography angiography
CVD	cardiovascular disease
DAD	delayed after-depolarization
DCM	dilated cardiomyopathy
DES	desmin
DVR	double ventricular responses
EAD	early after-depolarization
EAT	ectopic atrial tachycardia
ECG	electrocardiogram, electrocardiography
EP	electrophysiology
ER	early repolarization
ERP	effective refractory period
ERS	early repolarization syndrome
F	flutter waves
FBBB	functional bundle branch block
fQRS	fragmented QRS
FV	fasciculoventricular
GCV	great cardiac vein
HB	His bundle
HCM	hypertrophic cardiomyopathy
Health ABC	Health, Aging, and Body Composition
HF	heart failure
HHD	hypertensive heart disease
HPS	His-Purkinje system
HRT	heart rate turbulence
HRV	heart rate variability
IART	intra-atrial reentrant tachycardia
ICD	implantable cardioverter-defibrillator
IVCD	intraventricular conduction defect
IVF	idiopathic ventricular fibrillation
IVS	interventricular septum
IVT/VF	idiopathic ventricular tachycardia/VF
JLN	Jervell Lange-Nielsen
LAD	left-axis deviation
LAFB	left anterior fascicular block

LAO left anterior oblique
LB left bundle
LBB left bundle branch
LBBB left bundle branch block
LGE late gadolinium enhancement
LPFB left posterior fascular block
LPs late potentials
LQTS long QT syndrome
LV left ventricle/ventricular
LVEF left ventricular ejection fraction
LVESV LV end-systolic volume
LVH left ventricular hypertrophy
LVMI left ventricular mass index
LVOT left ventricular outflow tract

MELAS mitochondrial encephalopathy, lactic acidosis, and stroke-like episodes
MERRF myoclonic epilepsy and red-ragged fibers
MESA-RV Multiethnic Study of Atherosclerosis-Right Ventricle
MESA multiethnic study of atherosclerosis
MI myocardial infarction
MMA modified moving average
MRI magnetic resonance imaging
MTWA microvolt TWA
MV mitral valve

NEJM New England Journal of Medicine
NHANES III National Health and Nutrition Examination Survey
NSR normal sinus rhythm

ORT orthodromic reentrant tachycardia

PAC premature atrial complex
PAVB paroxysmal AV block
PCCD progressive cardiac conduction defect
PFO patent foramen ovale
PJRT permanent form of junctional reciprocating tachycardia
PM pacemaker
PV pulmonary vein
PVCs premature ventricular complexes
PWIs P-wave indices

QTc QT interval
RAO right anterior oblique
RAWP reverse AWP
RB right bundle
RBB right bundle branch
RBBB right bundle branch block
RCA right coronary artery
RF radiofrequency
RP refractory period
RV right ventricle/ventricular
RVH right ventricular hypertrophy
RVOT right ventricular outflow tract
RVOT-VT RV outflow tract-origin VT

SAECG signal-averaged ECG
SA sinoatrial
SCD sudden cardiac death
SCDHeFT Sudden Cardiac Death Heart Failure Trial
SD sudden death
SQTS short QT syndrome
STEMI ST-segment elevation myocardial infarction
SVT supraventricular tachycardia

TdP torsades de pointes
TDR transmural dispersion of repolarization
TOF tetralogy of Fallot
TTE transthoracic echocardiogram
TTN titin
TV tricuspid valve
TWA T-wave alternans
TWI T-wave inversions

UDMI Universal Definition of Myocardial Infarction

V ventricular
VAb aberrant ventricular conduction
VA ventriculoatrial
VAs ventricular arrhythmias
VA Veterans Affairs
VF ventricular fibrillation
VSD ventricular septal defect
VT ventricular tachycardia

WB Wenckebach block
WPW Wolff-Parkinson-White

CHAPTER

1

Normal Electrocardiograms Today

Galen Wagner, MD

A standard 12-lead ECG has 9 features that should be examined systematically[1]:

1. Rate and regularity;
2. P-wave morphology;
3. PR interval;
4. QRS complex morphology;
5. ST-segment morphology;
6. T-wave morphology;
7. U-wave morphology;
8. QTc interval; and
9. Cardiac rhythm.

The observations of these features should be initially considered to determine whether the recording is "normal" or "abnormal." This decision is challenged by the wide ranges of "normal limits" of each of the features. It is the purpose of this introductory chapter to provide the basis for making this determination, and to include common "variations from normal."

Much of the information provided by the ECG is contained in the morphologies of 3 principal waveforms: the P wave, the QRS complex, and the T wave, and of the "ST segment" between the QRS and T. It is helpful to develop a systematic approach to the analysis of these components by considering their (1) general contours, (2) durations, (3) positive and negative amplitudes, and (4) axes in the frontal and transverse planes.

RATE AND REGULARITY

The cardiac rhythm is rarely precisely regular. Even when electrical activity is initiated normally in the sinoatrial (SA) node, the rate is affected by variations in the sympathetic/parasympathetic balance of the autonomic nervous system. When an individual is at rest, minor variations in this balance are produced by the phases of the respiratory cycle. A glance at the sequence of cardiac cycles is sufficient to determine whether the cardiac rate is essentially regular or irregular. Normally, there are P waves preceding each QRS complex, by 120 to 200 ms, that can be considered to determine cardiac rate and regularity. When in the presence of certain abnormal cardiac rhythms, the numbers of P waves and QRS complexes are not the same. Atrial and ventricular rates and regularities must be determined separately. The morphology of the QRS complexes may change with increased atrial rate, because of "aberrant conduction" through incompletely recovered interventricular pathways.

When the cardiac rate is <100 beats per minute (bpm), it is sufficient to consider only the large squares on the ECG paper. However, when the rate is >100 bpm (tachycardia), small differences in the observed rate may alter the assessment of the cardiac rhythm, and the number of small squares must also be considered. If there is irregularity of the cardiac rate, the number of cycles over a particular interval of time

The ECG Handbook of Contemporary Challenges © 2015 Mohammad Shenasa, Mark E. Josephson, N.A. Mark Estes III
Cardiotext Publishing, ISBN: 978-1-935395-88-1

should be counted to determine the approximate cardiac rate.

P-WAVE MORPHOLOGY

At either slow or normal heart rates, the small, rounded P wave is clearly visible just before the taller, more peaked QRS complex. At more rapid rates, however, the P wave may merge with the preceding T wave and become difficult to identify. Four steps should be taken to define the morphology of the P wave, as follows:

(a) **General contour:** The P-wave contour is normally smooth and is either entirely positive or entirely negative in all leads except V_1 and possibly V_2. In the short-axis view provided by lead V_1, which best distinguishes left- versus right-sided cardiac activity, the divergence of right- and left-atrial activation typically produces a biphasic P wave.

(b) **P-wave duration:** The P-wave duration is normally <0.12 second.

(c) **Positive and negative amplitudes:** The maximal P-wave amplitude is normally no more than 0.2 mV in the frontal plane limb leads and no more than 0.1 mV in the transverse plane chest leads.

(d) **Axis in the frontal and transverse planes:** The P wave normally appears entirely upright in leftward and inferiorly oriented leads such as I, II, aVF, and V_4 to V_6. The normal limits of the P wave axis in the frontal plane are between 0 degrees and +75 degrees.[1]

PR INTERVAL

The PR interval measures the time required for an electrical impulse to travel from the atrial myocardium adjacent to the SA node to the ventricular myocardium adjacent to the fibers of the Purkinje network. This duration is normally from 0.10 to 0.21 second. A major portion of the PR interval reflects the slow conduction of an impulse through the atrioventricular (AV) node, which is controlled by the balance between the sympathetic and parasympathetic divisions of the autonomic nervous system. Therefore, the PR interval varies with the heart rate, being shorter at faster rates when the sympathetic component predominates, and vice versa. The PR interval tends to increase with age: childhood, 0.10 to 0.12 second; adolescence, 0.12 to 0.16 second; adulthood, 0.14 to 0.21 second.[1]

QRS COMPLEX MORPHOLOGY

To develop a systematic approach to waveform analysis, the following steps should be taken.

(a) **Contour:** The QRS complex is composed of higher frequency signals than are the P and T waves, thereby causing its contour to be peaked rather than rounded. In some leads (V_1, V_2, and V_3), the presence of any Q wave should be considered abnormal, whereas in all other leads (except rightward-oriented leads III and aVR), a "normal" Q wave is very small. The upper limit of normal for such Q waves in each lead is illustrated in Table 1.1.[2] The complete absence of Q waves in leads V_5 and V_6 should be considered abnormal. A Q wave of any size is normal in leads III and aVR, because of the rightward orientations of their positive electrodes. As the chest leads provide a panoramic view of the cardiac electrical activity, the initial R waves normally increase in amplitude and duration from lead V_1 to lead V_4. Expansion of this sequence with larger R waves in leads V_5 and V_6, typically occurs with left ventricular enlargement, and reversal of this sequence with decreasing R waves from lead V_1 to lead V_4 may indicate either right ventricular enlargement or loss of anterior left ventricular myocardium, as occurs with myocardial infarction.

(b) **Duration:** The duration of the QRS complex is termed the QRS interval, and it normally ranges from 0.07 to 0.11 second. The duration of the QRS complex tends to be slightly longer in males than in females.[3] The QRS interval is measured from the beginning of the first appearing Q or R wave to the end of the last appearing R, S, R′, or S′ wave. Multilead comparison is necessary to determine the true QRS duration, because either the beginning or the end of the QRS complex may be isoelectric (neither positive nor negative) in any single lead, causing a falsely shorter QRS duration. This isoelectric appearance occurs whenever the summation of ventricular electrical forces is perpendicular to the recording lead. The onset of the QRS complex is usually quite

Table 1.1. Normal Q-wave duration limits.

Limb leads		Precordial leads	
Lead	Upper limit(s)	Lead	Upper limit(s)
I	<0.03	V_1	Any Q[a]
II	<0.03	V_2	Any Q[a]
III	None	V_3	Any Q[a]
aVR	None	V_4	<0.02
aVL	<0.03	V_5	<0.03
aVF	<0.03	V_6	<0.03

[a]In these leads, any Q wave is abnormal.
Modified from Wagner GS, Freye CJ, Palmeri ST, et al. Evaluation of a QRS scoring system for estimating myocardial infarct size. I. Specificity and observer agreement. *Circulation*. 1982;65:345, with permission.

abrupt in all leads, but its ending at the junction with the ST segment (termed the J point) is often indistinct, particularly in the chest leads. However, the J point may be completely distorted by either slurring or notching of the final aspect of the QRS complex. This "J wave" has been typically considered to indicate "early repolarization," but could also be caused by "late depolarization" (Figure 1.1).[4] The J wave is usually a normal variant, but could be indicative of an abnormal ion channel and associated with risk of serious ventricular tachyarrhythmias.[5] A prominent J wave followed by ST-segment elevation and T-wave inversion, most prominent in lead V_1, has been termed "Brugada pattern" (Figure 1.2). Abnormality of these waveforms accompanied by ventricular tachyarrhythmias, termed the "Brugada syndrome," is predictive of ventricular fibrillation and sudden cardiac death.[6]

(c) **Positive and negative amplitudes:** The amplitude of the overall QRS complex has wide normal limits. It varies with age, increasing until about age 30 and then gradually decreasing. The amplitude is generally higher in males than in females, and varies among ethnic groups. The QRS amplitude is measured between the peaks of the tallest positive and negative waveforms in the complex. It is difficult to set an arbitrary upper limit for normal voltage of the QRS complex; peak-to-peak amplitudes as high as 4 mV are occasionally seen in normal individuals. Factors that contribute to higher amplitudes include youth, physical fitness, slender body build, intraventricular conduction abnormalities, and ventricular enlargement. An abnormally low QRS amplitude, that is, low voltage, occurs when the overall amplitude is no more than 0.5 mV in any of the limb leads and no more than 1.0 mV in any of the chest leads. The QRS amplitude is decreased by any condition that increases the distance between the myocardium and the recording electrode, such as a thick chest wall or various intrathoracic conditions.

(d) **Axis in the frontal and transverse planes:** The QRS axis represents the average direction of the total force produced by right- and left-ventricular depolarization. Although the Purkinje network facilitates the spread of the depolarization wave front from the apex to the base of the ventricles, the QRS axis is normally in the positive direction in the frontal plane leads (except aVR) because of the

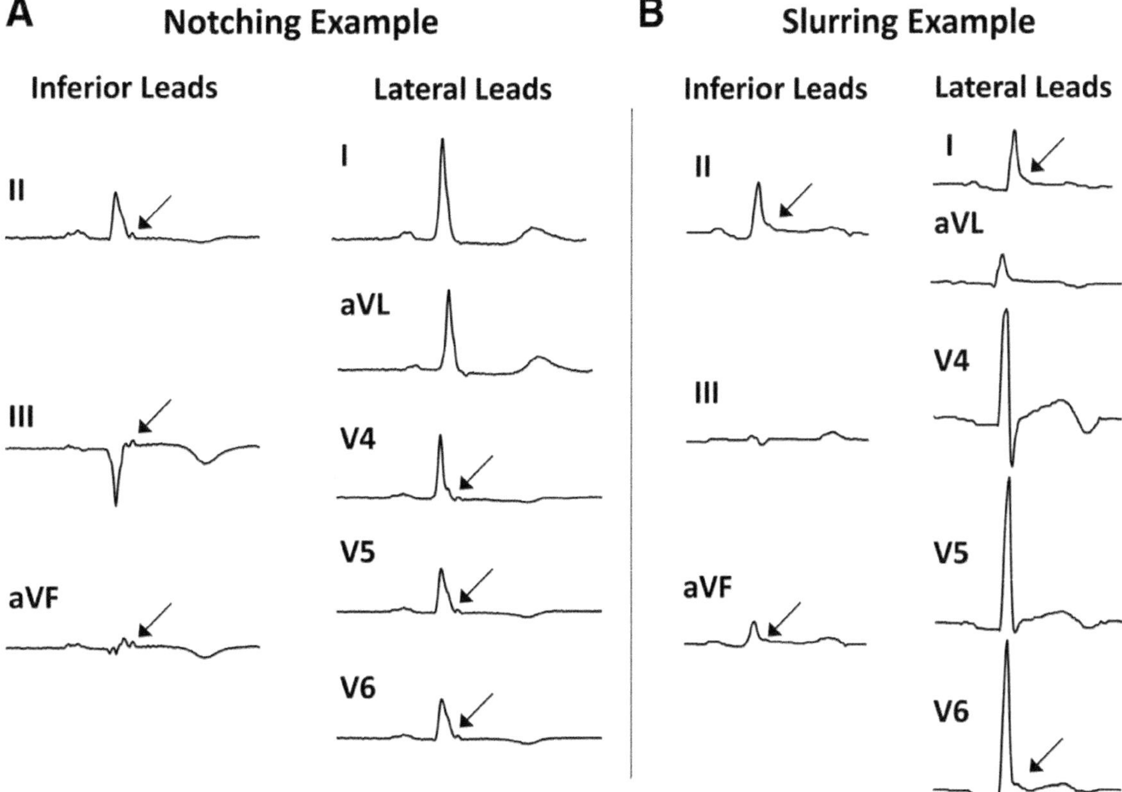

Figure 1.1. J-wave patterns on ECG. **A.** Example of notching pattern (arrows). **B.** Example of slurring pattern (arrows). (From Patel RB, Ng J, Reddy V, et al. Early repolarization associated with ventricular arrhythmias in patients with chronic coronary artery disease. *Circ Arrhythm Electrophysiol.* 2010;3:489–495, with permission.)

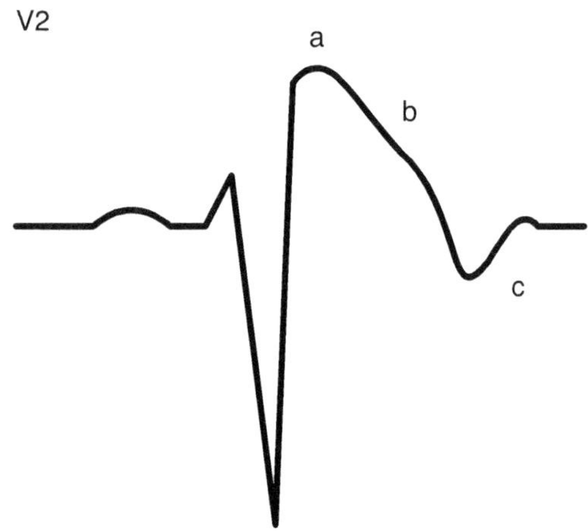

Figure 1.2. ECG characteristics of the type I Brugada pattern: a, J-point elevation > 2.0 mm; b, coved, downsloping ST segment; and c, T-wave inversion. (Modified from http://www.heartregistry.org.au/patients-families/genetic-heart-diseases/brugada-syndrome/.)

endocardial-to-epicardial spread of depolarization in the thicker walled left ventricle (LV). In the frontal plane, the full 360-degree circumference of the hexaxial reference system is provided by the positive and negative poles of the 6 limb leads; in the transverse plane, it is provided by the positive and negative poles of the 6 precordial leads (Figure 1.3). It should be noted that the leads in both planes are not separated by precisely 30 degrees. In the frontal plane, the scalene Burger triangle has been shown more applicable then the equilateral Einthoven triangle.[7] Of course, body shape and electrode placement determine the spacing between adjacent (contiguous) leads. Identification of the frontal-plane axis of the QRS complex would be easier if the 6 leads were displayed in their orderly sequence than in their typical classical sequence (Figure 1.4).

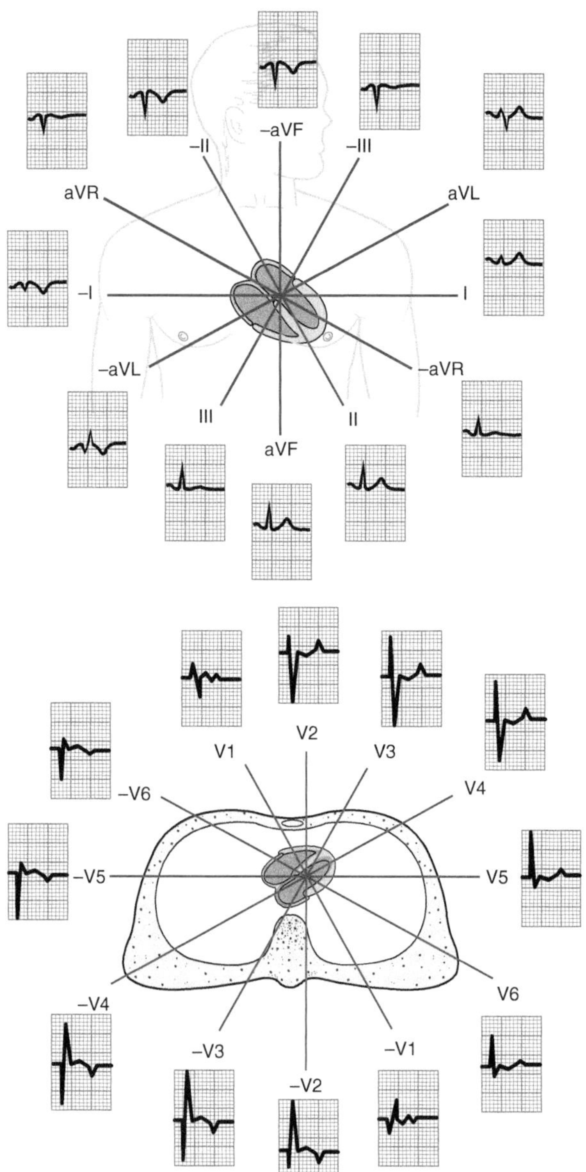

Figure 1.3. Clock faces. **Top.** Frontal plane, as seen from the front. **Bottom.** Transverse plane, as seen from below.

ST-SEGMENT MORPHOLOGY

The ST segment represents the period during which the ventricular myocardium proceeds through the preliminary 2 phases of repolarization: phases 1 and 2, following its depolarization in phase 0. These are the phases considered as "early repolarization." At its junction with the QRS complex (J point), the ST segment typically forms a distinct angle with the downslope of the R wave or upstroke of the S wave, and then proceeds nearly horizontally until it curves gently into the T wave. The length of the ST segment is influenced by factors that alter the duration of ventricular activation. Points along the ST segment are designated with reference to the number of milliseconds beyond the J point, such as "J + 20," "J + 40," and "J + 60." The first section of the ST segment is normally located at the same horizontal level as the baseline formed by the TP segment in the space between electrical cardiac cycles. Slight upsloping, downsloping, or horizontal depression of the ST segment may occur as a normal variant. Another normal variant of the ST segment appears when there is altered late depolarization or early repolarization within the ventricles. This causes displacement of the ST segment by as much as 0.1 mV in the direction of the following T wave. Occasionally, the ST segment in young males may show even greater elevation, especially in leads V_2 and V_3.[8] The appearance of the ST segment may also be altered when there is an abnormally prolonged QRS complex.

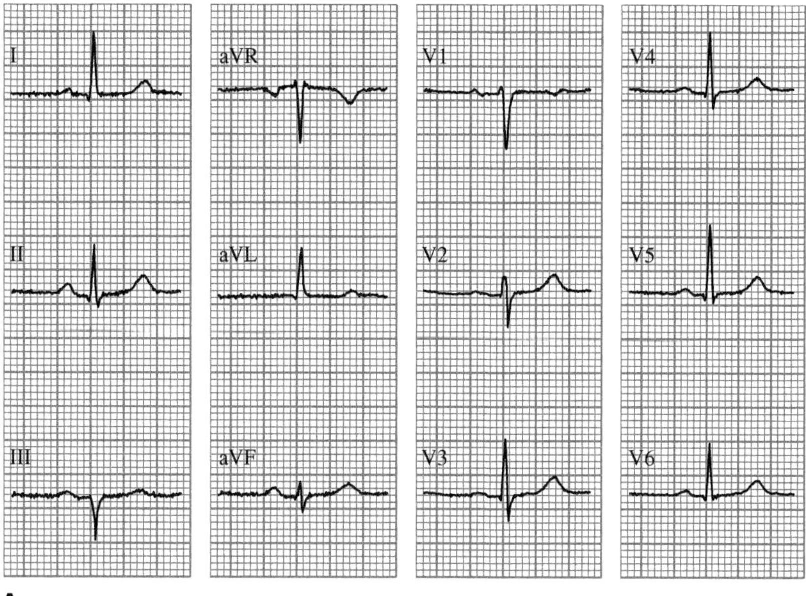

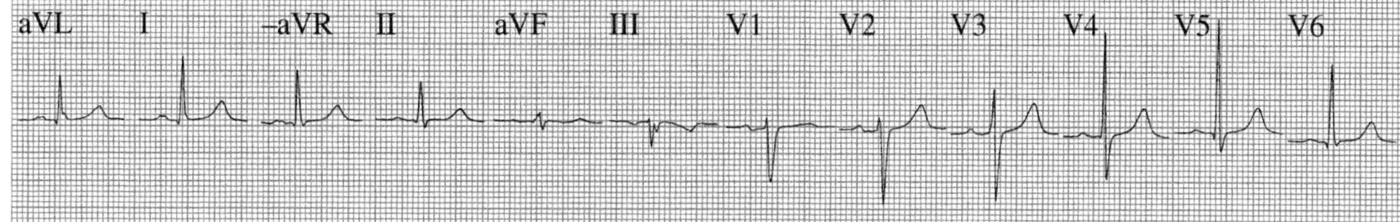

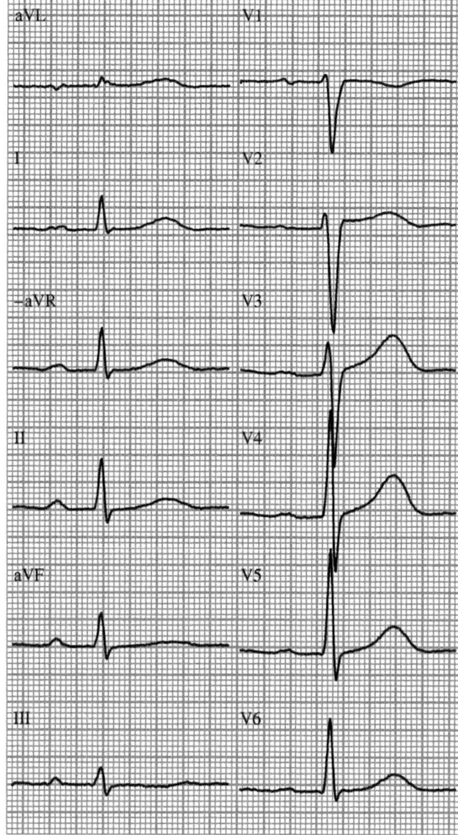

Figure 1.4. **A.** Classical display. **B.** Single horizontal display. **C.** Parallel vertical displays.

T-WAVE MORPHOLOGY

The steps for examining the morphology of the T wave are as follows:

(a) **Contour:** Both the shape and axis of the normal T wave resemble those of the P wave. The waveforms in both cases are smooth and rounded, and are positively directed in all leads except aVR, where they are negative, and V_1, where they are biphasic (initially positive and terminally negative). Slight "peaking" of the T wave may occur as a normal variant.

(b) **Duration:** The duration of the T wave itself is not usually measured, but it is instead included in the "QT interval."

(c) **Positive and negative amplitudes:** The amplitude of the T wave, like that of the QRS complex, has wide normal limits. It tends to diminish with age and is larger in males than in females. T-wave amplitude tends to vary with QRS amplitude and should always be greater than that of an accompanying U wave. T waves do not normally exceed 0.5 mV in any limb lead or 1.5 mV in any precordial lead. In females, the upper limits of T-wave amplitude are about two-thirds of these values. The T-wave amplitude tends to be lower at the extremes of the orderly views of the leads in both the frontal and transverse planes. The amplitude of the wave at these extremes does not normally exceed 0.3 mV in leads aVL and III or 0.5 mV in leads V_1 and V_6 (Table 1.2).[9]

(d) **Axis in the frontal and transverse planes:** The axis of the T wave should be evaluated in relation to that of the QRS complex. The rationale for the similar directions of the waveforms of these 2 ECG features, despite their representing the opposite myocardial electrical events of activation and recovery, is not entirely known. The methods for determining the axis of the QRS complex in the 2 ECG planes should be applied for determining the axis of the T wave. The term "QRS–T angle" is used to indicate the degrees between the axes of the QRS complex and the T wave in the frontal plane. The axis of the T wave tends to remain constant throughout life, whereas the axis of the QRS complex moves from a vertical toward a horizontal position. Therefore, during childhood, the T-wave axis is more horizontal than that of the QRS complex, but during adulthood, the T-wave axis becomes more vertical than that of the QRS complex. Despite these changes, the QRS–T angle does not normally exceed 45 degrees.[10]

Table 1.2. T-wave amplitude normal limits (mV).

Lead[a]	Males 40–49	Females 40–49	Males ≥50	Females ≥50
aVL	0.30	0.30	0.30	0.30
I	0.55	0.45	0.45	0.45
–aVR	0.55	0.45	0.45	0.45
II	0.65	0.55	0.55	0.45
aVF	0.50	0.40	0.45	0.35
III	0.35	0.30	0.35	0.30
V_1	0.65	0.20	0.50	0.35
V_2	1.45	0.85	1.40	0.70
V_3	1.35	0.85	1.35	0.85
V_4	1.15	0.85	1.10	0.75
V_5	0.90	0.70	0.95	0.70
V_6	0.65	0.55	0.65	0.50

[a]Cabrera sequence.

U-WAVE MORPHOLOGY

The U wave is normally either absent or present as a small, rounded wave following the T wave. It is normally oriented in the same direction as the T wave, has approximately 10% of the amplitude of the latter, and is usually most prominent in leads V_2 or V_3. The U wave is larger at slower heart rates, and both the U wave and the T wave diminish in size and merge with the following P wave at faster heart rates. The U wave is usually separated from the T wave, with the TU junction occurring along the baseline of the ECG. However, there may be fusion of the T and U waves, making measurement of the QT interval more difficult. The source of the U wave is uncertain.[11]

QTC INTERVAL

The QT interval measures the duration of electrical activation and recovery of the ventricular myocardium. The "tangential method" is currently used to determine the end of the T wave, and thereby the end of the QT interval. This is defined as a tangent line drawn along steepest portion of its T wave where it crosses the isoelectric line (Figure 1.5).[12] The QT interval varies inversely with the cardiac rate. To ensure complete recovery from one cardiac cycle before the next cycle begins, the duration of recovery decreases as the rate of activation increases. Therefore, the "normality" of the QT interval can be determined only by correcting for the cardiac rate. The corrected QT interval (QTc), rather than the measured QT interval is included in routine ECG analysis. Bazett developed the following method for performing this correction: RR is defined as the interval duration between 2 consecutive R waves measured

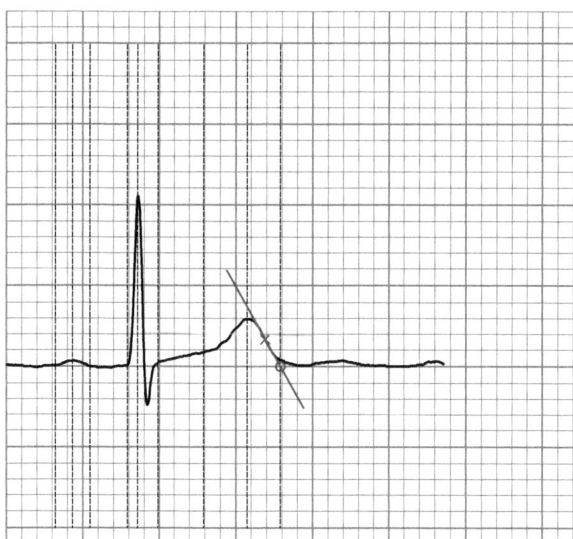

Figure 1.5. Tangential method used for determining end of the T wave.

in seconds.[13] The modification of Bazett's method by Hodges and coworkers, corrects more completely for high and low heart rates: QTc = QT + 0.00175 (ventricular rate −60).[14] The upper limit of QTc interval duration is approximately 0.46 second (460 ms). The QTc interval is slightly longer in females than in males, and increases slightly with age. Adjustment of the duration of electrical recovery to the rate of electrical activation does not occur immediately, but it requires several cardiac cycles. Thus, an accurate measurement of the QTc interval can be made only after a series of regular, equal cardiac cycles.[15,16]

CARDIAC RHYTHM

Assessment of the cardiac rhythm requires consideration of all 8 other electrocardiographic features. Certain irregularities of cardiac rate and regularity, P-wave morphology, and the PR interval may indicate abnormalities in cardiac rhythm; and certain irregularities of the other 5 ECG features may indicate the potential for development of abnormalities in cardiac rhythm.

(a) **Cardiac rate and regularity:** The normal cardiac rhythm is called sinus rhythm, because it is produced by electrical impulses formed within the SA node. Its rate is normally between 60 and 100 bpm. When <60 bpm, the rhythm is called sinus bradycardia, and when >100 bpm is called sinus tachycardia. However, the designation of "normal" requires consideration of the individual's activity level: sinus bradycardia with a rate as low as 40 bpm may be normal during sleep, and sinus tachycardia with a rate as rapid as 200 bpm may be normal during exercise. Indeed, a rate of 90 bpm would be "abnormal" during either sleep or vigorous exercise. Sinus rates in the bradycardia range may occur normally during wakefulness, especially in well-trained athletes whose resting heart rates range at 30 bpm and often <60 bpm even with moderate exertion. As indicated, normal sinus rhythm is essentially, but not absolutely, regular because of continual variation of the balance between the sympathetic and parasympathetic divisions of the autonomic nervous system. Loss of this normal heart rate variability may be associated with significant underlying autonomic or cardiac abnormalities.[17] The term "sinus arrhythmia" describes the normal variation in cardiac rate that cycles with the phases of respiration; the SA rate accelerates with inspiration and slows with expiration. Occasionally, sinus arrhythmia produces such marked irregularity that it can be confused with clinically important arrhythmias.

(b) **P-wave axis:** The normal frontal plane axis of the P wave was discussed in the section on "P-wave morphology." Alteration of this axis to either <+30 degrees or >+75 degrees may indicate that the cardiac rhythm is being initiated from a site low in the right atrium, AV node, or left atrium.[18] Vertical deviation of the P wave axis after age 45 has been associated with the development of pulmonary emphysema.[19]

(c) **PR interval:** An abnormal P-wave axis is often accompanied by an abnormally short PR interval, because the site of impulse formation has moved from the SA node to a position closer to the AV node. However, a short PR interval in the presence of a normal P-wave axis suggests either an abnormally rapid conduction pathway within the AV node or the presence of an abnormal bundle of cardiac muscle connecting the atria to the Bundle of His.

Such an abnormal bundle of cardiac muscle may connect the atrial to the ventricular myocardium as illustrated in Figure 1.6. This typically produces a notch or slur at the onset of the QRS complex, termed a "delta wave." This phenomenon is not in itself an abnormality of the cardiac rhythm; however, the pathway either within or bypassing the AV node that is responsible for the "ventricular preexcitation" creates the potential for electrical reentry into the atria, thereby producing a tachyarrhythmia. An abnormally long PR interval in the presence of a normal P-wave axis indicates delay of impulse transmission at some point along the normal pathway between the atrial and ventricular myocardium. When a prolonged PR interval is accompanied by an abnormal P-wave contour, it should be considered that the P wave

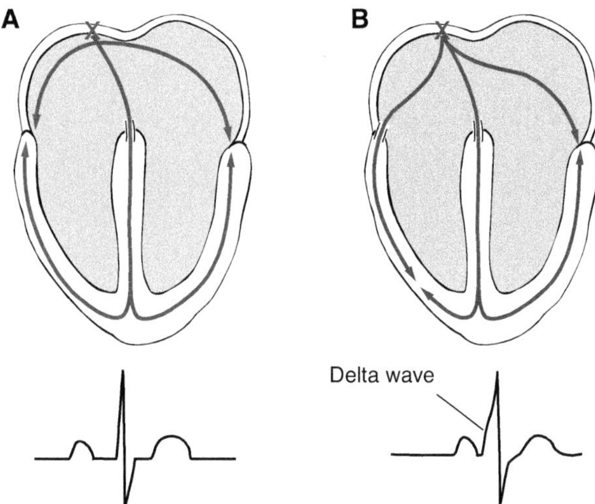

Figure 1.6. Anatomic basis for preexcitation. **A.** Normal condition. **B.** Abnormal congential anomaly. Pink X, sinoatrial node; pink lines, directions of electrical impulses; open channel, conductive pathway between atria and ventricles. (Modified from Wagner GS, Waugh RA, Ramo BW. *Cardiac Arrhythmias.* New York, NY: Churchill Livingstone; 1983:13, with permission).

may actually be associated with the preceding, rather than with the following, QRS complex because of reverse activation from the ventricles to the atria. This occurs when the cardiac impulse originates from the ventricles rather than the atria. In this situation, the P wave might only be identified as a distortion of the T wave. When the PR interval cannot be determined because of the absence of any visible P wave, there is obvious abnormality of the cardiac rhythm.

(d) **Morphology of the QRS complex:** Blockage of impulse conduction within the intraventricular conduction pathways is a common cause of abnormal QRS complex morphology. The cardiac rhythm remains normal when the conduction abnormality is confined to either the right or left bundle branch. However, if the process responsible spreads to the other bundle branch, the serious rhythm abnormality of partial (second degree) or even total (third degree) failure of AV conduction could suddenly occur. An abnormally prolonged QRS duration in the absence of a preceding P wave suggests that the cardiac rhythm is originating from the ventricles rather than from the atria.

(e) **ST segment, T wave, U wave, and QTc interval:** Marked elevation of the ST segment, an increase or decrease in T-wave amplitude, prolongation of the QTc interval, or an increase in U-wave amplitude are indications of underlying cardiac conditions that may produce serious abnormalities of cardiac rhythm.[20]

COMMON VARIATIONS FROM "NORMAL"

There are many conditions that cause variations of the waveforms recorded on the standard 12-lead ECG. These include: (a) technical artifacts that alter the baseline of the recording; (b) specific and nonspecific intraventricular conduction delays that alter the QRS complexes; (c) increases in either the sizes of, or tensions on, the myocardium of the right and left atrial and ventricular chambers; commonly termed "hypertrophy"; (d) nonspecific variations in the ST segments and T waves; and (e) electrolyte imbalances.

(a) **Technical artifacts that alter the baseline of the recording:** Differentiation between interpretation of the ECG as normal versus abnormal is more difficult, and sometime impossible, because of absence of an isoelectric baseline in the segments between ECG waveforms. These include the PR and ST segments in each cardiac cycle and the TP segment between cycles. These "artifacts" include both general absence of a horizontal baseline, termed "wandering baseline," and specific noncardiac waveforms from either skeletal muscles or extrinsic electrical currents. The former are typically caused by inadequate contact between the skin and recording electrodes, and the latter by either a noncardiac neuromuscular condition or an inadequate grounding of the cardiograph.[21]

(b) **Specific and nonspecific intraventricular conduction delays that alter the QRS complexes:** There are minor variations in the dimensions of the ECG waveforms for which no specific cause can be determined, and also major variations caused by incomplete or even complete interruptions in the transmissions of electrical impulses through the specialized conduction network, or "enlargements" in the cardiac chambers. The latter is considered in the following paragraph. Definitions of these ECG waveform variations have required recent changes because of the emergence of clinical therapeutic interventions that may either reduce the tension on the right or left ventricular myocardium,[22] or increase the synchrony of left ventricular contraction.[23] There has previously been common acceptance of the terms "incomplete" and "complete" right bundle branch blocks (RBBBs) and left bundle branch blocks (LBBBs) that do not really indicate abnormalities in these components of the specialized intraventricular conduction network. Slight normal delay in conduction in either the right or left bundle branch may indeed cause variations in the QRS complex waveforms, but these can also be caused by alterations within the right or left ventricular myocardium. Since the left bundle branch includes relatively discrete anterior and posterior fascicles, these "incomplete LBBBs" are more accurately termed left anterior fascicular block (LAFB) and left posterior fascular block (LPFB). Typically, a QRS duration of at least 120 ms has been considered the only criterion for either complete RBBB or complete LBBB; with differentiation determined by the direction of the terminal QRS waveform in standard lead V_1: positive for RBBB and negative for LBBB. However, it has been recently determined that interruption in conduction through the left bundle branch can produce such profoundly dyssynchronous ventricular contraction, that LV ejection is reduced and LV failure occurs; and that this can be clinically reversed by "resynchronization therapy" using optimally timed biventricular pacing. A similar prolongation in QRS duration by an LV intramyocardial delay does not produce such dyssynchrony.[24] The clinical challenge of documenting the specific ECG criteria of the LV conduction abnormality caused by block in the left bundle branch has led to development by Strauss et al of new strict criteria (Figure 1.7).[23] These reflect both gender-specific increases in QRS duration and timing-specific QRS waveform slurring or notching.

(c) **Increases in either the sizes of, or tensions on, the myocardium of the right and left atrial and ventricular cardiac chambers:** The right ventricles (RVs) and LVs respond to diastolic volume overloading by dilation, and systolic pressure overloading by hypertrophy. Typically, the representative ECG changes have been generally termed "ventricular hypertrophy".[25] However, dilation and hypertrophy have long been recognized to cause quite different waveform abnormalities.[26] Recent pharmacologic or mechanical clinical therapies that acutely reduce the systolic pressure overloading of either ventricle have been observed to produce such sudden resolution of these ECG changes, in which the decreased mass of myocardial hypertrophy could not yet have occurred.[27] This challenge has led to reconsideration of the typically accepted ECG criteria of both LVH and RVH.[28, 29] The criteria for "LVH" consider ECG aspects other than QRS waveform amplitudes, such as those included in the long-neglected Romhilt-Estes criteria: QRS duration and axis, P-wave morphology, and ST segment and T wave directions.[30] The criteria for "RVH" consider ratios of waveform spatial directions and depolarization/repolarization relationships.[31]

(d) **Nonspecific variations in the ST segments and T waves:** The rapidly emerging insights from continuous ECG monitoring have provided the understanding that many of the variations in the ST segments and T waves, previously considered "nonspecific" now have quite specific etiologies.[32]

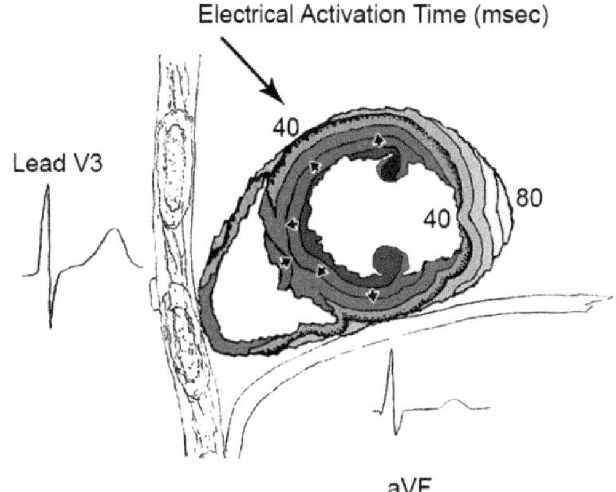

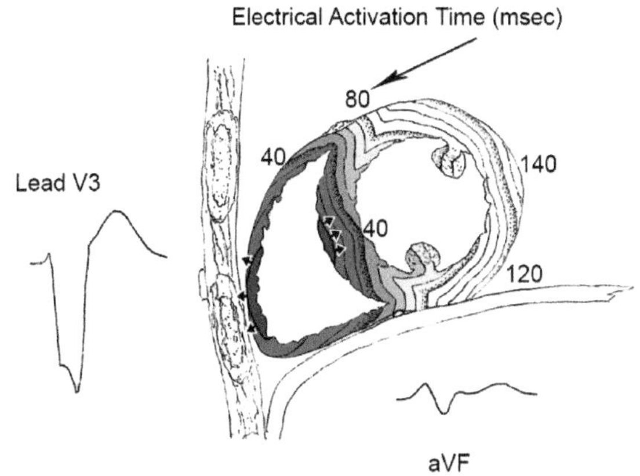

Figure 1.7. Ventricular activation in normal (A) and complete LBBB (B) activation. For reference, 2 QRS-T waveforms are shown in their anatomic locations in each image. Electrical activation starts at the *small arrows* and spreads in a wave front, with each colored line representing successive 0.01 second. Comparing A and B reveals the difference between normal and complete LBBB activation. In normal activation (A), activation begins within the left- and right-ventricular endocardium. In complete LBBB (B), activation only begins in the RV and must proceed through the septum for 0.04 to 0.05 second before reaching the LV endocardium. It then requires another 0.05 second for reentry into the left-ventricular Purkinje network and to propagate to the endocardium of the lateral wall. It then requires another 0.05 second to activate the lateral wall, producing a total QRS duration of 0.14 to 0.15 second. Any increase in septal or lateral wall thickness or left-ventricular endocardial surface area further increases QRS duration. Because the propagation velocity in human myocardium is 3 to 4 mm per 0.1 second, a circumferential increase in left-ventricular wall thickness by 3 mm will increase total QRS duration by 0.02 second in LBBB (0.1 second for the septum and 0.1 second for the lateral wall). (Reprinted with permission from Strauss DG, Selvester RH, Lima JAC, et al. ECG quantification of myocardial scar in cardiomyopathy patients with or without conduction defects: Correlation with cardiac magnetic resonance and arrhythmogensesis. *Circ Arrhythm Electrophysiol.* 2008;1:327–336.)

(e) **Electrolyte imbalances and hypothermia:** Either abnormally low (hypo) or high (hyper) serum levels of the electrolytes potassium and calcium may produce marked abnormalities of the ECG waveforms. Indeed, typical ECG changes may provide the first clinical evidence of the presence of these conditions.

Potassium

The terms hypokalemia and hyperkalemia are commonly used for alterations in serum levels of potassium. Because abnormalities in either of these conditions may be life threatening, an understanding of the ECG changes they produce is important. Hypokalemia may occur with other electrolyte disturbances (e.g., reduced serum magnesium levels), and is particularly dangerous in the presence of digitalis therapy. The typical ECG signs of hypokalemia may appear even when the serum potassium concentration is within normal limits; conversely, the ECG may be normal when serum levels of potassium are elevated. The typical ECG changes in hypokalemia are[33]:

- Flattening or inversion of the T wave.
- Increased prominence of the U wave.
- Slight depression of the ST segment.
- Increased amplitude and width of the P wave.
- Prolongation of the PR interval.
- Premature beats and sustained tachyarrhythmias.
- Prolongation of the QTc interval.

The characteristic reversal in the relative amplitudes of the T and U waves is the most characteristic change in waveform morphology in hypokalemia. The U-wave prominence is caused by prolongation of the recovery phase of the cardiac action potential. QTc prolongation can lead to the life-threatening torsades de pointes type of ventricular tachyarrhythmia.[34]

As in hypokalemia, there may be a poor correlation between serum potassium levels and the typical ECG changes of hyperkalemia.[33] The earliest ECG evidence of hyperkalemia usually appears in the T waves, and with increasing severity, the following ECG changes may occur:

- Increased amplitude and peaking of the T wave.
- Prolongation of the QRS interval.
- Prolongation of the PR interval.
- Flattening of the P wave.
- Loss of P wave.
- Sine wave appearance.

Calcium

The ventricular recovery time, as represented on the ECG by the QTc interval, is altered by the extremes of serum calcium levels. In hypocalcemia, the prolonged QT interval may be accompanied by terminal T-wave inversion in some leads. In hypercalcemia, the proximal limb of the T wave acutely slopes to its peak, and the ST segment may not be apparent.[35]

Temperature

Hypothermia has been defined as a rectal temperature <36° C or <97° F. At these lower temperatures, characteristic ECG changes develop. All intervals of the ECG (including the RR, PR, QRS, and QT intervals) may lengthen. Characteristic Osborn waves appear as deflections at the J point in the same direction as that of the QRS complex.[36]

REFERENCES

1. Wagner GS, Strauss DG. *Marriott's Practical Electrocardiolography*. 12th ed. Philadelphia, PA: Wolters Kluwer/Lippincott Williams & Wilkins; 2013.
2. Wagner GS, Freye CJ, Palmeri ST, et al. Evaluation of a QRS scoring system for estimating myocardial infarct size. I. Specificity and observer agreement. *Circulation.* 1982;65:342–347.
3. Macfarlane PW, Lawrie TDV, eds. *Comprehensive Electrocardiology. Vol. 3.* New York, NY: Pergamon Press; 1989:1442.
4. Froelicher V, Perez M. From bedside to bench. *J Electrocardiol.* 2013;46:114–115.
5. Gussak I, Antzelevitch CJ. Early repolarization syndrome: A decade of progress. *Electrocardiology.* 2013;46:110–113.
6. Brugada P, Brugada J. Right bundle branch block, persistent ST segment elevation, and sudden cardiac death: A distinct clinical and electrocardiographic syndrome. A multicenter report. *J Am Coll Card.* 1992;20:1391–1396.
7. Macfarlane PW, Lawrie TDV, eds. *Comprehensive Electrocardiology. Vol. 1.* New York, NY: Pergamon Press; 1989:296–305.
8. Macfarlane PW, Lawrie TDV, eds. *Comprehensive Electrocardiology. Vol. III.* New York, NY: Pergamon Press; 1989:1459.
9. Gambill CL, Wilkins ML, Haisty WK Jr, et al. T wave amplitudes in normal populations: Variation with electrocardiographic lead, gender, and age. *J Electrocardiol.* 1995;28:191–197.
10. Surawicz B. STT abnormalities. In: Macfarlane PW, Lawrie TDV, eds. *Comprehensive Electrocardiology. Vol. 1.* New York, NY: Pergamon Press; 1989:515.
11. Ritsema van Eck HJ, Kors JA, van Herpen G. The U wave in the electrocardiogram: a solution for a 100-year-old riddle. *Cardiovasc Res.* 2005;67:256–262.
12. Castellanos A, Inerian A Jr, Myerburg RJ. The resting electrocardiogram. In: Fuster V, Alexander RW, O'Rourke RA, eds. *Hurst's the Heart.* 11th ed. New York, NY: McGraw-Hill; 2004:99–300.

13. Bazett HC. An analysis of the time relations of electrocardiograms. *Heart.* 1920;7:353–370.
14. Hodges M, Salerno D, Erlien D. Bazett's QT correction reviewed. Evidence that a linear QT correction for heart is better. *J Am Coll Cardiol.* 1983;1:69.
15. Haarmark C, Graff C, Andersen MP, et al. Reference values of electrocardiogram repolarization variables in a healthy population. *J Electrocardiol.* 2010;43:31–39.
16. Rowlands D. Graphical representation of QT rate correction formulae: An aid facilitating the use of a given formula and providing a visual comparison of the impact of different formulae. *J Electrocardiol.* 2012;45:288–293.
17. Kleiger RE, Miller JP, Bigger JT, et al. The MultiCenter PostInfarction Research Group. Decreased heart rate variability and its association with increased mortality after acute myocardial infarction. *Am J Cardiol.* 1987;59:256–262.
18. Dilaveris P, Stefanadis C. Current morphologic and vectorial aspects of P-wave analysis. *J Electrocardiol.* 2007;42:395–399.
19. Chhabra L, Sareen P, Gandagule A, Spodick DH. Visual computed tomographic scoring of emphysema and its correlation with its diagnostic electrocardiographic sign: the frontal P vector. *J Electrocardiol.* 2012;45:136–140.
20. Rautaharju PM, Surawicz B, Gettes LS, et al. AHA/ACCF/HRS recommendations for the standardization and interpretation of the electrocardiogram. Part IV: The ST segment, T and U waves, and the QT interval: a scientific statement from the American Heart Association Electrocardiography and Arrhythmias Committee, Council on Clinical Cardiology; the American College of Cardiology Foundation; and the Heart Rhythm Society. *J Am Coll Cardiol.* 2009;53:982–991.
21. Kligfield P, Gettes LS, Bailey JJ, et al. Recommendations for the standardization and interpretation of the electrocardiogram. Part I: The electrocardiogram and its technology. *J Am Coll Cardiol.* 2007;49:1109–1127.
22. Bacharova L, Estes EH, Hill JA, et al.Changing role of ECG in the evaluation left ventricular hypertrophy. *J Electrocard.* 2012;45:609–611.
23. Strauss DG, Selvester RH, Wagner GS. Defining left bundle branch block in the era of cardiac resynchronization therapy. *Am J Cardiol.* 2011;107:927–934.
24. Risum N, Strauss DG, Sogaard P, et al. Left bundle-branch block: The relationship between electrocardiogram electrical activation and echocardiography mechanical contraction. *Am Heart J.* 2013;166:340–348.
25. Hancock EW, Deal BJ, Mirvis DM, et al. AHA/ACCF/HRS recommendations for the standardization and interpretation of the electrocardiogram. Part V: electrocardiogram changes associated with cardiac chamber hypertrophy: a scientific statement from the American Heart Association Electrocardiography and Arrhythmias Committee, Council on Clinical Cardiology; the American College of Cardiology Foundation; and the Heart Rhythm Society. *J Am Coll Cardiol.* 2009;53:992–1002.
26. Cabrera E, Monroy JR. Systolic and diastolic loading of the heart II: Electrocardiographic data. *Am Heart J.* 1952;43:669–686.
27. Estes EH, Kerivan L. An archeological dig: A rice-fruit diet reverses ECG changes in hypertension. *J Electrocardiol.* 2014;47:599–607.
28. Bacharova L. Left ventricular hypertrophy: Disagreements between increased left ventricular mass and ECG-LVH criteria: The effect of impaired electrical properties of myocardium. *J Electrocardiol.* 2014;47:625–629.
29. Bacharova L. What is recommended and what remains open in the American Heart Association recommendations for the standardization and interpretation of the electrocardiogram. Part V: electrocardiogram changes associated with cardiac chamber hypertrophy. *J Electrocardiol.* 2009;42:388–391.
30. Romhilt DW, Estes EH. A point score system for the ECG diagnosis of left ventricular hypertrophy. *Am Heart J.* 1968;75:792–799.
31. Butler PM, Leggett SI, Howe CM, et al. Identification of electrocardiographic criteria for diagnosis of right ventricular hypertrophy due to mitral stenosis. *Am J Cardiol.* 1986;57:639–643.
32. Wagner GS, Macfarlane P, Wellens H, et al. AHA/ACCF/HRS recommendations for the standardization and interpretation of the electrocardiogram. Part VI: Acute ischemia/infarction: A scientific statement from the American Heart Association Electrocardiography and Arrhythmias Committee, Council on Clinical Cardiology; the American College of Cardiology Foundation; and the Heart Rhythm Society. *J Am Coll Cardiol.* 2009;53:1003–1011.
33. Surawitz B. The interrelationships between electrolyte abnormalities and arrhythmias. *Cardiac Arrhythmias: Their Mechanisms, Diagnosis and Management.* Philadelphia, PA: JB Lippincott; 1980:83.
34. Krikler DM, Curry PVL. Torsades de pointes, an atypical ventricular tachycardia. *Br Heart J.* 1976;38:117–120.
35. Douglas PS, Carmichael KA, Palevsky PM. Extreme hypercalcemia and electrocardiographic changes. *Am J Cardiol.* 1984;53:674–679.
36. Okada M, Nishamura F, Yoshina H. The J wave in accidental hypothermia. *J Electrocardiol.* 1983;16:23–28.

CHAPTER

2

ECG Manifestations of Concealed Conduction

Mohammad-Reza Jazayeri, MD

INTRODUCTION

Concealed conduction (CC) is a common phenomenon that has fascinated both electrocardiographers and electrophysiologists for decades. This phenomenon occurs when an impulse partially propagates through a part of the conduction system without completing its course. Partial penetration of the conduction system is untraceable on the surface ECG, and its recognition is dependent upon its influence on the subsequent impulse(s). The ECG manifestation of CC could be as a simple conduction delay (block) or a complex event. Conceptually, any cardiac electrical activities that are not directly detectable on the surface ECG could be considered as "concealed." Occasionally, the intracardiac recordings and/or complex electrophysiologic maneuvers may be needed for verification of the occurrence of such a phenomenon or elucidation of its underlying mechanism(s).

HISTORICAL BACKGROUND

The seminal and ingenious work of Willem Einthoven[1,2] leading to the development of the ECG in early 1900s has indebted all physicians, scientists, and especially patients who benefit from this invention. Langendorf[3] introduced the term CC into the field of electrocardiography for the first time in 1948. However, others[4–7] had previously made observations on certain aspects of this concept during animal experimentations as early as 1894, even a few years before the introduction of ECG. With the advent of intracardiac signal recording and stimulation techniques, extensive animal studies and clinical investigations were undertaken and CC became a provocative concept being considered in both simple and most complex arrhythmias.[8–14] Over the past 65 years, CC has gained popularity among both electrocardiographers and electrophysiologists for the analysis and interpretation of cardiac arrhythmias.

ECG MANIFESTATIONS

CC can occur during propagation of the antegrade or retrograde impulses by exhibiting conduction delay or conduction block. It should be borne in mind that the coupling interval between the blocked impulse and its subsequent (rather than preceding) impulse is a crucial determinant of whether CC would occur and if so, how it would manifest.[15]

The ECG Handbook of Contemporary Challenges © 2015 Mohammad Shenasa, Mark E. Josephson, N.A. Mark Estes III
Cardiotext Publishing, ISBN: 978-1-935395-88-1

Concealment During Antegrade Conduction of Impulses

Premature Atrial Complex (PAC)

- In the vast majority of the blocked PACs, the site of CC is in the atrioventricular (AV) node.[11]
- CC of a blocked PAC exerts its impact on the subsequent atrial impulse as conduction delay or block. Two or more consecutive blocked PACs are termed as repetitive CC.[10]
- The PR-interval prolongation due to CC is mostly dependent on the coupling interval between the blocked impulse and the subsequent impulse and not on the prematurity of the former.[15]
- An impulse exerts greater conduction delay on a subsequent impulse if the former is fully propagated instead of being concealed.[15]

High-Rate Supraventricular Impulses

- Normally, the AV nodal conduction time (i.e., AH interval) progressively lengthens as the rate of impulses increases.
- Upon further rate acceleration, the AV node reaches its maximum ability to conduct in a 1:1 fashion and then a periodic block, also known as "Wenckebach block (WB)," ensues.[16]
- Upon further rate acceleration, AV nodal block of higher degrees (2:1, 3:1, etc.), which tend to be more stable, will ensue (Figure 2.1), and this is when CC comes into play.[17]
- Two types of unstable 2:1 behavior are worthy of mention:
  - The AV (PR) intervals of the conducted beats progressively prolong until this period ends with a higher-degree block. This phenomenon is called "alternate-beat Wenckebach periods (AWP)" (Figure 2.2).[18]
  - The AV (PR) intervals of the conducted beats progressively shorten until the period ends with a lesser-degree block. This phenomenon is called "reverse AWP (RAWP)" (see Figure 2.2).[19,20]
- In response to a sudden heart rate acceleration, functional 2:1 block in the His-Purkinje system (HPS),[21,22] functional bundle branch block (FBBB),[22,23] or functional fascicular block[22] may occur transiently or persistently. This is ordinarily expected if the onset of rapid pacing is preceded by a long or short-to-long cycle length (CL) sequence.
- The antegrade refractory period (RP) of the bundle branches (BBs) shortens as the rate is increased.[24]
- During atrial fibrillation (AF), the ventricular (V) response is typically characterized by irregular RR intervals. Although the exact reason for these irregularities is not well understood, several mechanisms, individually or in combination, may be implicated.
  - ***CC.*** Experimental studies in animals and humans have supported CC as being a major determinant of the ventricular rate during AF.[25–28]
  - ***The status of the autonomic nervous system.***[25,29] Fluctuations of the autonomic tone may be profoundly affecting the electrophysiology (EP) principles governing the V rate during AF.
  - ***The AV nodal refractoriness and conductivity.*** These intrinsic AV nodal properties have been proposed as one of the best determinants of the mean V rate during AF.[30]
  - ***Characteristics of the atrial impulses reaching the AV node.*** The degree of concealment in the AV

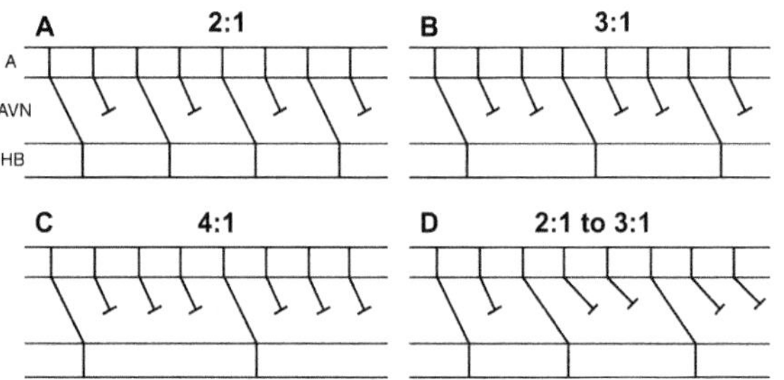

Figure 2.1. Various typical A:V ratios during rapid atrial impulses. These ladder diagrams represent different AV nodal responses to ultra rapid atrial impulses (i.e., AT or flutter). A: atrium; AVN: atrioventricular node; HB: His bundle. (Reproduced with permission.[70])

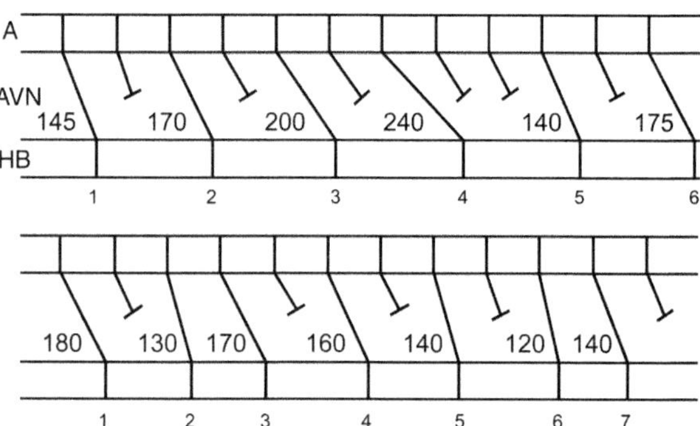

Figure 2.2. Different forms of Wenckebach periodicity during 2:1 conduction. The top panel depicts the AWP with progressive AV interval prolongation of the conducted impulse (1–4) until a higher-degree block ensues. The lower panel demonstrates the reverse AWP, in which the AV interval progressively shortens (3–6) until a lesser-degree block ensues. A: atrium; AVN: atrioventricular node; HB: His bundle. (Reproduced with permission.[70])

node depends upon the strength, form, number, direction, and sequence of the fibrillatory impulses approaching it.[31]

- ***Functional interaction(s) between dual or multiple atrionodal pathways (inputs).*** Indirect evidence supporting this hypothesis comes from the result of catheter ablation of the AV nodal slow pathway in patients with AV nodal reentry. These data clearly demonstrated that in patients with AV nodal reentry, a selective slow-pathway ablation may reduce the V rate during induced AF, particularly after dual-pathway physiology is completely abolished or the AV nodal effective refractory period (ERP) is lengthened postablation.[32,33]

ECG Perspectives Pertinent to Atrial Tachyarrhythmias

- The entire spectrum of the AV nodal conduction in response to rapid atrial impulses may be divided into 4 patterns, namely 1:1 conduction, Wenckebach periodicity, stable 2:1 (and less likely 3:1 or 4:1) conduction, and variable or unstable (AWB or RAWB) block.
- In regard to the relationship of the flutter waves (F) and the QRS complexes in 2:1 conduction pattern, it seems highly likely that first, the F wave closer to the midline between the 2 successive QRS complexes would be the conducted impulse; second, the same F wave exhibits an FR interval, which is usually equal to or longer than the PR interval during sinus beats. Since repetitive CC is an expected AV nodal behavior in response to rapid and successive atrial impulses, the irregularity of the V response during AF is predominantly caused by CC in the AV node rather than the HPS.
- Conversion of atrial tachycardia (AT) or flutter to AF is usually associated with a marked drop of V rate, which is predominantly a manifestation of enhanced AV nodal CC during AF (Figure 2.3).
- V pacing at relatively slower rates may suppress spontaneous V responses during AF. This is most likely related to the enhanced AV nodal concealment in response to V pacing.
- Long-to-short CL variations in the AV nodal outputs (i.e., H-H intervals) set the stage for the genesis of FBBB during AF (the Ashman phenomenon).
- Persistence of FBBB during conduction of several successive beats is not uncommon in AF, and it is due to a phenomenon known as the linking phenomenon.

Concealment During Retrograde Conduction

Premature Impulses

- Isolated ectopic junctional or ventricular beats are of 3 types:[34–37] (1) escape, (2) extrasystolic, and (3) parasystolic. The escape beat occurs after a constant interval (or pause) from the preceding sinus (or supraventricular) beat when the latter fails to reach the AV junction or ventricles. The extrasystoles are premature impulses occurring at constant coupling intervals, while parasystoles are characterized by constant discharges, which are independent of and asynchronous with the dominant rhythm. Any form of these beats can lead to CC if they fail to completely traverse the conduction system.
- If the occurrence of an extrasystole has no influence upon the timing of the next sinus beat, it will be sandwiched between 2 sinus beats, and thus termed "interpolated extrasystole"[36] (Figure 2.4). It is apparent that in order for the junctional or ventricular extrasystolic impulses (JEI and VEI, respectively) to become interpolated, they must have no retrograde conduction. In other words, they tend to block in the AV node and set the stage for the development of CC.

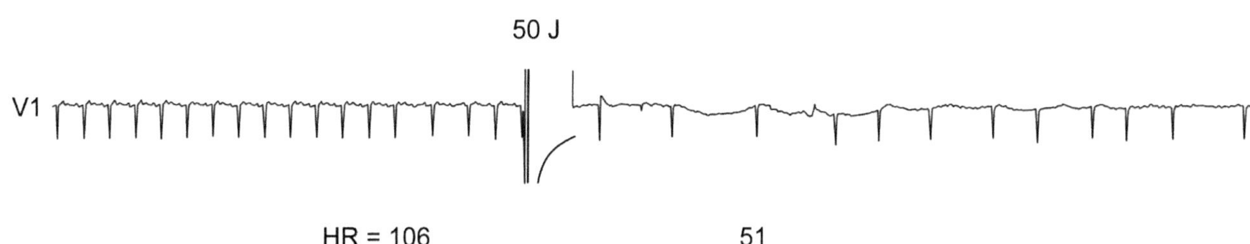

Figure 2.3. Different degrees of concealment during different atrial arrhythmias. A single, synchronized, transthoracic electrical countershock at 50 J converts atrial flutter to AF. Note a marked slowing of the V rate (51 vs. 106 beats per minute) that denotes a significant enhancement of the AV nodal concealed conduction during AF. (Reproduced with permission.[70])

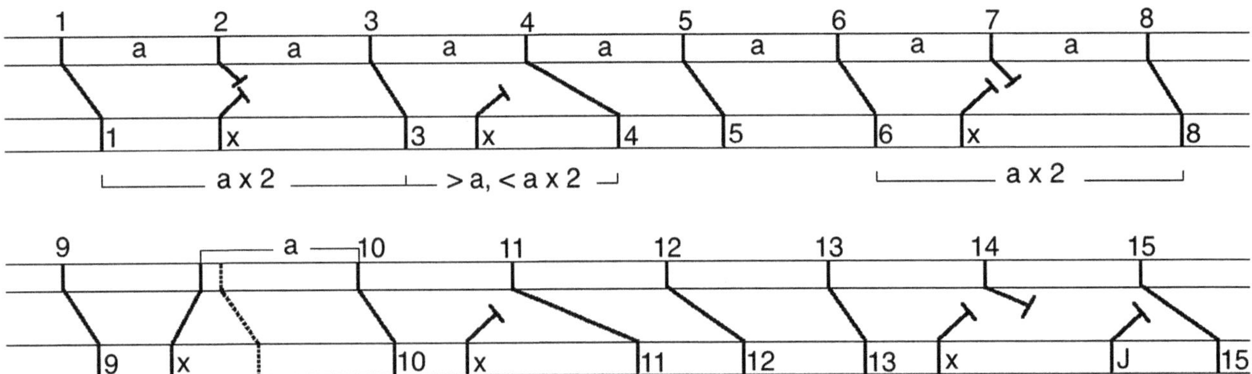

Figure 2.4. Potential influences of V extrasystoles upon conduction of sinus beats. This ladder diagram represents several presumptive situations, in which a single (isolated) V extrasystole (X) occurs during regular sinus rhythm (constant rate of "a") with normal conduction (1, 3, 5, 6, 8–10, 13). Except for the fourth X, all the other X impulses are "interpolated" with no retrograde conduction to the atrium. The first X occurs simultaneously with the sinus impulse (2). The retrograde concealment of the X in the conduction system completely blocks the sinus beat from reaching the ventricle. Most likely, the X would obscure the P wave and there would be a fully compensatory pause to follow. The second and third X impulses occur late in diastole and block retrogradely in the AV node, giving rise to CC. The subsequent sinus beats (4, 7) are conducted with either PR prolongation[4] or (pseudo) second-degree AV block (7). The 4th X conducts retrogradely to the atrium, which may or may not reset the subsequent sinus impulse. (10) The dotted lines represent the anticipated timing of the sinus beat if the X had not occurred. The fifth X, after blocking retrogradely in the AV node, is followed by extra long PR intervals of the subsequent 2 sinus beats (11, 12) (see Figure 1 in Fisch et al[49] and Figure VD8 page 487 in Pick and Langendorf[50]). The alternative explanation for the latter situation is as follows. The sixth X blocks retrograde in the AV node. The subsequent sinus impulse (14) is completely blocked and followed by a junctional escape beat (J), which in turn bocks retrogradely in the AV node and sets the stage for a prolonged PR interval of the subsequent sinus beat (15). (Reproduced with permission.[70])

- In the context of CC, the effect of both JEI and VEI is, for the most part, interchangeable. The HB has a shorter RP than the structures immediately adjacent to it (i.e., AV node and the BBs). Therefore, JEI would be undetectable on the surface ECG if it blocks in both antegrade and retrograde directions (concealed JEI) (Figure 2.5).[38]
- In patients with normal HPS, it seems highly unlikely that a single premature impulse would block retrogradely in the HPS during sinus rhythm.
- Couplets, triplets, or longer runs of consecutive impulses have a higher likelihood of retrograde conduction delay or block in the HPS.

High-Rate V Impulses

- Gradual increments in the V rate (i.e., incremental pacing) up to 200 bpm do not usually show any discernible delay in the HPS conduction.
- At least 20% of individuals with normal AV conduction, at rest and in nonmedicated state, have no retrograde ventriculoatrial (VA) conduction, which is almost always due to the retrograde AV nodal block.
- The AV node is almost always the site of block during incremental V pacing when the rate of pacing is slower than 200 bpm.
- The vast majority of adults with intact VA conduction exhibit Wenckebach periodicity at pacing rates of 90 to 150 bpm. Up to one-third of these

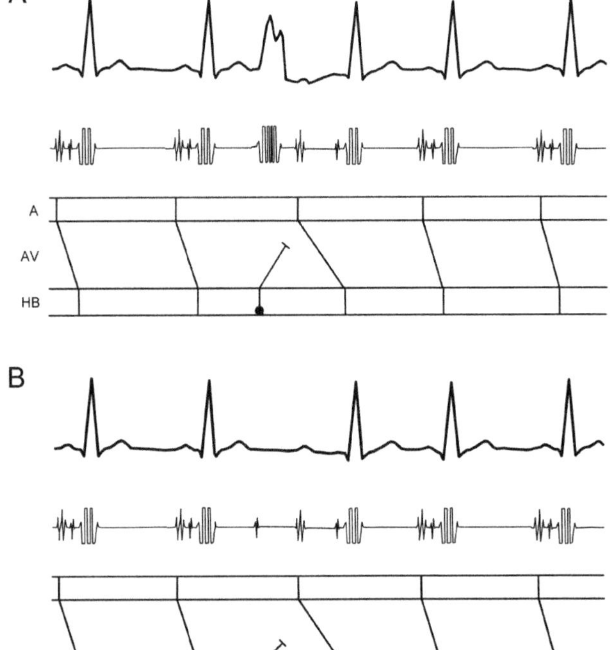

Figure 2.5. The effect of V and junctional extrasystoles on the subsequent sinus beats. These computer-generated tracings represent surface ECG leads, HB electrograms, and ladder diagrams. Panel **A** shows a V extrasystole blocking retrogradely in the AV node (CC) with resultant PR prolongation of the subsequent sinus beat. Panel **B** shows a similar situation created by a junctional extrasystole with bidirectional block. A: atrium; AV: atrioventricular; HB: His bundle. (Reproduced with permission.[70])

individuals have their Wenckebach periodicity interrupted by a ventricular echo beat due to atypical AV nodal reentry, which is almost always a single-beat phenomenon.

ECG Perspectives on the Impact of Retrograde CC on Conduction of Subsequent Antegrade Impulses

Manifestations of CC in response to appropriately-timed JEI or VEI are as follows.[39–57]

- PR interval prolongation (Figures 2.4–2.6).
- Pseudo first-degree AV block (due to concealed JEI) (see Figures 2.4 and 2.5).
- Pseudo second-degree AV block (due to concealed JEI) (see Figure 2.4).
- Pseudo BBB produced by extrasystoles arising in the BBs.
- Transient enhancement or resumption of conduction in the presence of first-degree, second-degree, or advanced AV block.
- Abrupt PR interval changes by shifting from a set of long to a set of short PR intervals or vice versa in the presence of dual or multiple AV nodal pathways (Figure 2.7).
- Promoting double ventricular responses (DVR) due to sequential conduction of the sinus beats over the fast and the slow pathways in the presence of antegrade dual or multiple AV nodal pathways (Figures 2.8 and 2.9).
- Concealed reciprocation (reentry) in the presence of an AV junctional reentrant circuit.

CC DURING COLLISION OF ANTEGRADE AND RETROGRADE IMPULSES

- Antegrade and retrograde impulses may penetrate a pathway simultaneously or sequentially. Depending upon the timing of their arrival, collision of these opposing impulses may occur at different sites along the AV node–HPS axis.[58–61]
- This phenomenon may facilitate conduction and shorten the refractoriness of the corresponding tissue(s) in both antegrade and retrograde directions.[58,59,62]
- In the absence of VA conduction at baseline, collision of impulses may facilitate the retrograde conduction and allow the subsequent V impulse to conduct to the atrium.[61]
- By the same token, in the presence of second-degree or more advanced AV block, an appropriately timed (spontaneous or induced) JEI or VEI may facilitate the antegrade propagation of the next atrial impulse temporarily and thereby allow its conduction.[50]

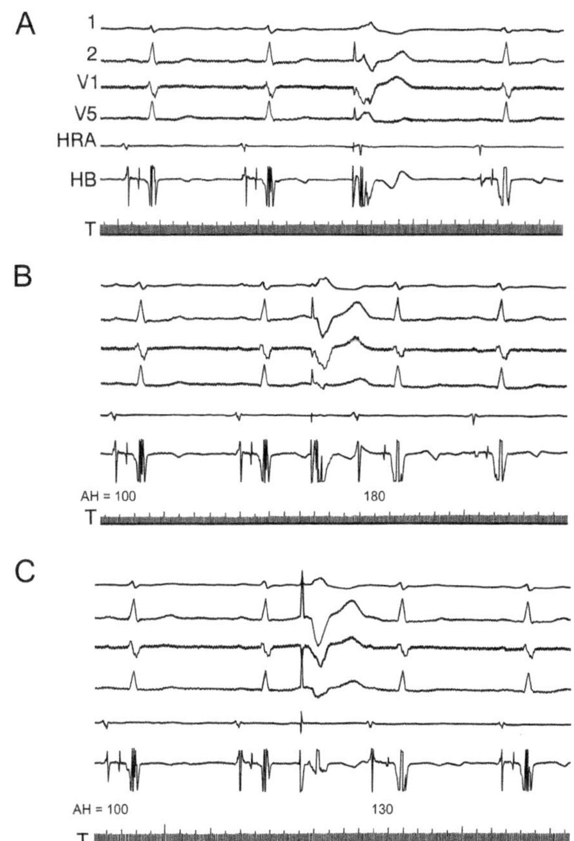

Figure 2.6. Interpolated paced V complexes. A single paced ventricular beat (PVB) is introduced during sinus rhythm at different timing. Note that the PVB has no retrograde conduction. In panel A, the PVB occurs late in diastole and obscures the sinus beat. In panel B, the PVB is introduced early in diastole, and as a result of its CC to the AV node, the subsequent sinus beat is conducted with a prolonged AH interval (180 ms vs. 100 ms during normal conduction). Panel C shows a similar scenario to that in panel B, but the PVB is even earlier in diastole as compared to that in the latter. Consequently, the ensuing concealment has a lesser impact on the subsequent AH interval (130 ms). It becomes apparent that there is an inverse relationship between the timing of the PVB, relative to the subsequent sinus beat, and the magnitude of AH (or PR) prolongation of that beat. HRA: high right atrial electrogram; HB: His bundle electrogram; T: timelines. (Reproduced with permission.[70])

Transseptal CC

- Conduction of impulses across the interventricular septum (i.e., transseptal conduction) occurs in certain situations that will be outlined below. This phenomenon, however, must be considered "concealed" because there is no direct evidence on the surface ECG that would suggest its presence.
- Block of one BB during antegrade conduction of impulses will lead to the transseptal activation (also known as the retrograde invasion) of the same BB via the contralateral BB.[63–65]

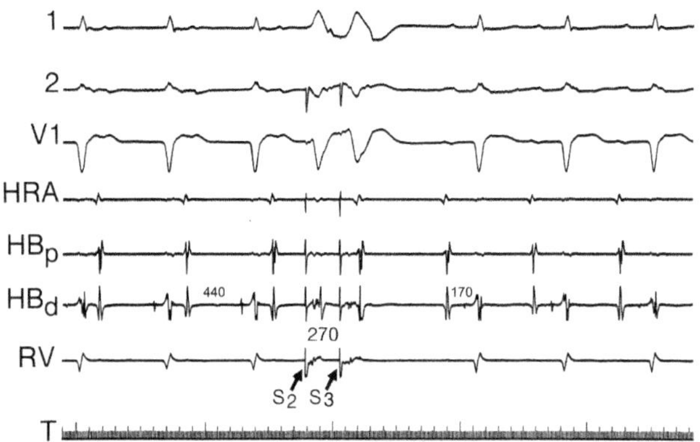

Figure 2.7. Impact of CC on dual AV nodal pathways. Two PVB are introduced during sinus rhythm with a coupling interval of 270 ms. Note that there is no retrograde conduction for these 2 PVBs. This patient has dual AV nodal pathways with 2 sets (short and long) of PR intervals during sinus rhythm. The 2 conducted sinus beats on the left have long PR intervals (AH intervals of 440 ms), which are switched to the shorter PR interval (AH interval of 170 ms) by this ventricular couplet. This is due to CC of these PVBs in the AV node, which inhibited conduction in the slow pathway and facilitated conduction in its faster counterpart. Under the same circumstance, a shift of conduction from the short- to the long-PR set is also feasible (see Figures 86-26 of Fischr[54]). HRA: high right atrial electrogram; HBp and HBd: proximal and distal HB electrograms; RV: right ventricular electrogram; T: timelines. (Reproduced with permission.[70])

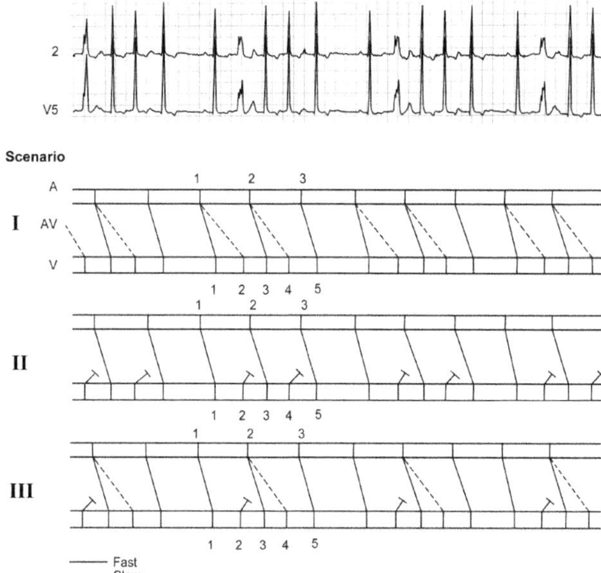

Figure 2.8. ECG diagnosis of DVR. Top panel shows a pattern of group beating in 2 ECG leads (II and V_5). The bottom ladder diagrams represent 3 possible scenarios elucidating the potential underlying mechanism of this group beating. A close examination of the ECG lead II shows regular sinus P waves. The QRS complexes outnumber the P waves 5 to 3 in each group. The second QRS complex in each group is consistently wider than the others. Because all groups are identical, the one that is numbered will be commented on. In scenario I, the first and second sinus beats are conducted sequentially over both fast and slow pathways (FP and SP, respectively), a phenomenon also known as DVR. The second QRS complex exhibits FBBB due to its preceding long-to-short CL sequence. The third sinus impulse is conducted normally. In scenario II, the first, third, and fifth QRS complexes are normally conducted sinus beats. The second and fourth QRS complexes are extrasystoles, both arising from the AV junction with the second one exhibiting FBBB for the same reason outlined above. Alternatively, the second complex is a ventricular extrasystole and the fourth one is a junctional extrasystolic impulse (JEI). In scenario III, the first and third sinus beats are conducted normally with the second complex being an (junctional or V) extrasystole, which in turn by blocking retrogradely in the AV node, facilitates the genesis of a DVR. Figure 2.9 by using an HB electrogram, discloses the precise mechanism of this arrhythmia. (Reproduced with permission.[70])

- As an obligatory component of the reentrant circuit, the transseptal conduction plays a vital role in the following arrhythmias.
  - Orthodromic reentrant tachycardia (ORT) in the presence of antegrade BBB, ipsilateral to the accessory pathway (AP).
  - Antidromic reentrant tachycardia (ART) in the presence of retrograde BBB, ipsilateral to the AP.
  - BB reentrant ventricular tachycardia.

Aberrant Ventricular Conduction (VAb)[22]

Development

- VAb[22] occurs when a supraventricular impulse arrives at the HPS during its RP. This phenomenon can occur in any portion of the intraventricular conduction system; that is, main His bundle (HB), right bundle (RB), and left bundle (LB) or its fascicles.
- VAb patterns are contingent upon the RPs of different components of the HPS, which are all CL dependent.
- VAb may occur as a result of: (1) physiological (functional) behavior; (2) an acceleration-dependent (also known as tachycardia-dependent or rate-related) block (Figure 2.10); or (3) a fatigue phenomenon.
- VAb caused by conduction delay in the BBs has similar electrocardiographic features to that resulted from complete BBB, and therefore the mechanism is not readily discernable by ECG or even EP studies. Thus, both terms of conduction delay and block may be used interchangeably in this situation.
- Because of the longer RP of the RB, FRBBB is more common than FLBBB.
- VAb preceded by a "long-to-short" CL variation is known as the Ashman phenomenon.[66] Because

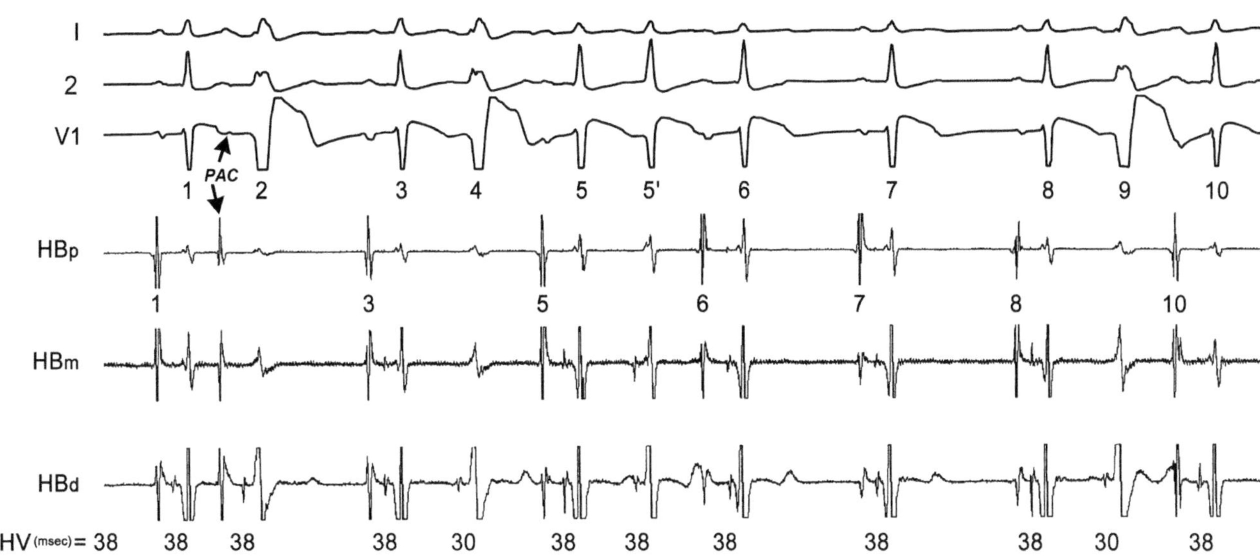

Figure 2.9. HB recording for accurate diagnosis of a DVR. This is obtained from the same patient as in Figure 2.8. During an electrophysiologic study, the patient had spontaneous runs of nonsustained tachycardia, almost the same group of beats that he had demonstrated earlier, but with less frequency. The QRS complexes (1, 3, 7, 8) are normally conducted sinus beats. The QRS complex (2) is a conducted PAC with functional left bundle branch block (FLBBB). The QRS complexes (4, 8) are JEI conducted with FLBBB. Note that the HV intervals of these 2 complexes are slightly shorter than those during normally conducted sinus beats (30 vs. 38 ms), indicating that they probably originated within the HB stem below the recording site. The sinus beat (5) following the first JEI is conducted sequentially over 2 antegrade AV nodal pathways giving rise to a DVR. It becomes apparent that scenario III in Figure 2.8 illustrated the correct mechanism of the grouped beats in this patient. Therefore, without a HB recording, it would have been impossible to determine the exact mechanism of this group beating. HBp, HBm, and HBd: proximal, medial, and distal HB electrograms. (Reproduced with permission.[70])

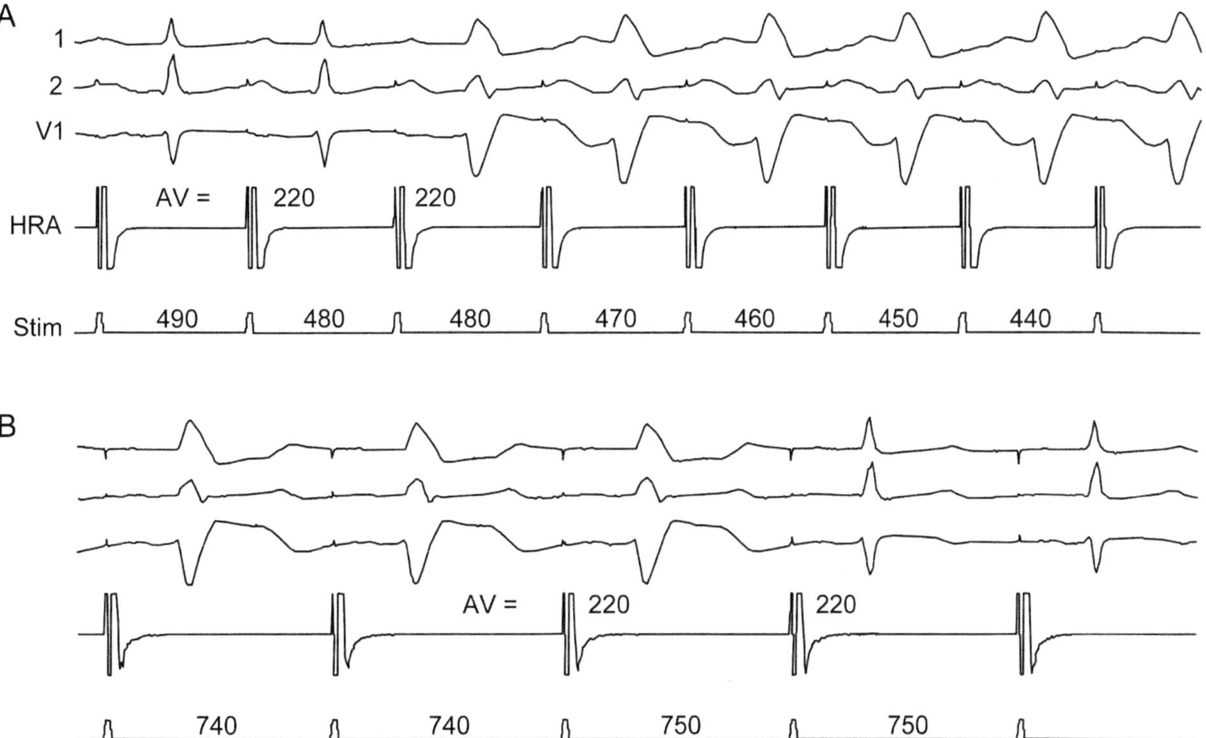

Figure 2.10. Acceleration-dependent BB block. A segment of incremental atrial pacing at CL of 490 to 440 ms is shown in Panel **A**. Note the development of left LBBB in the third conducted complex, which persists to the end of the panel. Panel **B** shows a segment of decremental pacing CL of 740 to 750 ms, which results in the resolution of LBBB. It should be mentioned that, shortly after the development of LBBB, incremental pacing was reversed without interruption to decremental pacing. Note that there is a 270 ms-window between the development and resolution of LBBB, which implies a mechanism by which BBB has maintained. Linking by interference[70] is the most likely mechanism for such a phenomenon.

of the higher prevalence of CL variations of the impulses arriving at the HPS during AF, the Ashman phenomenon (Figure 2.11) is more common during AF than any other supraventricular arrhythmia.

- Alternating VAb patterns[67–69] may occur during atrial bigeminy (i.e., successive long-short-long cycles). These patterns are: RBBB alternating with no VAb, RBBB alternating with RBBB, RBBB alternating with LBBB, and bilateral BB alternating with bilateral BB. Concealed transseptal activation of the blocked BB via its contralateral BB plays a major role in displaying these patterns. For instance, in the most fascinating pattern where RBBB alternates with LBBB (Figure 2.12), the first BB manifesting block is activated retrogradely via its contralateral BB. Thus, the CL of activation and hence the RP of the blocked BB (distal to the site of block) for the next cycle is shorter than those of the contralateral BB. The likelihood of the contralateral BB being the site of FBBB during conduction of the subsequent beat, ending the next short cycle, is therefore higher than that of the ipsilateral BB. Obviously, several other factors may also be important in facilitating the occurrence of this phenomenon. These include the prematurity of the impulses ending the short cycles, the length of the long CLs separating the short cycles, differential RPs of BBs, and the AV nodal functional RP.

Maintenance

Once FBBB develops, it may become persistent, at least for several cycles. Repetitive retrograde (transseptal) penetration of the distal portion of the blocked BB via its contralateral BB (i.e., linking by interference[70]) is the mechanism of FBBB maintenance. Similarly, concealed retrograde interfascicular conduction may also maintain functional fascicular block (as an isolated FB or in combination with FRBBB) for several successive beats.[71]

Resolution

FBBB may be resolved spontaneously or by premature impulses.[22,43] Migration of the site of block to a more distal location with shorter RP[72] or gradual shortening of the refractoriness due to accommodation[73–76] are 2 mechanisms that are worthy of mention in spontaneous resolution of FBBB. Peeling back refractoriness[77] is the putative mechanism of FBBB resolution mediated by premature impulses.

DVR and CC

DVR is a phenomenon that has also been termed as "1:2 response". DVR is characterized by 2 sets of V activation in response to a single atrial impulse. This could be a spontaneous or laboratory-induced phenomenon. DVR may develop in the presence of dual or multiple (AV nodal or accessory) pathways capable of conducting in the antegrade direction[22,78–81] with different conduction properties. Ordinarily, the retrograde concealment in the pathway with slower conduction would not permit complete propogation of the impulse and the genesis of DVR. Therefore for DVR to occur, CC must at least partially resolve.[70]

Impact of CC on Different Forms of Tachycardia

Reentrant Tachycardias

For any anatomic reentrant process to occur, a reentrant circuit[82] is required in which (1) a unidirectional block allows the impulses to circulate in only one

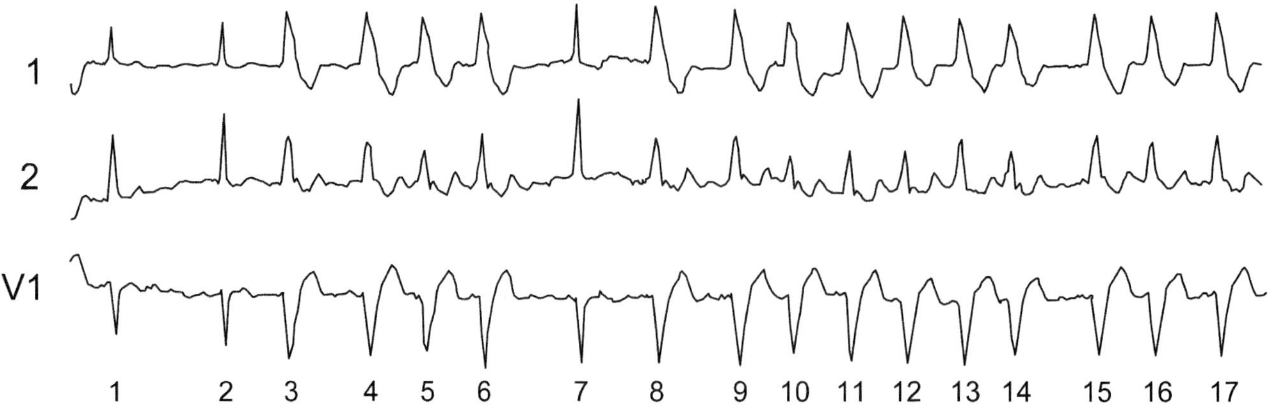

Figure 2.11. Ashman's phenomenon during AF. ECG leads show a segment of AF with narrow (1, 2, 7) as well as wide QRS complexes (3–6, 8–17). The wide QRS complexes are due to functional (left) FBBB. The occurrence of FBBB is preceded by long-to-short CL variations, a process also known as the Ashman's phenomenon. The maintenance of FBBB is due to "linking by interference."[70] (Reproduced with permission.[70])

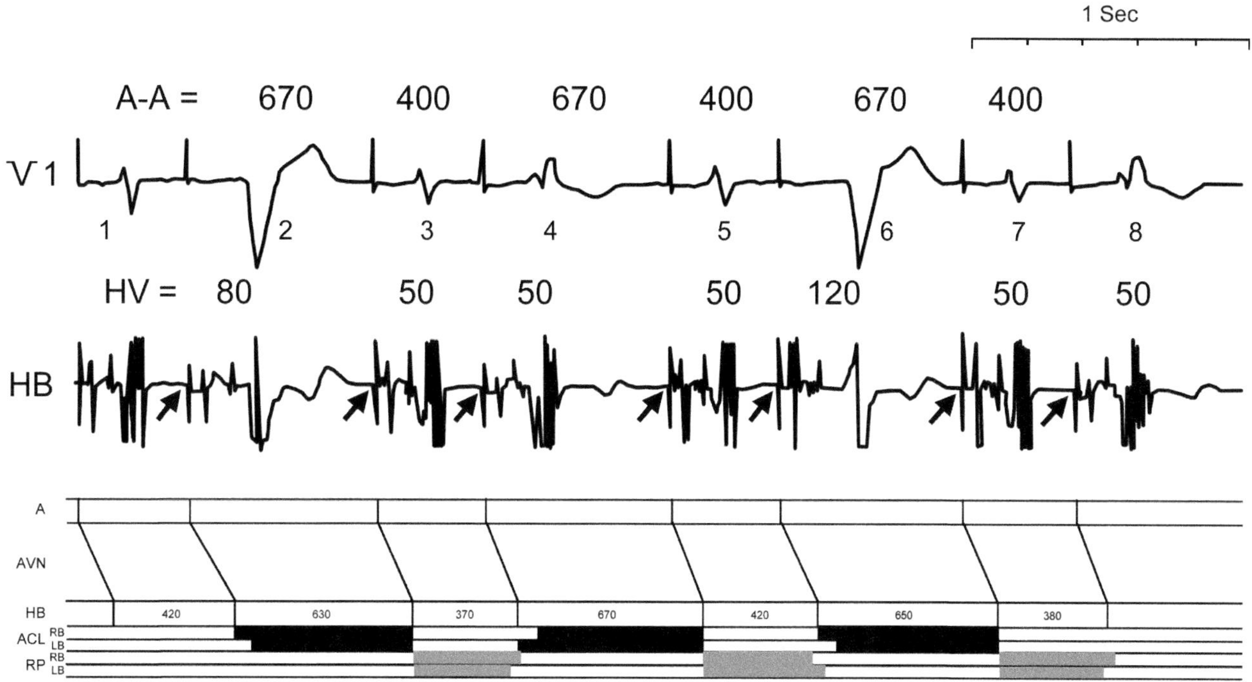

Figure 2.12. Alternating FBBB during atrial bigeminy. Tracings from top to bottom are surface ECG leads V_1 and His-bundle electrogram (HB). A ladder diagram placed at the bottom depicts the relative activation timing of the atria (A), AV node (AVN), and HB, as well as the activation cycle lengths (ACL) and RPs of the RB and LB. This is a segment of paced bigeminal atrial rhythm, which shows a series of alternating long and short cycles. For all practical purposes, the atrial impulses ending the short cycles behave as premature (A2) beats. The A2 impulses conduct with alternating functional LB and RB block. Note that the retrograde CC of each blocked bundle via the contralateral bundle sets the stage for the occurrence of functional block in the latter during antegrade conduction of the subsequent A2. Also note the HV interval is markedly prolonged with functional LB block (80 and 120 ms) as compared to the other complexes (50 ms), which indicates significant conduction delay along the HB-RB axis. (Adapted with permission.[22])

direction; and (2) in a spatial or temporal sense, the circuit must be long or slow enough to permit the reentrant wavefront to circulate without encountering any refractory tissue along the way. It becomes apparent that the initial (unidirectional) block is pivotal for the initiation of the reentrant tachycardia. Additionally, the site of the initial block is equally important for both the initiation of reentry and the direction in which, the reentrant impulses circulate. For instance, in the presence of an AP, the antegrade block of a PAC in the AP, and its conduction over the NP would initiate ORT and conversely, the antegrade block of a PAC in the NP and its conduction over the AP would initiate true ART. Similarly, the retrograde block of a premature V impulse in the NP and its conduction over the AP would set the stage for the initiation of ORT, whereas the opposite situation may fulfill the prerequisite(s) of the initiation of ART. More specifically, in both ORT and ART, the AV node is usually the weakest link for the initiation and maintenance of reentry.[22,83] Thus, during ORT initiation by premature V impulse, the site of retrograde block in the HPS is more likely to permit ORT to occur than if the AV node was the site of CC.[84,85] On the other hand, induction of ART by A2 usually requires a proximal AV nodal block. Therefore, by the time the impulse has completed its course over the AP, V muscle, the HPS, and the distal AV node, the proximal AV node would have enough time to regain its excitability. Termination of a reentrant process by CC is also a common occurrence. This is primarily accomplished when a part of the reentrant circuit becomes refractory by premature impulses.[86–89]

Tachycardias with V > A

The main characteristic of these tachycardias is the presence of AV discordance. Technically, the term AV dissociation may not be quite suitable or descriptive for the situation. They have also been termed as pseudotachycardia,[90] abrupt doubling of the V rate,[91] or 1:2 tachycardia.[92] Occasionally, the A:V ratio is variable and not necessarily in a constant 1:2 relationship. Two prototypes have been identified.

- ***Nonreentrant Supraventricular (AV Nodal or Junctional) Tachycardia.*** This tachycardia is a persistent form of a DVR phenomenon in which successive dual AV nodal responses produce a run of tachycardia (Figure 2.13).[91,93–98] The occurrence

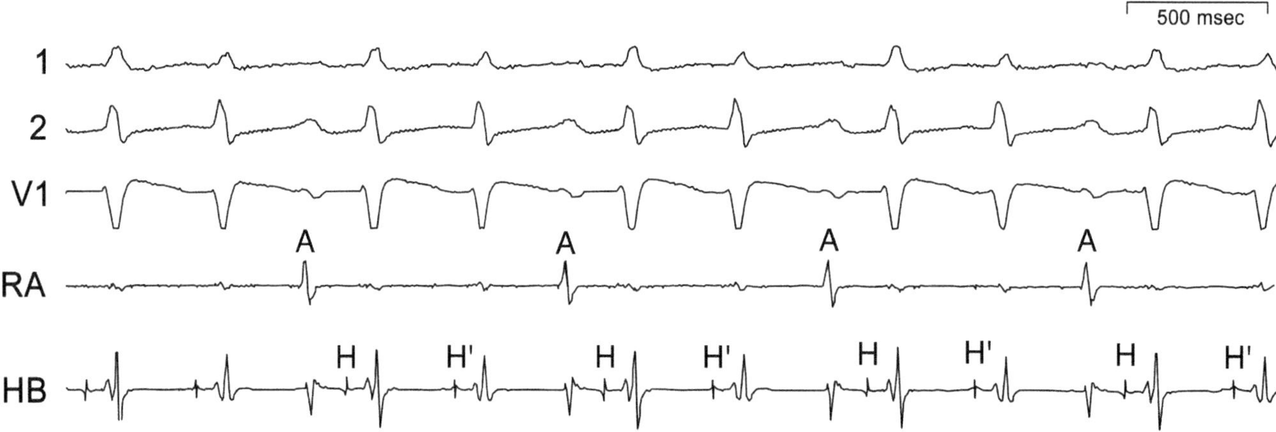

Figure 2.13. Nonreentrant supraventricular tachycardia (SVT). A segment of SVT is shown in a patient with dual AV nodal pathways. The QRS complexes outnumber the sinus P waves 2 to 1. Each atrial impulse (A) is conducted to the HB sequentially via a fast pathway (H) and a slow pathway (H'). RA: right atrial electrogram. (Reproduced with permission.[70])

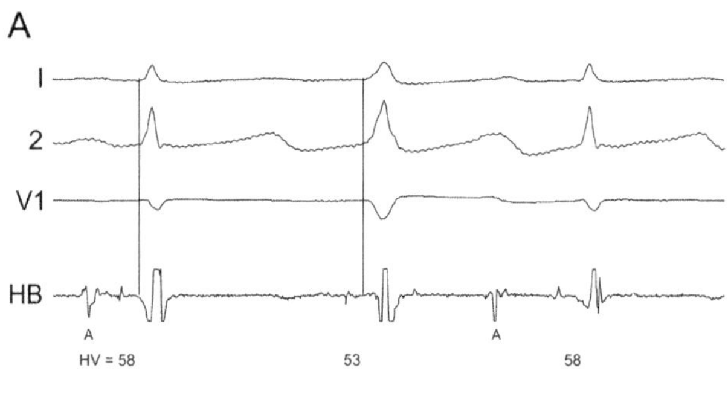

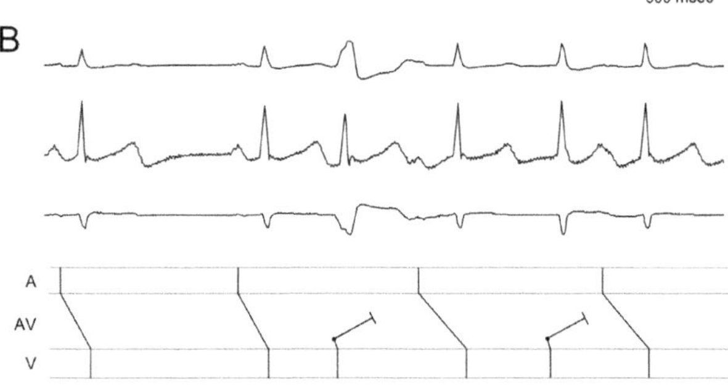

Figure 2.14. Abrupt doubling of ventricular rate due to interpolated extrasystoles. Panel **A** shows an interpolated JEI sandwiched between 2 sinus beats (SB). The HV interval of 53 ms (vs. 58 ms during SB) is in favor of the middle complex being JEI rather than a supraventricular impulse of a different origin, such as the second component of a DVR. Panel **B** shows a segment of tachycardia produced by the JEIs alternating with the SB. Note that the JEIs block retrogradely in the AV node (i.e., CC), which is crucial for the genesis of this rather unusual form of tachycardia. It should be pointed out that in the presence of retrograde ventriculoatrial conduction, the JEI would not have been interpolated, sandwiched between 2 successive SB, and therefore this tachycardia would not have occurred. (Reproduced with permission.[70])

of this tachycardia depends upon a very delicate balance between the conduction properties and recovery of excitability of the AV nodal pathways. The underlying atrial drive could be sinus rhythm, ectopic atrial rhythm, or AT.

- ***Sinus Beats Alternating with Interpolated Premature Impulses.***[91,99] An interpolated impulse (VEI or JEI) is sandwiched between 2 conducted sinus beats (Figure 2.14). For this to occur, the extrasystole must lack retrograde VA conduction to the atrium. This is usually furnished by retrograde AV nodal block (CC) of the interpolated impulse, which in turn might also lengthen the PR interval of the subsequent sinus beat. Successive occurrence of the interpolated impulse in a bigeminal fashion gives rise to tachycardia if the underlying sinus rhythm is 50 bpm or faster.

REFERENCES

1. Moukabary T. Willem Einthoven (1860–1927): Father of electrocardiography. *Cardiol J.* 2007;14:316–317.
2. Rosen M. The electrocardiogram 100 years later: Electrical insights into molecular messages. *Circulation.* 2002;106:2173–2179.
3. Langendorf R. Concealed A-V conduction; the effect of blocked impulses on the formation and conduction of subsequent impulses. *Am Heart J.* 1948;35:542–552.
4. Englemann TW. Beobachtungen und Versuche am suspendieren Herzen. *Pfluegers Arch.* 1894;56:149–202.
5. Ashman R. Conductivity in compressed cardiac muscle. *Am J Physiol.* 1925;74:121–139.
6. Drury AN. Further observations upon intraauricular block produced by pressure or cooling. *Heart.* 1925;12:143–169.

7. Lewis T, Master AM. Observations upon conduction in the mammalian heart. A-V conduction. *Heart.* 1925;12:209–269.
8. Langendorf R, Pick A. Concealed conduction further evaluation of a fundamental aspect of propagation of the cardiac impulse. *Circulation.* 1956;13:381–399.
9. Moe GK, Abildskov JA, Mendez C. An experimental study of concealed conduction. *Am Heart J.* 1964;67:338–356.
10. Langendorf R, Pick A, Edelist A, et al. Experimental demonstration of concealed AV conduction in the human heart. *Circulation.* 1965;32:386–393.
11. Moore EN. Microelectrode studies on concealment of multiple premature atrial responses. *Circ Res.* 1966;18:660–672.
12. Moore EN. Microelectrode studies on retrograde concealment of multiple premature ventricular responses. *Circ Res.* 1967;20:88–98.
13. Moore EN, Knoebel SB, Spear JF. Concealed conduction. *Am J Cardiol.* 1971;28:406–413.
14. Damato AN, Lau SH. Concealed and supernormal atrioventricular conduction. *Circulation.* 1971;43:967–970.
15. Wu D, Denes P, Dhingra RC, et al. Quantification of human atrioventricular nodal concealed conduction utilizing S1S2S3 stimulation. *Circ Res.* 1976;39:659–665.
16. Denes P, Levy L, Pick A, et al. The incidence of typical and atypical A-V Wenckebach periodicity. *Am Heart J.* 1975;89:26–31.
17. McKinnie J, Avitall B, Caceres J, et al. Electrophysiologic spectrum of concealed intranodal conduction during atrial rate acceleration in a model of 2:1 atrioventricular block. *Circulation.* 1989;80:43–50.
18. Castellanos A, Interian A Jr, Cox MM, et al. Alternating Wenckebach periods and allied arrhythmias. *Pacing Clin Electrophysiol.* 1993;16:2285–2300.
19. Young M, Gelband H, Castellanos A, et al. Reverse alternating Wenckebach periodicity. *Am J Cardiol.* 1987;80:90–94.
20. Castellanos A, Fuenmayor AJ, Huikuri H, et al. Dynamics of atrioventricular nodal conduction ratios of reverse alternating Wenckebach periods. *Am J Cardiol.* 1989;64:1047–1049.
21. Damato AN, Varghese J, Caracta AR, et al. Functional 2:1 A-V Block within the His-Purkinje system. Simulation of type II second-degree A-V block. *Circulation.* 1973;47:534–542.
22. Jazayeri MR, Sra JJ, Akhtar M. Wide QRS complexes. Electrophysiologic basis of a common electrocardiographic diagnosis. *J Cardiovasc Electrophysiol.* 1992;3:365–393.
23. Denker S, Shenasa M, Gilbert CJ, et al. Effects of abrupt changes in cycle length on refractoriness of the His-Purkinje system in man. *Circulation.* 1983;67:60–68.
24. Chiale PA, Sanchez RA, Franco DA, et al. Overdrive prolongation of refractoriness and fatigue in the early stages of human bundle branch disease. *J Am Coll Cardiol.* 1994;23:724–732.
25. Moe GK, Abildskov JA. Observations on the ventricular dysrhythmia associated with atrial fibrillation in the dog. *Circ Res.* 1964;14:447–460.
26. Moore EN. Observations on concealed conduction in atrial fibrillation. *Circ Res.* 1967;21:201–208.
27. Moore EN, Spear JF. Electrophysiological studies on atrial fibrillation. *Heart Vessels Suppl.* 1987;2:32–39.
28. Cohen SI, Lau SH, Berkowitz WD, et al. Concealed conduction during atrial fibrillation. *Am J Cardiol.* 1970;25:416–419.
29. van den Berg MP, Haaksma J, Brouwer J, et al. Heart rate variability in patients with atrial fibrillation is related to vagal tone. *Circulation.* 1997;96:1209–1216.
30. Toivonen L, Kadish A, Kou W, et al. Determinants of the ventricular rate during atrial fibrillation. *J Am Coll Cardiol.* 1990;16:1194–1200.
31. Bootsma BK, Hoelsen AJ, Strackee J, et al. Analysis of R-R Intervals in patients with atrial fibrillation at rest and during exercise. *Circulation.* 1970;41:783–794.
32. Blanck Z, Dhala AA, Sra J, et al. Characterization of atrioventricular nodal behavior and ventricular response during atrial fibrillation before and after a selective slow-pathway ablation. *Circulation.* 1995;91:1086–1094.
33. Markowitz SM, Stein KM, Lerman BB. Mechanism of ventricular rate control after radiofrequency modification of atrioventricular conduction in patients with atrial fibrillation. *Circulation.* 1996;94:2856–2864.
34. Schamroth L, Marriott HJ. Concealed ventricular extrasystoles. *Circulation.* 1963;27:1043–1049.
35. Schamroth L. Genesis and evolution of ectopic ventricular rhythm. *Br Heart J.* 1966;28:244–257.
36. Schamroth L. Interpolated extrasystoles. *S Afr Med J.* 1967;41:919–922.
37. Schamroth L, Surawicz B. Concealed interpolated A-V junctional extrasystoles and A-V junctional parasystole. *Am J Cardiol.* 1971;27:703–707.
38. Rosen KM, Ehsani AA, Sinno MZ, et al. Simultaneous block proximal and distal to His bundle. An example of concealed "concealed conduction." *Arch Intern Med.* 1973;131:588–590.
39. Katz LN, Langendorff R, Cole SL: An unusual effect of interpolated ventricular premature systoles. *Am Heart J.* 1944;28:167–176.
40. Langendorf R, Mehlman JS. Blocked (nonconducted) A-V nodal premature systoles imitating first and second degree A-V block. *Am Heart J.* 1947;34:500–506.
41. Marriott HJL, Bradley SM. Main-stem extrasystoles. *Circulation.* 1957;16:544–547.
42. Rosen KM, Rahimtoola SH, Gunnar RM. Pseudo A-V block secondary to premature nonpropagated His bundle depolarizations. documentation by His bundle electrocardiography. *Circulation.* 1970;42:367–373.
43. Chung EK. A reappraisal of concealed atrioventricular conduction. *Am Heart J.* 1971;82:408–416.
44. Massumi RA, Ertem GE, Vera Z. Aberrancy of junctional escape beats. Evidence for origin in the fascicles of the left bundle branch. *Am J Cardiol.* 1972;29:351–359.
45. Massumi RA, Hilliard G, DeMaria A, et al. Paradoxic phenomenon of premature beats with narrow QRS in the presence of bundle-branch block. *Circulation.* 1973;47:543–553.
46. Cannom DS, Gallagher JJ, Goldreyer BN, et al. Concealed bundle of His extrasystoles simulating nonconducted atrial premature beats. *Am Heart J.* 1972;83:777–779.

47. Lindsay AE, Schamroth L. Atrioventricular junctional parasystole with concealed conduction simulating second degree atrioventricular block. *Am J Cardiol.* 1973;31:397–399.
48. Castellanos A, Befeler B, Myerburg RJ. Pseudo AV block produced by concealed extrasystoles arising below the bifurcation of the His bundle. *Br Heart J.* 1974;36:457–461.
49. Fisch C, Zipes DP, McHenry PL. Electrocardiographic manifestations of concealed junctional ectopic impulses. *Circulation.* 1976;53:217–223.
50. Pick A, Langendorf R. Specific mechanisms of various disorders of impulse formation, conduction, and their combinations. In: Pick A, Langendorf R, eds. *Interpretations of Complex Arrhythmias.* Philadelphia, PA: Lea and Febiger; 1979:367–578.
51. Camous JP, Baudouy M, Guarino L, et al. Effects of an interpolated premature ventricular contraction on the AV conduction of the subsequent premature atrial depolarization. An apparent facilitation. *J Electrocardiol.* 1980;13:353–357.
52. Fisch C. Concealed conduction. *Cardiol Clin.* 1983;1:63–74.
53. Fisch C. Concealed conduction at the AV nodal level. In: Mazgalev T, Dreifus LS, Michelson EL, eds. *Electrophysiology of Sinoatrial and Atrioventricular Nodes.* New York, NY: Alan R. Liss, Inc; 1988:287–300.
54. Fisch C. Concealed conduction. In: Jalife J, Zipes DP, eds. *Cardiac Electrophysiology: From Cell to Bedside.* Philadelphia, PA: WB Saunders; 1995:961–969.
55. Damato AN, Varghese PJ, Lau SH, et al. Manifest and concealed reentry. A mechanism of AV nodal Wenckebach phenomenon. *Circ Res.* 1972;30:283–292.
56. Gallagher JJ, Damato AN, Varghese PJ, et al. Manifest and concealed reentry: A mechanism of A-V nodal Wenckebach in man. *Circulation.* 1973;47:752–757.
57. Langendorf R, Pick A. Manifestations of concealed reentry in the atrioventricular junction. *Eur J Cardiol.* 1973;1:11–21.
58. Shenasa M, Denker S, Mahmud R, et al. Atrioventricular nodal conduction and refractoriness after intranodal collision from antegrade and retrograde impulses. *Circulation.* 1983;67:651–660.
59. Lehmann MH, Mahmud R, Denker S, et al. Retrograde concealed conduction in the atrioventricular node: Differential manifestations related to level of intranodal penetration. *Circulation.* 1984;70:392–401.
60. Mahmud R, Lehmann M, Denker S, et al. Atrioventricular sequential pacing: Differential effect on retrograde conduction related to level of impulse collision. *Circulation.* 1983;68:23–32.
61. Mahmud R, Denker S, Lehmann MH, et al. Effect of atrioventricular sequential pacing in patients with no ventriculoatrial conduction. *J Am Coll Cardiol.* 1984;4:273–4277.
62. Li H, Yee R, Thakur RK, et al. The effect of variable retrograde penetration on dual AV nodal pathways: Observations before and after slow pathway ablation LDD. *Pacing Clin Electrophysiol.* 1997;20:2146–2153. C2
63. Moe GK, Mendez C, Han J. Aberrant A-V impulse propagation in the dog heart. A study of functional bundle branch block. *Circ Res.* 1965;16:261–286.
64. Moe GK, Mendez C. Functional block in the intraventricular conduction system. *Circulation.* 1971;43:949–954.
65. Wellens HJJ, Durrer D. Supraventricular tachycardia with left aberrant conduction due to retrograde invasion into the left bundle branch. *Circulation.* 1968;38:474–479.
66. Gouaux JL, Ashman R. Auricular fibrillation with aberration simulating ventricular paroxysmal tachycardia. *Am Heart J.* 1947;34:366–373.
67. Cohen SI, Lau SH, Scherlag BJ, Damato AN. Alternate patterns of premature ventricular excitation during induced atrial bigeminy. *Circulation.* 1969;39:819–829.
68. Denker S, Lehmann M, Mahmud R, et al. Effects of alternating cycle lengths on refractoriness of the His-Purkinje system. *J Clin Invest.* 1984;74:559–570.
69. Stark S, Farshidi A. Mechanism of alternating bundle branch aberrancy with atrial bigeminy. Electrocardiographic-electrophysiologic correlate. *J Am Coll Cardiol.* 1985;5:1491–1495.
70. Jazayeri MR. Concealed conduction and allied concepts. *Card Electrophysiol Clin.* 2014;6:377–418.
71. Jazayeri MR, Caceres J, Tchou P, et al. Electrophysiologic characteristics of sudden QRS axis deviation during orthodromic tachycardia. Role of functional fascicular block in localization of accessory pathway. *J Clin Invest.* 1989;83:952–959.
72. Myerburg RJ. The gating mechanism in the distal atrioventricular conducting system. *Circulation.* 1971;43:955–960.
73. Akhtar M, Gilbert C, Al-Nouri M, et al. Site of conduction delay during functional block in the His-Purkinje systemin man. *Circulation.* 1980;61:1239–1248.
74. Lehmann MH, Denker S, Mahmud R, et al. Postextrasystolic alterations in refractoriness of the His-Purkinje system and ventricular myocardium in man. *Circulation.* 1984;69:1096–1102.
75. Lehmann MH, Denker S, Mahmud R, et al. Functional His-Purkinje system behavior during sudden ventricular rate acceleration in man. *Circulation.* 1983;68:767–775.
76. Miles WM, Prystowsky EN. Alteration of human right bundle branch refractoriness by changes in duration of the atrial drive train. *Circulation.* 1986;73:244–248.
77. Moe GK, Childers RW, Merideth J. Appraisal of "supernormal" A-V conduction. *Circulation.* 1968;38:5–28.
78. Wu D, Denes P, Dhingra R, et al. New manifestations of dual A-V nodal pathways. *Eur J Cardiol.* 1975;2:459–466.
79. Akhtar M, Damato AN, Lau SH, et al. Clinical uses of His bundle electrocardiography. Part III. *Am Heart J.* 1976;91:805–809.
80. Josephson ME, Seides SF, Damato AN. Wolff-Parkinson-White syndrome with 1:2 atrioventricular conduction. *Am J Cardiol.* 1976;37:1094–1096.
81. Jazayeri MR, Keelan ET, Jazayeri MA. Atrioventricular nodal reentrant tachycardia: Current understanding

and controversies. In: Shenasa M, Hindricks G, Borggrefe M, et al., eds. *Cardiac Mapping.* 4th ed. New York, NY: Wiley-Blackwell Publishing Ltd; 2012.
82. Mines GR. On circulating excitations in heart muscles and their possible relation to tachycardia and fibrillation. *Trans R Soc Can.* 1914;8:43–52.
83. Lehmann MH, Tchou P, Mahmud R, et al. Electrophysiological determinants of antidromic reentry induced during atrial extrastimulation. Insights from a pacing model of Wolff-Parkinson-White syndrome. *Circ Res.* 1989;65:295–306.
84. Akhtar, M, Shenasa M, Schmidt DH. Role of retrograde His Purkinje block in the initiation of supraventricular tachycardia by ventricular premature stimulation in the Wolff-Parkinson-White syndrome. *J Clin Invest.* 1981;67:1047–1055.
85. Akhtar M, Lehmann MH, Denker ST, et al. Electrophysiologic mechanisms of orthodromic tachycardia initiation during ventricular pacing in the Wolff-Parkinson-White syndrome. *J Am Coll Cardiol.* 1987;9:89–100.
86. Moe GK, et al. Experimentally induced paroxysmal A-V nodal tachycardia in the dog. *Am Heart J.* 1963;65:87–92.
87. Massumi RA, Kistin AD, Tawakkol AA. Termination of reciprocating tachycardia by atrial stimulation. *Circulation.* 1967;36:637–643.
88. Barold SS, Linhart JW, Samet P, Lister JW. Supraventricular tachycardia initiated and terminated by a single electrical stimulus. *Am J Cardiol.* 1969;24:37–41.
89. Ross, DL, Farre J, Bar FW, et al. Spontaneous termination of circus movement tachycardia using an accessory pathway. Incidence, site of block and mechanisms. *Circulation.* 1981;63:1129–1139.
90. Massumi RA. Atrioventricular junctional rhythms. In: Mandel WJ, ed. *Cardiac Arrhythmias. Their Mechanisms, Diagnosis, and Management.* Philadelphia, PA: JB Lippincott; 1987:235–260.
91. Massumi R, Shehata M. Doubling of the ventricular rate by interpolated junctional extrasystoles resembling supraventricular tachycardia. *Pacing Clin Electrophysiol.* 2010;33:945–949.
92. Germano JJ, Essebag V, Papageorgiou P, et al. Concealed and manifest 1:2 tachycardia and atrioventricular nodal reentrant tachycardia: Manifestations of dual atrioventricular nodal physiology. *Heart Rhythm.* 2005;2:536–539.
93. Csapo G. Paroxysmal nonreentrant tachycardias due to simultaneous conduction in dual atrioventricular nodal pathways. *Am J Cardiol.* 1979;43:1033–1045.
94. Buss J, Kraatz J, Stegaru B, et al. Unusual mechanism of PR interval variation and nonreentrant supraventricular tachycardia as manifestation of simultaneous anterograde fast and slow conduction through dual atrioventricular nodal pathways. *Pacing Clin Electrophysiol.* 1985;8:235–241.
95. Kim SS, Lal R, Ruffy R. et al. Paroxysmal nonreentrant supraventricular tachycardia due to simultaneous fast and slow pathway conduction in dual atrioventricular node pathways. *J Am Coll Cardiol.* 1987;10:456–461.
96. Li HG, Klein GJ, Natale A, et al. Nonreentrant supraventricular tachycardia due to simultaneous conduction over fast and slow AV node pathways: Successful treatment with radiofrequency ablation. *Pacing Clin Electrophysiol.* 1994;17:1186–1193.
97. Arena G, Bongiorni MG, Soldati E, et al. Incessant nonreentrant atrioventricular nodal tachycardia due to multiple nodal pathways treated by radiofrequency ablation of the slow pathways. *J Cardiovasc Electrophysiol.* 1999;10:1636–1642.
98. Yokoshiki H, Sasaki K, Shimokawa J, et al. Nonreentrant atrioventricular nodal tachycardia due to triple nodal pathways manifested by radiofrequency ablation at coronary sinus ostium. *J Electrocardiol.* 2006;39:395–399.
99. Massumi RA. Interpolated His bundle extrasystoles. An unusual cause of tachycardia. *Am J Med.* 1970;49:265–270.

CHAPTER

3

P-Wave Indices and the PR Interval—Relation to Atrial Fibrillation and Mortality

Konstantinos N. Aronis, MD and
Jared W. Magnani, MD, MS

INTRODUCTION

Atrial fibrillation (AF) has a rising prevalence with concomitant related morbidity and mortality. Increased attention to AF risk assessment and prevention has yielded advances in AF epidemiology and genetics. Simultaneously, the ECG has garnered renewed attention in these efforts, particularly because of its low cost, widespread accessibility and the application of software-based algorithms for quantifying atrial conduction. In population- and community-based studies, the PR interval has been related to AF. P-wave indices (PWIs)—measures of atrial electrical conduction derived from the 12-lead ECG—have been recognized as intermediate risk markers for AF. A literature is likewise emerging describing the association of PWIs with other adverse outcomes, that is, stroke and mortality. This chapter reviews the derivation, quantification, and clinical significance of PWIs. We describe the present epidemiology of PWIs and their relation to adverse outcomes. Our primary focus is on AF, as PWIs have been described as intermediate endophenotypes for AF risk. We conclude by identifying future directions and applications of PWIs.

BACKGROUND

Electroanatomical Significance of the P Wave and Definitions of PWIs

The electrocardiographic P wave is visualized on the ECG and represents atrial conduction. An extensive history of ECG analysis has incorporated P-wave characteristics in ECG interpretation. P-wave amplitude ≥0.25 mV in lead II is a criterion for right atrial enlargement (P-pulmonale). P-wave duration ≥120 ms with prominent notching in lead II and 0.4 ms interval between notches has been used for left atrial enlargement (P-mitrale). A leftward P-wave axis (−30° to −45°) or increased P-wave terminal force ≥4 μV·ms (Morris' index) is suggestive of left atrial enlargement.[1]

A fundamental premise in P-wave analysis is their correlation with atrial electrophysiologic activity. The electrophysiologic significance of P-wave measurements is borne out by intracardiac studies describing altered atrial electrical function. Individuals with sinus node dysfunction have altered atrial electrophysiology (EP), as demonstrated by increased atrial conduction time, atrial refractory periods, and P-wave duration.[2] Atrial fractionation increases with aging,[3] and intracardiac studies demonstrate the progressive increase in P-wave duration accompanying age-related changes in atrial electrical function. Atrial conduction is further altered in hypertension, sleep-disordered breathing, and heart failure.[6–8] Other diverse insults, such as pressure or volume overload, ischemia, and inflammation promote fibrotic and degenerative changes of the atria. Such insults yield an array of changes to the atrial ultra-structure, cellular uncoupling, and tissue fibrosis. The net result is alteration of the electrophysiologic properties of the atria and development of atrial conduction disease.[9–12] A more complete synthesis of atrial electrical remodeling has been well summarized elsewhere.[13] In summary, atrial remodeling is a complex and heterogeneous process consisting of adaptive and progressive atrial electrical and structural modification. PWIs have relevance as noninvasive surrogates for the modification to atrial electrical integrity. As a surrogate, they have broad applicability in community- and population-based investigations in which intracardiac studies would not be practical or feasible.

PWIs are defined by their direct measurement on the surface ECG. P-wave duration is most readily measured and as a result has had more extensive use than other PWIs. P-wave duration (ms) is defined from onset at the termination of the T-P isoelectric segment to off-set at the isoelectric PR interval (see Figure 3.1). P-wave area (μV·ms) is measured as the area underneath the positive or negative deflection demarcating the P wave (see Figure 3.1). As a continuous measure, P-wave duration and area may be described as median, maximum, and by specific lead. P-wave terminal force (μV·ms) is specific to right precordial lead V_1 (see Figure 3.1). It is quantified as the product of the negative P-wave deflection in lead V_1 (μV) and the duration (ms) from onset of the negative deflection to its nadir. P-wave dispersion has been defined as the difference between the maximum and minimum duration across the 12 leads. However, we would assert that P-wave dispersion is an electrocardiographic measurement with limited physiologic correlation; the P wave is a low-amplitude signal, and low-duration P waves may be the result of ECG vectors rather than atrial electrical activity. We include the PR interval in this chapter because of its relation to PWIs; the P wave comprises a large portion of the PR interval.

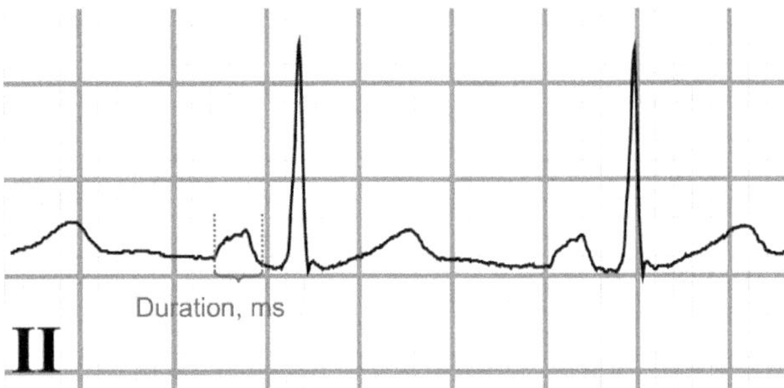

Figure 3.1. P-wave duration as quantified from P-wave on-set to off-set and is measured in ms.

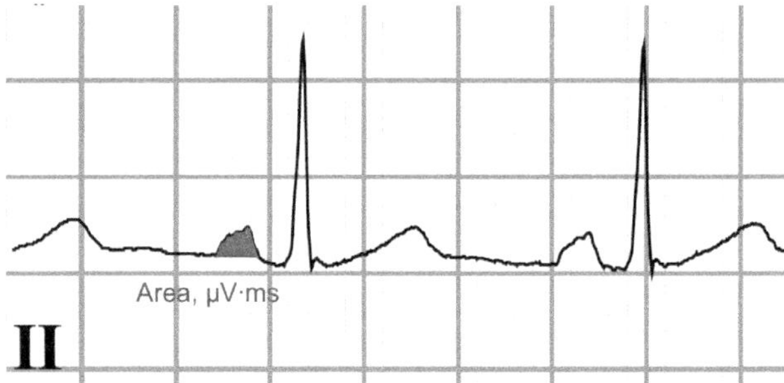

Figure 3.2. The shaded area of the P wave represents P-wave area, as the sum of the area under the positive phase of this P wave. Total P-wave area may include the component of the lead inferior to the isoelectric line and may be lead-specific. P-wave area is measured as μV·ms, and for practical purposes is only feasibly obtained using contemporary, automated, quantitative digital electrocardiography.

Measurement and Reproducibility

Studies have used a range of approaches for measurement and reproducibility of PWIs. Measurements have been made employing printed ECGs using a caliper or from reproductions in digital format. Approaches for studies using printed ECGs include increasing the sweep speed and voltage from the standard 25 mm/s and 1 mV/cm to 50 mm/s and

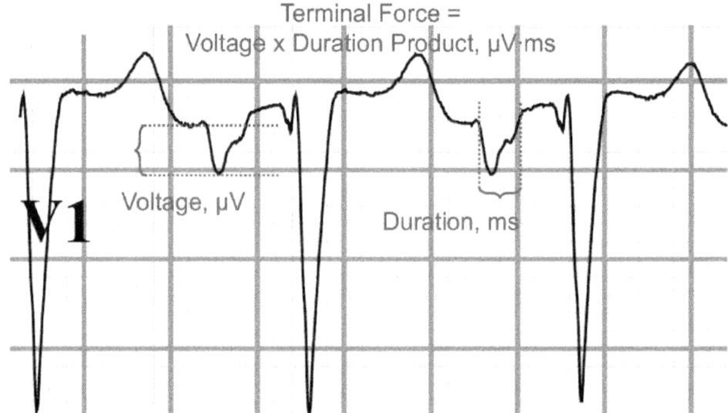

Figure 3.3. Two components used for the quantification of P-wave terminal force: a measure specific to lead V_1 and obtained as the product of the voltage of the negative phase of the P wave and its duration, reported as μV·ms.

2 mV/cm to enhance the visualization of P-wave dimensions. There are a few reports of employing digital magnification.[16] In general, PWIs, whether manual or digital caliper measurement using a high resolution computer screen, have been demonstrated as superior and associated with improved quality control assessments such as variability.[16] The literature has further debated the number of ECG leads required for reliability, use of simultaneous versus sequential lead recordings, and resolution threshold for P-wave signal acquisition.[19] Measurements of PWIs utilizing automated computer algorithms (General Electric 12SL software, for example) alleviate the burden and limitations of manual image processing and quantification.[20] Use of software algorithms facilitates the accurate measurement of PWIs in large studies.

Reproducibility assessment is essential for validating the integrity of measurement approaches and has been ascertained with variable results. P-wave duration with digital caliper measurement has had excellent intra-observer reproducibility (80%) and a moderate inter-observer reproducibility (54%).[21] PR interval, P-wave area, and P-wave terminal force have reproducibility that ranges from moderate to excellent (46%–97%).[22] Both the intra- and the inter-observer reproducibility of PWIs can be improved approximately by 50% with the use of digitally acquired ECG images instead of paper ECGs.[16] The advantage of automated measurement using digitized ECGs is evident: software algorithms are consistent and have been cited having reproducibility that is essentially 100%.[20]

EPIDEMIOLOGY AND ASSOCIATIONS WITH AF RISK FACTORS

Epidemiology: Normative Distribution and Associations with Sex, Age, and Race

The distribution of PWIs in different cohorts is summarized in Table 3.1. A meta-analysis of the control groups of 80 studies with 6827 participants free

Table 3.1. **Distributions of PWIs in referent cohorts and selected studies (only studies sample size ≥100 included).**

Author	Design	N	Maximum P-wave duration (ms)	P-wave area (μV·ms)	P-wave terminal forces in lead V_1 (μV·ms)
Nussinovitch et al[23]	Meta-analysis	All: 6827	99.3 ± 11.5 [64 ± 9.4–125 ± 15]	N/A	N/A
Gialafos et al[24]	Cohort	All: 1353	96 ± 11 [62–142]	N/A	N/A
Magnani et al[29]	Cohort (Framingham)	All: 295 Men:152 Women:143	103 [94–110]* 105 [96–112]* 100 [91–107]*	N/A	N/A
Soliman et al[30]	Cohort (MESA)	WM: 231 WW: 357 AAM: 95 AAW: 112	Middle 104 ± 14 Senior 111 ± 13 Middle 98 ± 13 Senior 105 ± 13 Middle 108 ± 13 Senior 112 ± 14 Middle 103 ± 10 Senior 106 ± 9	N/A	1507 ± 1519 1932 ± 1810 1350 ± 1510 2143 ± 1849 1954 ± 1900 2766 ± 1604 2049 ± 1424 2431 ± 1964
Yildiz et al[32]	Cross-sectional	All: 984 Men: 810 Women:174	112.8 ± 16.4 109.9 ± 12.7	N/A	N/A
Dilaveris et al[117]	Cross-sectional	All: 40	101.0 ± 10.0	N/A	N/A
Aytemir et al[14]	Cross-sectional	All: 70	101.0 ± 11.0	N/A	N/A
Guray et al[73]	Cross-sectional	All: 47	102.0 ± 13.0	N/A	N/A
Dagli et al[41]	Cross-sectional	All: 60	64.0 ± 10.2	N/A	N/A

Results are reported as mean ± standard deviation [range], * signifies [25th–75th interquartile range]. *N*: number of subjects in the reference or control cohort; MESA: Multiethnic study of atherosclerosis; WM: white men, WW: white women, AAM: African-American men, AAW: African-American women, Middle: middle aged subjects (45–65 years old), Senior: Senior subjects (>65 years old).

of diabetes, hypertension, coronary artery disease or other cardiovascular, lung, connective tissue or thyroid disease, yielded a mean P-wave duration of 99.3 ± 11.5 ms (ranging from 64 ± 9.4 to 125 ± 2 ms).[23] A large community-based study of healthy male subjects identified a mean P-wave duration was 96 ms.[24] The normal distributions of P-wave area and terminal force have not been thoroughly described.

Abnormal levels of PWIs have not been formally defined. A P-wave duration cutoff of ≥110 or ≥120 ms has been used in the literature. Applying these cutoffs to a cohort of healthy young individuals, only 9.1% and 1.2%, respectively, had abnormal P-wave duration.[25] These rates increase up to 41% and 47% in inpatient cohorts and 56% in patients prior to coronary artery bypass grafting (CABG). The prevalence of P-wave duration ≥110 ms in adults ≥65 years old has been estimated to be 59%.[28]

Data from Framingham demonstrate a positive and linear relationship of P-wave duration, and PR interval with age in healthy individuals. Linear regression analysis estimates that for each 10 years of age, P-wave duration increases on average by 2.6 ms and the PR interval by 2.3 ms.[29] Similar results have been reported in the multiethnic study of atherosclerosis (MESA). Individuals older than 65 years had an average P-wave duration that was longer by 5.8 ms, P-wave terminal force by 682.4 μV·ms, and PR interval by 5.1 ms, compared to younger individuals.[30]

Women demonstrate lower values in all PWIs. In Framingham, women had an average shorter P-wave duration by 3.7 ms and PR interval by 5.7 ms compared to men.[29] In MESA, women had shorter P-wave duration by 6.1 ms, P-wave terminal force by 99.9 μV·ms, and PR interval by 9.6 ms.[30] Similar results have been reported in other studies performed in healthy individuals of a much younger population (mean age, 19 years old).

Ethnic and racial differences of PWIs have been observed in limited studies. African Americans have longer PWIs compared to Caucasians, while Hispanics have lower PR interval compared to Caucasians.[30] The underlying mechanisms of these ethnic and racial differences have not been established yet. Their significance in development of AF remain also to be elucidated.

AF Risk Factors

Clinical risk factors of AF include hypertension, type 2 diabetes mellitus[35] and the metabolic syndrome, obesity,[36] obstructive sleep apnea,[37] ischemic heart disease,[38] mitral valve (MV) disease,[39] and congenital heart diseases (CHDs).[40] In this section, we will describe the most significant evidence examining associations of these risk factors with PWIs and the role of PWIs as an intermediate marker of AF risk in the setting of these risk factors. Table 3.2 summarizes the selected studies evaluating the associations of PWIs with different AF risk factors.

Hypertension

Hypertension results in left ventricular hypertrophy, diastolic dysfunction, elevated filling pressures, hemodynamic and structural changes in the left atrium, and ultimately heterogeneity in atrial conduction.[6] Atrial conduction heterogeneity can be captured by the PWIs. There is a significant correlation between P-wave duration and atrial volume in patients with hypertension.[41] P-wave duration is increased in prehypertensive subjects compared to normotensive, representing an intermediately increased AF risk in prehypertension.[42] Individuals with persistently elevated BP overnight have longer P-wave duration than those with reduced blood pressure overnight.[43] Persistently, elevated blood pressure may have proportionate effects on atrial electrical function, potentially predisposing patients to a higher AF risk. P-wave area is significantly larger in hypertensive compared to normotensive subjects.[44] P-wave terminal force is positively correlated with systolic, diastolic, and pulse pressure in the MESA, while there is no association between blood pressure and PR interval or P-wave duration.[45] Further studies are required, evaluating for any additive contribution of abnormal PWIs in AF stratification in hypertensive patients.

Blood pressure control with antihypertensive medication decreases P-wave duration[46–51] and P-wave area.[44] Most of the studies utilize a renin-angiotensin-aldosterone inhibitor but β-blockers have also been used with similar results. Nitroprusside reduces P-wave duration in the setting of hypertensive emergency treatment.[48] The follow-up period in these studies ranges from days (in the setting of hypertensive emergency) up to one year.[49] It is unknown whether this improvement in PWIs is mediated by atrial unloading from treatment of hypertension, or by a direct effect of the medications on the atria, reversing the hypertension-induced atrial remodeling.

Ischemic Heart Disease

Ischemic heart disease is a well-established risk factor for AF. Mechanisms for the development of AF in ischemic heart disease may include: (1) direct atrial ischemia resulting in fibrosis and increased refractory period heterogeneity[54] and (2) inflammation originating from atherosclerotic coronary arteries and expanding to the atrial tissue.[38] Myocardial ischemia results in myocardial stiffness, elevated left ventricular filling pressures, increased atrial stretch, and altered

Table 3.2. Associations of PWIs with AF Risk Factors.

Risk Factor	Author	Design	N	Results
Hypertension	Cagirci et al[42]	Case-control	156	P-dur is increased in prehypertensive subjects compared with normotensive subjects.
	Fodor et al[44]	Case control Single-arm interventional (uncontrolled)	104 84	P-area is significantly larger in hypertensive compared to normotensive subjects. P-area decreases after 5 years with hypertension treatment compared to pretreatment values.
	Alonso et al[45]	Cross-sectional	3180	PWTF is positively correlated with systolic, diastolic, and pulse pressure.
	Karaca et al[48]	Single-arm interventional (uncontrolled)	102	P-dur decreases after rapid regulation of blood pressure with nitroprusside in patients presenting with hypertensive urgency.
	Celik et al[50]	Double-arm interventional (uncontrolled)	100	P-dur decreases after treatment with telmisartan and ramipril in patients with HTN. P-dur reduction in the telmisartan arm is greater compared to the ramipril arm.
	Baykan et al[56]	Cohort	147	P-dur is significantly higher in patients that develop AF in the setting of acute anterior wall MI. P-dur does is not associated with AF after multivariate adjustments.
	Turgut et al[57]	Cohort	100	P-dur improves within 2 hours after IV administration of metoprolol in patients with acute coronary syndrome.
	Celik et al[58]	Cohort	125	P-dur decreases after PCI compared to the preintervention, in patients with AMI. P-dur decreases more in patients where a higher coronary flow was achieved after PCI.
LV Dysfunction	Tsai et al[109]	Cross-sectional	270	P-dur and P-area are mildly but independently correlated with echocardiographic left atrial volume index (β = 0.22–0.34) and LV diastolic dysfunction (OR = 1.01–1.03).
	Magnani et al[64]	Cohort	2722	PR interval is independently associated with incident heart failure over 10 years (HR: 1.13, 95%CI: 1.02–1.25 for each SD of PR increment). Subjects with a PR interval >200 ms have an increased 10-year risk of incident heart failure by 46%.
	Zeng et al.[67]	Cross-sectional	136	P-area is correlated with left atrial diameter in patients with MS. P-area ≥4 mV·ms has 85.8% sensitivity and 93.7% specificity for left atrial enlargement. P-area had a better sensitivity than P-wave duration (43.3%) in diagnosing left atrial enlargement.
	Guray et al[73]	Case-control	109	P-dur is longer in patients with ASD compared to controls. P-dur is significantly correlated with mean Qp:Qs in patients with ASD.

(*Continued*)

Table 3.2. (*Continued*)

Risk Factor	Author	Design	N	Results
	Yavuz et al[75]	Case-control Cohort	101 50	P-dur is higher in children with ASD compared to controls. P-dur decreases, within the first year after surgical closure of ASD, to values comparable to healthy controls.
Obesity, diabetes, and the metabolic syndrome	Mangani et al[78]	Cross-sectional	14,433	PR interval, P-dur, and PWTF are increased in all high-BMI categories compared to normal weight individuals. PWIs prolongation is observed in patients with the metabolic syndrome. PWIs are prolonged in patients with HTN. P-dur is positively correlated with waist circumference.
	Mangani et al[64]	Cohort	2722	PR interval prolongs as BMI increases. The multivariable adjusted OR for PR >200 ms is 1.22 (95%CI: 1.07–1.39) for each 1 SD BMI increment.
	Yazici et al[82]	Case-control	116	P-dur is prolonged in patients with DM.
Obstructive sleep apnea	Cagirci et al[87]	Cross-sectional	126	P-dur is higher in patients with more severe OSA (as quantified by the apnea-hypoxia index) compared to the ones with less severe.
Hyperthyroidism	Gen et al[94]	Case-control	140	P-dur is elevated in patients with endogenous and exogenous subclinical hyperthyroidism compared with euthyroid controls. P-dur is not different between patients with endogenous and exogenous subclinical hyperthyroidism.
	Aras et al[95]	Case-control	190	P-dur is significantly higher in patients with overt hyperthyroidism and documented AF compared to patients with overt hyperthyroidism but no AF. P-dur is elevated in patients with subclinical hyperthyroidism compared with euthyroid controls. P-dur is associated with of AF.
Miscellaneous proinflammatory diseases	Yavuzkir et al[103]	Case-control	123	P-dur is significantly increased in patients with rheumatoid arthritis compared to healthy controls. P-dur is positively correlated with C-reactive protein levels in patients with rheumatoid arthritis.
	Bacaksiz et al[107]	Case-control	119	P-dur is increased in patients with psoriasis vulgaris.

Only studies with sample size ≥ 100 are shown. P-dur: P-wave duration, P-area: P-wave area, PWTF: P-wave terminal force, AF: atrial fibrillation, PCI: percutaneous coronary intervention, IV: intravenous, NYHA: New York Heart Association, LV: left ventricular, HR: hazard ratio, 95%CI: 95% confidence interval, SD: standard deviation, MS: mitral valve stenosis, ASD: atrial septal defect, BMI: body mass index, DM: diabetes mellitus, OSA: obstructive sleep apnea, HTN: hypertension, AMI: acute myocardial infarction, OR: odds ratio.

hemodynamics, generating a suitable substrate for development of AF. In a small study ($n = 90$), P-wave duration increased after anterior wall myocardial infarction (MI), and this increase was independently associated with the severity of left ventricular diastolic dysfunction.[55] P-wave duration was significantly higher in patients that develop AF in a small study of 147 acute anterior wall MI cases.[56] However, in the same study P-wave duration was not independently associated with AF after multivariable adjustments.[56] P-wave area and P-wave terminal force have not been studied in coronary artery disease. Studies examining abnormal PWIs in the setting of coronary artery disease have not been conducted to our knowledge. Administration of intravenous β-blockers[57] or revascularization with angioplasty during acute myocardial infarction (AMI) has been shown to decrease P-wave duration. The significance of this decrease of P-wave duration in the short- and long-term prognosis and risk of AF remain to be explored.

Left Ventricular Dysfunction and Heart Failure

AF prevalence is high in patients with heart failure and has been estimated to range between 13% and 27%, increasing in parallel with the severity of the disease.[60] The association between heart failure and AF is complex and not entirely elucidated. AF and heart failure share common risk factors, such as age, hypertension, diabetes, and obesity, as well as valvular, ischemic, and nonischemic structural heart disease. From a pathophysiological standpoint, AF is linked to heart failure through a vicious circle as each disease is able to initiate, perpetuate, and advance the other.[60] A case report demonstrated decreased P-wave duration with resolution of decompensated heart failure.[61] In a small study (n = 72), P-wave duration was elevated in patients with congestive heart failure (CHF).[62] Treatment with 6 months of metoprolol significantly reduced P-wave duration in a small cohort of patients with CHF (n = 42).[63] PR interval is independently associated with a higher 10-year risk of incident heart failure in a cohort of 2722 older adults (HR: 1.13, 95%CI: 1.02–1.25 for each SD of PR increase). Subjects with a PR interval >200 ms have an increased 10-year risk of incident heart failure by 46%.[64] The prognostic significance of abnormal PWIs in mortality of patients with heart failure remains to be determined.

MV Disease

MV disease and particularly mitral stenosis strongly predispose patients to the development of AF.[39] The left atrial pressure overload generated from the stenotic MV orifice can initiate a maladaptive left atrial remodeling response, ultimately leading to AF. P-wave duration is prolonged in patients with mitral stenosis and has been proposed to constitute an intermediate AF phenotype.[65] P-wave duration increases in parallel with the progression of mitral stenosis; P-wave duration is inversely associated with MV area (r = –0.61) and positively correlated with left atrial size (r = 0.57) and mean MV gradient (r = 0.41, n = 30).[66] P-wave area exhibits a strong correlation with left atrial diameter in patients with mitral stenosis (r = 0.74, n = 136).[67] P-wave area ≥4 ms·mV has 85.8% sensitivity and 93.7% specificity in discriminating left atrial enlargement in patients with mitral stenosis.[67] Percutaneous mitral balloon valvuloplasty significantly improves P-wave duration even within the first 72 hours[65] and up to 6 months[68] after the intervention. Administration of β-blockers for 1 month decreased P-wave duration in patients with rheumatic mitral stenosis.[69] Whether this translates into future AF risk reduction remains to be determined. PWIs are also elevated in different MV diseases, namely mitral annulus calcification[70] and severe mitral regurgitation.[71]

Atrial Septal Defect (ASD)

ASD is the third most common form of CHD in adults. The prevalence of AF in patients with ASD has been reported to be 13.8% to 15.6%.[40] In patients with ASD, P-wave duration is significantly prolonged.[72–74] P-wave duration increases linearly with atrial septal defect size and is higher in patients with right atrial enlargement.[74] Surgical or percutaneous transvenous[76] closure of the ASD normalizes P-wave duration and PR interval after 6 months from the procedure. This has been proposed to reflect a reversal of the electromechanical alterations of the atria induced by the ASD. The association of prolonged P-wave duration with postoperative AF has been evaluated in small cohorts.[72]

Obesity, Diabetes, and the Metabolic Syndrome

Obesity is a disease with rapidly increasing incidence and prevalence and is a major risk factor for the development of AF.[36] Body mass index (BMI) is part of the 2 major prediction models for new-onset AF. Data from the Atherosclerosis Risk in Communities (ARIC) study demonstrate that the PR interval, P-wave duration, and terminal force are increased in all high-BMI categories compared with normal BMI. Both sexes have similar increments in the PWIs and PR intervals across BMI categories. African Americans have longer PR interval and P-wave duration, but not P-wave terminal force, compared to Caucasians.[78] PR interval is also positively associated with BMI in a biracial cohort of older adults.[64] Limited data exist on the associations of PWIs and obesity in different ethnic backgrounds.[79] Weight loss, either through lifestyle modification and medical management[80] or via bariatric surgery,[81] results in a reduction in P-wave duration by 8 to 10 ms (n = 30–40). Whether this improvement of the PWIs is further translated to a reduction of the AF incidence has not yet been determined.

Subjects with the metabolic syndrome have increased PR interval, P-wave duration, and terminal force compared to healthy participants in ARIC.[78]

Subjects with diabetes have longer P-wave duration compared to nondiabetic individuals.[82] Prolongation of the P-wave duration has also been observed in prediabetic individuals[83] and in women with polycystic ovary syndrome,[84] which is a different clinical entity characterized by insulin resistance and metabolic aberrations. The presence of diabetic autonomic neuropathy is associated with further prolongation of P-wave duration by 11 ms compared to diabetics without neuropathy (n = 100).[85] Studies evaluating whether abnormal PWIs could confer any additional AF risk in patients with obesity, diabetes, and the metabolic syndrome have not been published yet.

Obstructive Sleep Apnea

Obstructive sleep apnea is the most common sleep disorder, with a prevalence of up to 15%, and has been associated with AF, increasing the AF risk by up to 2.8-fold in some cohorts.[37] Obstructive sleep apnea is associated with prolonged P-wave duration.[86–88] The severity of the disease, as quantified with the apnea-hypoxia index, is positively correlated with prolongation of P-wave duration. Studies evaluating the effect of obstructive sleep apnea in P-wave area and terminal force are yet to be performed. It is unknown whether abnormal PWIs could confer any additional AF risk in patients with obstructive sleep apnea. In a computational study, artificial neural networks integrating P-wave duration and the time interval from the peak of the P wave to the onset of the R wave were able to accurately detect obstructive sleep apnea.[89]

Miscellaneous Diseases

Clinical and sub-clinical hyperthyroidism have been associated with incident and prevalent AF. Small studies have demonstrated prolongation of P-wave duration in hyperthyroid patients[90–92] as well as in subjects with sub-clinical disease (n = 50–190).[93–95] This prolongation has been shown to be associated with pAF in patients with hyperthyroidism.[95] Hyperthyroid patients had reduced P-wave duration by 7.5 to 13.2 ms, following treatment to euthyroidism with propylthiouracil[90-92] or methimazole (n = 50–62).[91] The mechanisms that mediate the intra-atrial conduction delay in hyperthyroidism remains unknown.

The prevalence of AF in patients with end-stage kidney disease on hemodialysis is estimated to be up to 27.0%.[96] Limited data exist on P-wave duration in hemodialysis and yield conflicting results. Four studies report an increase in P-wave duration[97–100] during or after a hemodialysis session, and 2 demonstrated no change (n = 17–47).

Systemic inflammation could directly affect the atria, leading to local inflammation, electroanatomical remodeling, and potentially predisposing to AF. Several diseases have been associated with systemic inflammation. Although the association of AF with these diseases is not well established, there is emerging evidence demonstrating a positive relationship between systemic inflammatory diseases and PWI prolongation. Rheumatoid arthritis, one of the most common systemic inflammatory diseases, is associated with a significant increase in P-wave duration. Patients with Behçet's disease, a chronic systemic disease associated with recurrent oral and genital ulceration and relapsing uveitis, have increased P-wave duration. P-wave duration prolongation has also been described in adults with psoriasis vulgaris, a cutaneous inflammatory disease.[107] Studying the associations between the molecular pathophysiology of these diseases and the longitudinal changes of PWIs could provide novel insights into the inflammatory mechanisms of atrial remodeling and AF.

ASSOCIATION WITH AF

PWIs as an Intermediate Endophenotype for AF

The structural and electrical changes of the atria in response to different exposures have been proposed to be an intermediate step in the development of AF. PWIs measured on the surface ECG can capture these atrial changes.[108] P-wave duration and P-wave area are correlated with left atrial enlargement (β = 0.34 and 0.30 accordingly, n = 270)[109] and a P-wave area ≥24 ms·mV has been proposed to be an ECG criterion of left atrial enlargement.[67] This section describes the associations of PWIs with AF. It also examines the evidence pertaining whether PWIs are risk factors for AF or surrogate markers of traditional AF risk factors. Selected studies evaluating the associations of PWI with incidence and prevalence of AF as well as stroke and mortality, are summarized in Table 3.3.

Incident AF

The largest longitudinal epidemiologic datasets examining the prospective associations of PWIs with incident AF come primarily from Framingham and ARIC. Participants of Framingham in the fifth highest percentile of P-wave duration had a higher risk of developing AF over 15.8 years, independently of other AF risk factors (HR of 2.51, 95%CI: 1.13–5.57, n = 1555).[110] Data from ARIC demonstrate that P-wave duration, mean area, and terminal force as well as PR interval are independently associated with higher incidence of AF over 7 years (HRs 1.23–2.00 for each 1 SD of PWIs increase, n = 15,429).[20] In a prospective study

Table 3.3. Associations of PWIs with AF, Stroke, and Mortality.

Outcome	Author	Design	N	Results
Incident AF	Magnani et al[110]	Cohort (Framingham)	1550 Median follow-up: 15.8 years	The upper 5th percentile of P-dur has a multivariable-adjusted HR of 2.51 (95%CI: 1.13–5.57) for incident AF and 1.11 (95% CI: 0.87–1.40) for mortality. For each 1 SD increase in P-dur the multivariable adjusted HR for incident AF is 1.15 (95%CI: 0.90–1.47) and for mortality 1.02 (95%CI: 0.96–1.08).
	Soliman et al[20]	Cohort (ARIC)	15,429 Follow-up: 7.0 ± 1.5 years	The multivariable-adjusted HR for incident AF is 1.79 (95%CI: 1.51–2.14) for each 1 SD increase in P-dur. The multivariable-adjusted HR for incident AF is 1.17 (95%CI: 1.01–1.41) for each 1 SD increase in P-area. The multivariable-adjusted HR for incident AF is 1.23 (95%CI: 1.04–1.46) for each 1 SD increase in PWTF. The multivariable-adjusted HR for incident AF is 1.41 (95%CI: 1.20–1.65) for each 1 SD increase in PR interval.
	Magnani et al[64]	Cohort (Health ABC)	2722 Follow-up: 10 years	PR interval is independently associated with incident AF. PR increase by 1 SD (29 ms) is associated with 13% increase in AF risk (95%CI: 1.04–1.23). There is no effect modification by race.
	Cheng et al[112]	Cohort (Framingham)	7575 Follow-up: 20 years	PR interval is an independent risk factor of AF. PR interval >200 ms is associated with a 2-fold increase in AF risk (HR: 2.06, 95% CI: 1.36–3.12). Each 20-ms increase in PR interval is associated with an adjusted AF HR of 1.11 (95%CI: 1.02–1.22).
	De Sisti et al[113]	Cohort	140 Follow-up 27.6 ± 17.8 months	P-dur ≥120 ms is independently associated with incident AF in patients that received a PPM for sinus node dysfunction. P-dur ≥120 ms is associated with 30-month AF-free rates of 13% compared to 56% in patients with P-dur <120 ms. Abnormal P-wave morphology is associated with 30-months AF-free rates of 28% compared to 74% in patients with normal P wave.
	Padeletti et al[115]	Cohort	660 Mean follow-up: 19 months	P-dur >100 ms (the median for this cohort) is independently associated with AF-related hospitalizations and more frequent cardioversions in patients that receive a dual-chamber PPM.
	Snoeck et al[114]	Cohort	320 Follow-up: 5 years	P-dur in lead V_1 at the time of a PPM implantation is associated with higher 5-year AF incidence, in patients that received a PPM for sick sinus syndrome or AV block.
	Healey et al[116]	Cohort	485 Follow-up: 2 years	Prolonged sensed or paced P-dur is associated with higher incidence of induced AF during electrophysiologic testing (23.5% vs. 13.6%) in patients with a dual-chamber PPM.

(Continued)

Table 3.3. (*Continued*)

Outcome	Author	Design	N	Results
	Kristensen et al[160]	Cohort	109 Follow-up: 1.5 years	P-dur measured before and during PPM implantation are not associated with subsequent AF development.
Prevalent AF	Aytemir et al[14]	Case-control	160	P-dur is higher in patients with a history of pAF compared to controls. P-dur ≥106 ms discriminates patients with pAF with a sensitivity of 83%, a specificity of 72%, and a PPV of 79%
	Dilaveris et al[117]	Case-control	100	P-dur is higher in patients with idiopathic pAF compared to controls. P-dur ≥110 ms discriminates patients with AF with a sensitivity of 88% and a specificity of 75%.
	Dogan et al[118]	Cross-sectional	400	P-dur is higher in patients with pAF when compared with patients without AF.
	De Bacquer et al[122]	Nested case-control	160	P-dur is an independent AF risk factor. The joint occurrence of longer P-dur and morphologic changes in P wave are associated with AF development over 10 years, with an adjusted OR of 13.4 (95%CI: 3.3–46.6).
Recurrence of AF	Salah et al[132]	Cohort	198 Mean follow-up: 9 ± 3 months	P-dur is prolonged in patients that experience AF recurrence after successful PVI. P-dur >125 ms has 60% sensitivity, 90% specificity, 72% PPV and 83.7% NPV in diagnosing recurrent AF after successful PVI. Prolonged PWTF was associated with AF recurrence after successful PVI. P-dur and PWTF were not associated with AF recurrence in multivariable models.
	Caldwell[134]	Cohort	100	P-dur prolongation is associated with greater AF recurrence rates. P-dur was not associated with AF recurrence in multivariable models.

Only studies with sample size ≥ 100 are shown. P-dur: P-wave duration, P-area: P-wave area, PWTF: P-wave terminal force, AF: atrial fibrillation, HR: hazards ratio, 95%CI: 95% confidence interval, ARIC: Atherosclerosis Risk in Communities study, Health ABC: Health, Aging, and Body Composition Study, PPM: permanent pacemaker, PPV: positive predictive value, NPV: negative predictive value, OR: odds ratio, pAF: paroxysmal atrial fibrillation, DCCV: direct current cardioversion, PVI: pulmonic vein isolation.

of patients with baseline P-wave terminal force ≥60 ms 0.2 mV the area, duration, and amplitude of the initial portion of P wave on lead V_1 were independently associated with development of AF over 43 months (HR 4.02, 95%CI 1.25–17.8, $n = 78$).[111]

In the biracial Health, Aging, and Body Composition (Health ABC) study of older adults, PR interval was independently associated with higher incidence of AF. For every 1 SD (29 ms) increase in PR interval, there was an associated 13% increase in the 10-year AF risk.[64] In Framingham, prolonged PR interval >200 ms was associated with a 2-fold increase in AF risk.[112] Prolongation of the PR interval is a part of the Framingham AF 10-year risk prediction score.[33] This prediction score has also been validated in African Americans.[34] The extent to which the contribution of P-wave duration in the PR interval is associated with AF risk remains to be determined.

The associations of PWIs with incident AF have also been studied in cohorts of patients with implantable permanent pacemakers. In small- to medium-sized cohorts of patients that undergo pacemaker implantation, prolonged P-wave duration is independently associated with higher incidence of AF, AF-related hospitalizations and cardioversions (n = 140–660; see Table 3.3).[115] Prolonged sensed or paced P-wave duration was associated with higher incidence of AF induced during electrophysiologic testing (23.5% vs. 13.6%) in a cohort of patients that received a dual-chamber pacemaker (n = 485). Of note, the other electrophysiologic properties of the atria, such as the sinus node recovery time, the atrial effective refractory period (ERP), and the rate-adaptive shortening of the atrial ERP were similar between cases and controls.[116]

Both community-based and pacemaker studies demonstrate that prolonged PWIs are independently associated with higher incidence of AF, suggesting that PWIs have a direct value in AF risk prediction, rather than simply reflecting the cumulative risk from the traditional AF risk factors. Whether incorporation of the PWIs in new or current AF prediction models will improve the models remains to be determined.

Prevalent AF

P-wave duration is significantly elevated in patients with pAF. The cutoffs of P-wave duration ≥106 ms and ≥110 ms have been used to identify patients with pAF with sensitivity of 83% and 88% and specificity of 72% and 75%, respectively. Prolonged P-wave duration has also been associated with AF in cohorts of patients with stroke,[118] structural heart disease,[119] hypertrophic cardiomyopathy,[120] and Wolff-Parkinson-White syndrome status post-accessory pathway ablation (see Table 3.3).[121] In a case-control study, nested within the Belgian Interuniversity Research on Nutrition and Health survey, P-wave duration was a significant independent AF risk factor (OR: 13.4, 95%CI: 3.3–46.6).[122] P-wave duration is prolonged by 11 ms in patients with AF present for >48 hours, compared to patients with AF present ≤48 hours (n = 96).[123] P-wave duration remains positively associated with duration of AF and left atrial size after multivariable adjustments.[123] Prolonged P-wave duration is also associated with higher rates of exercise-induced AF during exercise stress testing.[124]

Pulmonary Vein (PV) Isolation

PV isolation is a procedure where the PVs are electrically isolated from the left atrium, either percutaneously or surgically, with the use of radiofrequency (RF) energy, cryoablation, or direct electrocautery. PV isolation has been shown to be an effective method of nonpharmacologic treatment of AF.[125] In small cohorts (n = 29–50), P-wave duration and terminal force decrease within the first 7 days to 6 months following PV isolation.[126–128] The rate of interatrial block decreases from 93.3% to 68.9%, after PV isolation, but no further reduction is observed after 3 months.

AF Recurrence Following Cardioversion or PV Isolation

The association of PWIs with recurrent AF after direct current cardioversion or PV isolation has also been studied. Prolonged P-wave duration ≥142 ms immediately after external cardioversion for AF is associated with higher AF recurrence 1 month after the procedure (OR: 0.33, 95%CI: 0.13–0.87).[129] The sensitivity and specificity of PWIs in identifying AF recurrence after external cardioversion have been reported to be 64.6% and 62.1%, respectively.[129] PWIs have also been studied after internal cardioversion for AF. Prolonged P-wave duration on lead II and attenuated P-wave amplitude on the ECG obtained after a successful internal cardioversion are associated with a higher 48-hour AF relapse rate.[130] Patients cardioverted for sustained ventricular tachycardia and developed AF postcardioversion had a higher P-wave duration compared to AF-free patients, in a small case-control study (n = 58).[131] Differences in PWIs after cardioversion suggest that after restoration of sinus rhythm, the atria may get into different states of interatrial conduction delay that predispose patients to AF recurrence, but the exact mechanisms remain to be determined. Further studies are required to evaluate whether PWIs are independently associated with AF recurrence.

Prolonged P-wave duration and terminal force[132] on the ECG obtained after successful PV isolation are associated with higher AF recurrence (n = 31–198). The mean follow-up period in these studies ranges from 9[132] to 16 months.[133] The positive predictive value of prolonged PWIs in AF development for different cutoffs ranges between 72%[132] and 85.7%.[134] In multivariable models, PWIs has failed to be independently associated with AF recurrence after PV isolation, but the sample size of these studies was relatively small (100–198 subjects). The associations of PWIs with AF recurrence after PV isolation need to be tested in larger studies. The timing after PV isolation when PWIs should be obtained might be important, since PV isolation causes local inflammation from the ablation lesions that might affect impulse propagation in the left atrium.

Postoperative AF

The occurrence of postoperative AF can be as high as 7% to 40% after CABG.[135] The associations of PWIs with postoperative AF and atrial flutter were first introduced in 1981. Total P-wave duration was measured from simultaneous recordings of leads I, II, and III. Patients with total P-wave duration >110 ms had higher rates of AF or atrial flutter compared to patients with total P-wave duration ≤110 ms (37.5% vs. 14.3%, n =

99).[136] In a small cohort, P-wave duration decreased immediately after open heart surgery (n = 16) and subsequently increased until postoperative day 3 to its maximum duration (n = 20). Day 3 after surgery is the timeframe of greatest risk for postoperative AF.[137] Patients that develop postoperative AF demonstrated a more pronounced postoperative P-wave duration decline (by 2.9 ms) compared to those without AF (n = 300).[138] The presence of P-wave duration ≥100 ms in lead II, on the preoperative ECG, is independently associated with postoperative AF, increasing the risk by 2.9-fold compared to individuals with a P-wave duration ≤100 ms.[139] The high incidence and short time required for the development of postoperative AF could have some utility in further studying the pathophysiologic cascade, from preoperative AF risk to changes in PWIs and development of AF.

Progression from Paroxysmal to Permanent AF

AF is a progressive disease, with pAF transitioning to persistent AF and ultimately permanent AF. Long-standing, disorganized, electrical atrial activity due to AF could further contribute to the electroanatomical atrial remodeling, resulting in a vicious cycle leading to permanent AF. PWIs could potentially reflect these changes and could be utilized to risk stratify patients for AF progression. In a small study of patients with pAF, P-wave duration was independently associated with progression to persistent AF (HR: 5.49, 95% CI: 2.38–12.7, n = 71).[140]

ASSOCIATIONS WITH OTHER OUTCOMES: STROKE AND MORTALITY

Stroke

Given the strong association of AF with stroke, it would be reasonable to investigate the associations of PWIs with stroke. Paroxysmal AF might be challenging to capture in epidemiologic studies, or to diagnose in the clinical setting. The role of PWIs as an intermediate AF phenotype could be helpful in identifying patients at risk for stroke. Data from ARIC demonstrate that prolongation of all PWIs is associated with higher incidence of stroke; however, only mean (HR: 1.11, 95%CI: 1.02–1.20) and maximum P-wave area (HR: 1.13, 95%CI: 1.05–1.23) as well as P-wave terminal force (HR: 1.22, 95%CI: 1.14–1.31) were independently associated with stroke incidence over 7 years.[20] The associations of PWIs with stroke are weaker compared to AF,[20] which is consistent with the theoretical model of AF risk factors leading to atrial remodeling and abnormal PWIs and subsequently to AF that predisposes to stroke. PWIs have also been studied in patients with cryptogenic stroke and patent foramen ovale (PFO). P-wave duration is elevated in patients with PFO that suffer a stroke compared to controls, suggesting that atrial arrhythmias might be involved in the pathophysiology of the stroke.[141] Further studies are required to evaluate whether prolonged PWIs in patients with stroke could be a marker of pAF. Whether initiation of oral anticoagulation therapy in patients with cryptogenic stroke and abnormal PWIs (as a surrogate marker of undetected pAF) could improve clinical outcomes remains to be determined.

Mortality

PWIs prolong with aging, constitute an intermediate phenotype of AF, and are associated with stroke. PWIs are affected by multiple disease processes that are associated with increased mortality risk. There is an increased interest in studying the associations of PWIs with of mortality outcomes, with most of the evidence being derived from Framingham and the third National Health and Nutrition Examination Survey (NHANES III). PR interval ≥200 ms is associated with an increase in absolute risk of mortality by 2.05% per year (HR: 1.08, 95%CI: 1.02–1.13, for each 20 ms increase in PR) in Framingham.[112] In NHANES III, although both P-wave amplitude and P-wave duration in lead II were associated with all-cause mortality, only P-wave duration was independently associated with all-cause and cardiovascular mortality over 8.6 years [HR (95%CI): 1.06 (1.00–1.12) and 1.13 (1.04–1.23), respectively].[142] P-wave area and terminal force were not studied in the NHANES III cohort. PR interval was not associated with mortality in this NHANES III cohort.[142] The Health ABC[64] and the Finnish Social Insurance Institution's Coronary Heart Disease Study[143] also failed to demonstrate a significant association between prolonged PR interval and all-cause mortality.

The observed inconsistency in the associations of PR interval with mortality across different cohorts has not been fully explained yet. It has been proposed that the association of PR interval with mortality is primarily dictated by the level of contribution of the P-wave duration to the PR interval.[144] The contribution of the P-wave duration to the PR interval's associations with AF has not been studied to date. In a small study of heart failure patients, P-wave terminal force ≥40 mm·ms was independently associated with cardiac death or hospitalization over 6.5 years (HR: 2.72, 95%CI: 1.24–5.99, n = 185).[145] Abnormal P-wave axis (normal P-wave axis 0°–75°) was independently associated with all-cause and cardiovascular mortality over 8.6 years in the NHANES III study [HR (95%CI): 1.24 (1.13–1.36) and 1.19 (1.03–1.38), respectively].[146]

The Role of Genetics

AF risk has recently been demonstrated to have a genetic contribution. Genetic loci associated with increased AF risk include variants on chromosome 4q25 near the *PITX2* gene, on 16q22.3 near the *ZFHX3* (*ATBF1*) gene, on 1q21 in the *KCNN3* gene, and on 7q36.1 in the *KCNH2* gene.[147–152] The PR interval also has a significant heritable component that has been reported to range between 30% and 50%.[153–156] Since the PR interval is closely associated with AF, stroke, and mortality, there is an increasing interest in identifying genetic loci that might explain the variations in the PR interval and studying whether these loci could account for AF risk. In subjects of European ancestry, genetic associations with PR have been identified on the 3p22.2 locus, and specifically in proximity to sodium channel genes *SCN10A* and *SCN5A*.[157] The *SCN10A* gene codes for the sodium channel NaV1.8 that is expressed in the peripheral nervous system, and its role in the heart remains to be determined.[158] *SCN5A* encodes for the primary voltage-gated sodium channel NaV1.5, mutations of which have also been associated with AF, QT prolongation, the Brugada syndrome, and others.[159] Weaker, yet significant, associations were described in 6 other loci near genes *CAV1-CAV2*, *NKX2-5* (*CSX1*), *SOX5*, *WNT11* (*ARHGAP24*), *MEIS1*, and *TBX5-TBX3*. Common genetic associations shared by both the PR interval and increased risk of AF suggest common pathways by which PR variants may mediate AF risk. The genetic associations of PWIs have not yet been reported to our knowledge.

Future Directions in Epidemiology and Clinical Investigations

Despite the increased scientific interest and great progress in the investigation of PWIs and AF, outstanding questions remain (see Table 3.4). In this section, we select major directions for future research that we think that merit consideration. First, more robust studies are essential to relate PWIs to invasive electrophysiologic studies of atrial electrical function. PWIs are noninvasive and easily measured. Improving our understanding of the relation of PWIs and intracardiac studies will provide insight into the

Table 3.4. **Future Directions for the Investigation of PWIs.**

Area	Specific direction
Methods	1. Standardization of methods by which PWIs are acquired. 2. Validation of PWIs against invasive electrophysiologic testing. 3. Comparisons of PWIs with other noninvasive measurements, such as the signal-averaged ECG. 4. Correlations of PWIs with atrial structural and functional characteristics obtained with advanced imaging techniques.
Epidemiology	1. Better description of the distributions of P-wave area and terminal force. 2. Standardization of abnormal or cut-off values, in different ethnic and racial groups, for meaningful planning and comparison between studies. 3. Evaluation for longitudinal changes of PWIs as individuals age; description of the trajectory in the "life course" of P waves. 4. Evaluation of the role of genetics and environmental factors in the longitudinal changes of PWIs. 5. Determine the role of genetics in explaining the differences of PWIs distributions across different ethnic and racial population.
AF Risk Factors	1. Confirm the associations between PWIs and AF risk factors in larger, prospective studies. 2. Evaluate for the longitudinal adaptation of the P wave to different insults. 3. Determine factors associated with this adaptation and study their prognostic significance. 4. Determine whether there is a genetic component the P-wave adaptation. 5. Evaluate whether abnormal PWIs in the presence of these AF risk factors convey any incremental AF risk or are just surrogate markers of the underlying atrial electroanatomical remodeling. 6. Evaluate whether interventions that improve PWIs translate in AF risk reduction.
AF and other outcomes	1. Determine for any potential role of different patterns of P-wave changes across time in providing additional information regarding AF risk. 2. Evaluate whether incorporation of PWIs in new or current AF prediction models will improve the classification and discriminant capacity city of the models. 3. Evaluate whether PWIs, could be used as screening tools in asymptomatic populations. 4. Study the functional significance of the polymorphisms associate with AF and PR prolongation.

physiologic relevance of PWIs. Second, studies are required evaluating the associations of PWIs with parameters of atrial structure and function obtained by advanced imaging techniques. Cardiac magnetic resonance imaging can quantify atrial fibrosis. Different echocardiography techniques can quantify atrial strain. Studying the associations of PWIs with parameters such as atrial fibrosis and strain could provide insights on how changes of the atrial substrate are reflected on the surface ECG.

Third, more studies are required characterizing the normative distributions of PWIs. Although the normative distribution of P-wave duration has adequately been described, the distributions of P-wave area and terminal force have not been thoroughly studied. Ethnic and racial distributions of PWIs have had limited exploration. Determination of normal distributions is essential for meaningful comparison between studies. Only a few studies have been conducted in racial and ethnic minorities or individuals not of European descent; the relevance of PWIs across races and ethnicities has not been well ascertained.

Fourth, studies assessing for longitudinal changes or PWIs are necessary. A strong positive association between PWIs and age has been established from the epidemiology of PWIs. However, PWIs have not been longitudinally studied. The changes of PWIs as individuals get older and what could determine different trajectories in the "life course" of P-waves remain largely unknown. Different patterns of P-wave changes across time could provide additional information on the risk of AF and other clinical outcomes. The role of genetics, as well as the influence of environmental factors in the longitudinal changes of P-waves, merit further research.

Fifth, most of the evidence on the associations of PWIs with AF risk factors has been derived from small to moderate-sized cross-sectional or case-control studies. These studies cannot assess for confounding or effect modification and need to be confirmed in larger, prospective studies. Studies are also needed evaluating for any additive contribution of PWIs to AF risk in the setting of other exposures. The longitudinal adaptation of P-wave to AF risk factors remains largely unknown. Improvement of PWIs has been described with treatment of different diseases that are associated with AF risk. It remains unknown whether these improvements further translate to AF risk reduction. Last, although the PR interval is part of major AF prediction models, whether the incorporation of PWIs in new or current AF prediction models will improve the models' classification and discrimination remains to be determined. Given the low cost associated with obtaining PWIs, studies evaluating their use as screening tools in asymptomatic populations need to be performed.

CONCLUSION

Over the past decades, there has been a tremendous paradigm shift in the utility and information derived from the P wave. First-degree atrioventricular (AV) block was once considered "innocent," and P-wave morphology was primarily utilized for the diagnosis of atrial enlargement. In the modern era of cardiovascular medicine, there is an increasing understanding that PR interval and P-wave morphology have provided important, noninvasive insight on atrial electrical function. The current literature-driven prototype around PR interval and PWIs is that genetic substrate and acquired AF risk factors result in atrial electro-anatomical adaptation that can be captured in abnormal PWIs. Abnormal PWIs constitute an intermediate phenotype of AF preceding the development of clinical AF and ultimately result in increased stroke rates and overall mortality. Further research is necessary to better understand the exact mechanisms of the atrial adaptation to different exposures and how this adaptation translates in risk for clinical outcomes. To achieve this, a deeper understanding of how PWIs are related to atrial electrical and mechanical function is required.

REFERENCES

1. Robert O, Bonow DLM, Zipes DP, Libby P. Electrocardiography. In: *Braunwald's Heart Disease—A Textbook of Cardiovascular Medicine.* 9th ed. Philadelphia, PA: Elsevier, Inc.; 2011.
2. Sanders P, Morton JB, Kistler PM, et al. Electrophysiological and electroanatomic characterization of the atria in sinus node disease: Evidence of diffuse atrial remodeling. *Circulation.* 2004;109:1514–1522.
3. Roberts-Thomson KC, Kistler PM, Sanders P, et al. Fractionated atrial electrograms during sinus rhythm: Relationship to age, voltage, and conduction velocity. *Heart Rhythm.* 2009;6:587–591.
4. Kojodjojo P, Kanagaratnam P, Markides V, Davies DW, Peters N. Age-related changes in human left and right atrial conduction. *J Cardiovasc Electrophysiol.* 2006;17:120–127.
5. Kistler PM, Sanders P, Fynn SP, et al. Electrophysiologic and electroanatomic changes in the human atrium associated with age. *J Am Coll Cardiol.* 2004;44:109–116.
6. Medi C, Kalman JM, Spence SJ, et al. Atrial electrical and structural changes associated with longstanding hypertension in humans: Implications for the substrate for atrial fibrillation. *J Cardiovasc Electrophysiol.* 2011;22:1317–1324.
7. Stevenson IH, Roberts-Thomson KC, Kistler PM, et al. Atrial electrophysiology is altered by acute hypercapnia but not hypoxemia: implications for promotion of atrial fibrillation in pulmonary disease and sleep apnea. *Heart Rhythm.* 2010;7:1263–1270.

8. Sanders P, Morton JB, Davidson NC, et al. Electrical remodeling of the atria in congestive heart failure: Electrophysiological and electroanatomic mapping in humans. *Circulation.* 2003;108:1461–1468.
9. Anyukhovsky EP, Sosunov EA, Plotnikov A, et al. Cellular electrophysiologic properties of old canine atria provide a substrate for arrhythmogenesis. *Cardiovasc Res.* 2002;54:462–469.
10. Everett THT, Wilson EE, Verheule S, et al. Structural atrial remodeling alters the substrate and spatiotemporal organization of atrial fibrillation: A comparison in canine models of structural and electrical atrial remodeling. *Am J Physiol Heart Circ Physiol.* 2006;291:H2911–H2923.
11. Ohtani K, Yutani C, Nagata S, et al. High prevalence of atrial fibrosis in patients with dilated cardiomyopathy. *J Am Coll Cardiol.* 1995;25:1162–1169.
12. Sinno H, Derakhchan K, Libersan D, et al. Atrial ischemia promotes atrial fibrillation in dogs. *Circulation.* 2003;107:1930–1936.
13. Kumar S, Teh AW, Medi C, et al. Atrial remodeling in varying clinical substrates within beating human hearts: relevance to atrial fibrillation. *Prog Biophys Mol Biol.* 2012;110:278–294.
14. Aytemir K, Ozer N, Atalar E, et al. P wave dispersion on 12-lead electrocardiography in patients with paroxysmal atrial fibrillation. *Pacing Clin Electrophysiol.* 2000;23:1109–1112.
15. Kose S, Aytemir K, Can I, et al. Seasonal variation of P-wave dispersion in healthy subjects. *J Electrocardiol.* 2002;35:307–311.
16. Dilaveris P, Batchvarov V, Gialafos J, Malik M. Comparison of different methods for manual P wave duration measurement in 12-lead electrocardiograms. *Pacing Clin Electrophysiol.* 1999;22:1532–1538.
17. Agarwal YK, Aronow WS, Levy JA, Spodick DH. Association of interatrial block with development of atrial fibrillation. *Am J Cardiol.* 2003;91:882.
18. Dilaveris PE, Gialafos JE. P-wave duration and dispersion analysis: methodological considerations. *Circulation.* 2001;103:E111.
19. Censi F, Calcagnini G, Corazza I, et al. On the resolution of ECG acquisition systems for the reliable analysis of the P-wave. *Physiol Meas.* 2012;33:N11–N17.
20. Soliman EZ, Prineas RJ, Case LD, Zhang ZM, Goff DC Jr. Ethnic distribution of ECG predictors of atrial fibrillation and its impact on understanding the ethnic distribution of ischemic stroke in the atherosclerosis risk in communities (ARIC) study. *Stroke.* 2009;40:1204–1211.
21. Magnani JW, Mazzini MJ, Sullivan LM, et al. P-wave indices, distribution and quality control assessment (from the Framingham heart study). *Ann Noninvasive Electrocardiol.* 2010;15:77–84.
22. Snyder ML, Soliman EZ, Whitsel EA, Gellert KS, Heiss G. Short-term repeatability of electrocardiographic P wave indices and PR interval. *J Electrocardiol.* 2014;47:257-263.
23. Nussinovitch U. Meta-analysis of P-wave dispersion values in healthy individuals: the influence of clinical characteristics. *Ann Noninvasive Electrocardiol.* 2012;17:28–35.
24. Gialafos EJ, Dilaveris PE, Synetos AG, et al. P wave analysis indices in young healthy men: data from the digital electrocardiographic study in Hellenic air force servicemen (DEHAS). *Pacing Clin Electrophysiol.* 2003;26:367–372.
25. Gialafos E, Psaltopoulou T, Papaioannou TG, et al. Prevalence of interatrial block in young healthy men <35 years of age. *Am J Cardiol.* 2007;100:995–997.
26. Jairath UC, Spodick DH. Exceptional prevalence of interatrial block in a general hospital population. *Clin Cardiol.* 2001;24:548–550.
27. Asad N, Spodick DH. Prevalence of interatrial block in a general hospital population. *Am J Cardiol.* 2003;91:609–610.
28. Ninios I, Pliakos C, Ninios V, Karvounis H, Louridas G. Prevalence of interatrial block in a general population of elderly people. *Ann Noninvasive Electrocardiol.* 2007;12:298–300.
29. Magnani JW, Johnson VM, Sullivan LM, et al. P-wave indices: derivation of reference values from the Framingham heart study. *Ann Noninvasive Electrocardiol.* 2010;15:344–352.
30. Soliman EZ, Alonso A, Misialek JR, et al. Reference ranges of PR duration and P-wave indices in individuals free of cardiovascular disease: The Multi-Ethnic Study of Atherosclerosis (MESA). *J Electrocardiol.* 2013;46:702–706.
31. Yildiz M, Aygin D, Pazarli P, et al. Assessment of resting electrocardiogram, P wave dispersion and duration in different genders applying for registration to the school of physical education and sports—results of a single centre Turkish trial with 2093 healthy subjects. *Cardiol Young.* 2011;21:545–550.
32. Yildiz M, Pazarli P, Semiz O, et al. Assessment of P-wave dispersion on 12-lead electrocardiography in students who exercise regularly. *Pacing Clin Electrophysiol.* 2008;31:580–583.
33. Schnabel RB, Sullivan LM, Levy D, et al. Development of a risk score for atrial fibrillation (Framingham heart study): A community-based cohort study. *Lancet.* 2009;373:739–745.
34. Schnabel RB, Aspelund T, Li G, et al. Validation of an atrial fibrillation risk algorithm in whites and African Americans. *Arch Intern Med.* 2010;170:1909–1917.
35. Huxley RR, Alonso A, Lopez FL, et al. Type 2 diabetes, glucose homeostasis and incident atrial fibrillation: the atherosclerosis risk in communities study. *Heart.* 2012;98:133–138.
36. Magnani JW, Hylek EM, Apovian CM. Obesity begets atrial fibrillation: A contemporary summary. *Circulation.* 2013;128:401–405.
37. Digby GC, Baranchuk A. Sleep apnea and atrial fibrillation. *Curr Cardiol Rev.* 2012;8:265–272.
38. Guvenc TS, Ilhan E, Hasdemir H, Satilmis S, Alper AT. A novel explanation for the cause of atrial fibrillation seen in atherosclerotic coronary artery disease: "Downstream inflammation" hypothesis. *Med Hypotheses.* 2010;74:665–667.
39. Shiu MF. Mitral valve disease. *Eur Heart J.* 1984;5(suppl A):131–134.
40. Oliver JM, Gallego P, Gonzalez A, et al. Predisposing conditions for atrial fibrillation in atrial septal defect

with and without operative closure. *Am J Cardiol.* 2002;89:39–43.
41. Dagli N, Karaca I, Yavuzkir M, Balin M, Arslan N. Are maximum P wave duration and P wave dispersion a marker of target organ damage in the hypertensive population? *Clin Res Cardiol.* 2008;97:98–104.
42. Cagirci G, Cay S, Karakurt O, et al. P-wave dispersion increases in prehypertension. *Blood Press.* 2009;18:51–54.
43. Ermis N, Acikgoz N, Cuglan B, et al. Comparison of atrial electromechanical coupling interval and P-wave dispersion in non-dipper versus dipper hypertensive subjects. *Blood Press.* 2011;20:60–66.
44. Fodor JG, Heyden S, Chockalingam A, Logan AG, Hames CG. The P-wave in the electrocardiogram of hypertensive patients before and after therapy. *Can J Cardiol.* 1986;2:264–267.
45. Alonso A, Soliman EZ, Chen LY, Bluemke DA, Heckbert SR. Association of blood pressure and aortic distensibility with P wave indices and PR interval: The Multi-Ethnic Study of Atherosclerosis (MESA). *J Electrocardiol.* 2013;46:359 e351–e356.
46. Aksoy S, Gurkan U, Oz D, et al. The effects of blood pressure lowering on P-wave dispersion in patients with hypertensive crisis in emergency setting. *Clin Exp Hypertens.* 2010;32:486–489.
47. Korkmaz H, Onalan O, Akbulut M, Ozbay Y. Nebivolol and quinapril reduce P-wave duration and dispersion in hypertensive patients. *Indian Pacing Electrophysiol J.* 2009;9:158–166.
48. Karaca I, Durukan P, Dagli N, et al. The effect of rapid blood pressure control on P-wave dispersion in hypertensive urgency. *Adv Ther.* 2008;25:1303–1314.
49. Guntekin U, Gunes Y, Tuncer M, Simsek H, Gunes A. Comparison of the effects of quinapril and irbesartan on P-wave dispersion in hypertensive patients. *Adv Ther.* 2008;25:775–786.
50. Celik T, Iyisoy A, Kursaklioglu H, et al. The comparative effects of telmisartan and ramipril on P-wave dispersion in hypertensive patients: a randomized clinical study. *Clin Cardiol.* 2005;28:298–302.
51. Fogari R, Derosa G, Ferrari I, et al. Effect of valsartan and ramipril on atrial fibrillation recurrence and P-wave dispersion in hypertensive patients with recurrent symptomatic lone atrial fibrillation. *Am J Hypertens.* 2008;21:1034–1039.
52. Ozben B, Sumerkan M, Tanrikulu AM, et al. Perindopril decreases P wave dispersion in patients with stage 1 hypertension. *J Renin Angiotensin Aldosterone Syst.* 2009;10:85–90.
53. Tuncer M, Gunes Y, Guntekin U, Gumrukcuoglu HA, Eryonucu B. Short-term effects of cilazapril and atenolol on P-wave dispersion in patients with hypertension. *Adv Ther.* 2008;25:99–105.
54. Turgut O, Tandogan I, Yilmaz MB, Yalta K, Aydin O. Association of P wave duration and dispersion with the risk for atrial fibrillation: Practical considerations in the setting of coronary artery disease. *Int J Cardiol.* 2010;144:322–324.
55. Yilmaz R, Demirbag R, Durmus I, et al. Association of stage of left ventricular diastolic dysfunction with P wave dispersion and occurrence of atrial fibrillation after first acute anterior myocardial infarction. *Ann Noninvasive Electrocardiol.* 2004;9:330–338.
56. Baykan M, Celik S, Erdol C, et al. Effects of P-wave dispersion on atrial fibrillation in patients with acute anterior wall myocardial infarction. *Ann Noninvasive Electrocardiol.* 2003;8:101–106.
57. Turgut O, Yilmaz MB, Yilmaz A, et al. Acute coronary syndrome: short-term effects of early intravenous metoprolol on maximum P wave duration and P wave dispersion. *Adv Ther.* 2007;24:14–22.
58. Celik T, Iyisoy A, Kursaklioglu H, et al. Effects of primary percutaneous coronary intervention on P wave dispersion. *Ann Noninvasive Electrocardiol.* 2005;10:342–347.
59. Akdemir R, Ozhan H, Gunduz H, et al. Effect of reperfusion on P-wave duration and P-wave dispersion in acute myocardial infarction: primary angioplasty versus thrombolytic therapy. *Ann Noninvasive Electrocardiol.* 2005;10:35–40.
60. Anter E, Jessup M, Callans DJ. Atrial fibrillation and heart failure: treatment considerations for a dual epidemic. *Circulation.* 2009;119:2516–2525.
61. Proietti R, Mafrici A, Spodick DH. Dynamic variations of P-wave duration in a patient with acute decompensated congestive heart failure. *Cardiol J.* 2012;19:95–97.
62. Gunes Y, Tuncer M, Guntekin U, Akdag S, Gumrukcuoglu HA. The effects of trimetazidine on P-wave duration and dispersion in heart failure patients. *Pacing Clin Electrophysiol.* 2009;32:239–244.
63. Camsari A, Pekdemir H, Akkus MN, et al. Long-term effects of beta blocker therapy on P-wave duration and dispersion in congestive heart failure patients: a new effect? *J Electrocardiol.* 2003;36:111–116.
64. Magnani JW, Wang N, Nelson KP, et al. Electrocardiographic PR interval and adverse outcomes in older adults: The Health, Aging, and Body Composition study. *Circ Arrhythm Electrophysiol.* 2013;6:84–90.
65. Demirkan B, Guray Y, Guray U, et al. The acute effect of percutaneous mitral balloon valvuloplasty on atrial electromechanical delay and P-wave dispersion in patients with mitral stenosis. *Herz.* 2013;38:210–215.
66. Guntekin U, Gunes Y, Tuncer M, et al. Long-term follow-up of P-wave duration and dispersion in patients with mitral stenosis. *Pacing Clin Electrophysiol.* 2008;31:1620–1624.
67. Zeng C, Wei T, Zhao R, et al. Electrocardiographic diagnosis of left atrial enlargement in patients with mitral stenosis: The value of the P-wave area. *Acta Cardiol.* 2003;58:139–141.
68. Tarastchuk JC, Guerios EE, Perreto S, et al. Changes in P-wave after percutaneous mitral valvuloplasty in patients with mitral stenosis and left atrial enlargement. *Arq Bras Cardiol.* 2006;87:359–363.
69. Erbay AR, Turhan H, Yasar AS, et al. Effects of long-term beta-blocker therapy on P-wave duration and dispersion in patients with rheumatic mitral stenosis. *Int J Cardiol.* 2005;102:33–37.
70. Pekdemir H, Cansel M, Yagmur J, et al. Assessment of atrial conduction time by tissue doppler echocardiography and P-wave dispersion in patients

with mitral annulus calcification. *J Electrocardiol.* 2010;43:339–343.

71. Elbey MA, Oylumlu M, Akil A, et al. Relation of interatrial duration and P wave terminal force as a novel indicator of severe mitral regurgitation. *Eur Rev Med Pharmacol Sci.* 2012;16:1576–1581.
72. Guray U, Guray Y, Mecit B, et al. Maximum P wave duration and P wave dispersion in adult patients with secundum atrial septal defect: the impact of surgical repair. *Ann Noninvasive Electrocardiol.* 2004;9:136–141.
73. Guray U, Guray Y, Yylmaz MB, et al. Evaluation of P wave duration and P wave dispersion in adult patients with secundum atrial septal defect during normal sinus rhythm. *Int J Cardiol.* 2003;91:75–79.
74. Ho TF, Chia EL, Yip WC, Chan KY. Analysis of P wave and P dispersion in children with secundum atrial septal defect. *Ann Noninvasive Electrocardiol.* 2001;6:305–309.
75. Yavuz T, Nisli K, Oner N, et al. The effects of surgical repair on P-wave dispersion in children with secundum atrial septal defect. *Adv Ther.* 2008;25:795–800.
76. Javadzadegan H, Toufan M, Sadighi AR, Chang JM, Nader ND. Comparative effects of surgical and percutaneous repair on P-wave and atrioventricular conduction in patients with atrial septal defect–ostium secundum type. *Cardiol Young.* 2013;23:132–137.
77. Chamberlain AM, Agarwal SK, Folsom AR, et al. A clinical risk score for atrial fibrillation in a biracial prospective cohort (from the atherosclerosis risk in communities [aric] study). *Am J Cardiol.* 2011;107:85–91.
78. Magnani JW, Lopez FL, Soliman EZ, et al. P wave indices, obesity, and the metabolic syndrome: The atherosclerosis risk in communities study. *Obesity (Silver Spring).* 2012;20:666–672.
79. Liu T, Fu Z, Korantzopoulos P, et al. Effect of obesity on P-wave parameters in a chinese population. *Ann Noninvasive Electrocardiol.* 2010;15:259–263.
80. Duru M, Seyfeli E, Kuvandik G, Kaya H, Yalcin F. Effect of weight loss on P wave dispersion in obese subjects. *Obesity (Silver Spring).* 2006;14:1378–1382.
81. Russo V, Ammendola E, De Crescenzo I, et al . Severe obesity and P-wave dispersion: the effect of surgically induced weight loss. *Obes Surg.* 2008;18:90–96.
82. Yazici M, Ozdemir K, Altunkeser BB, et al. The effect of diabetes mellitus on the P-wave dispersion. *Circ J.* 2007;71:880–883.
83. Karabag T, Aydin M, Dogan SM, et al. Prolonged P wave dispersion in pre-diabetic patients. *Kardiol Pol.* 2011;69:566–571.
84. Erdogan E, Akkaya M, Turfan M, et al. Polycystic ovary syndrome is associated with P-wave prolongation and increased P-wave dispersion. *Gynecol Endocrinol.* 2013;29:830–833.
85. Bissinger A, Grycewicz T, Grabowicz W, Lubinski A. The effect of diabetic autonomic neuropathy on P-wave duration, dispersion and atrial fibrillation. *Arch Med Sci.* 2011;7:806–812.
86. Jazi MH, Amra B, Yazdchi MR, et al. P wave duration and dispersion in holter electrocardiography of patients with obstructive sleep apnea. *Sleep Breath.* 2014;18:549-554.
87. Cagirci G, Cay S, Gulsoy KG, et al. Tissue doppler atrial conduction times and electrocardiogram interlead P-wave durations with varying severity of obstructive sleep apnea. *J Electrocardiol.* 2011;44:478–482.
88. Can I, Aytemir K, Demir AU, et al. P-wave duration and dispersion in patients with obstructive sleep apnea. *Int J Cardiol.* 2009;133:e85–e89.
89. Lweesy K, Fraiwan L, Khasawneh N, Dickhaus H. New automated detection method of OSA based on artificial neural networks using P-wave shape and time changes. *J Med Syst.* 2011;35:723–734.
90. Guntekin U, Gunes Y, Simsek H, Tuncer M, Arslan S. P wave duration and dispersion in patients with hyperthyroidism and the short-term effects of antithyroid treatment. *Indian Pacing Electrophysiol J.* 2009;9:251–259.
91. Berker D, Isik S, Canbay A, et al. Comparison of antithyroid drugs efficacy on P wave changes in patients with Graves' disease. *Anadolu Kardiyol Derg.* 2009;9:298–303.
92. Katircibasi MT, Deniz F, Pamukcu B, Binici S, Atar I. Effects of short-term propylthiouracil treatment on P wave duration and P wave dispersion in patients with overt hypertyroidism. *Exp Clin Endocrinol Diabetes.* 2007;115:376–379.
93. Cetinarslan B, Akkoyun M, Canturk Z, et al. Duration of the P wave and P wave dispersion in subclinical hyperthyroidism. *Endocr Pract.* 2003;9:200–203.
94. Gen R, Akbay E, Camsari A, Ozcan T. P-wave dispersion in endogenous and exogenous subclinical hyperthyroidism. *J Endocrinol Invest.* 2010;33:88–91.
95. Aras D, Maden O, Ozdemir O, et al. Simple electrocardiographic markers for the prediction of paroxysmal atrial fibrillation in hyperthyroidism. *Int J Cardiol.* 2005;99:59–64.
96. Genovesi S, Pogliani D, Faini A, et al. Prevalence of atrial fibrillation and associated factors in a population of long-term hemodialysis patients. *Am J Kidney Dis.* 2005;46:897–902.
97. Tezcan UK, Amasyali B, Can I, et al. Increased P wave dispersion and maximum P wave duration after hemodialysis. *Ann Noninvasive Electrocardiol.* 2004;9:34–38.
98. Szabo Z, Kakuk G, Fulop T, et al. Effects of haemodialysis on maximum P wave duration and P wave dispersion. *Nephrol Dial Transplant.* 2002;17:1634–1638.
99. Severi S, Pogliani D, Fantini G, et al. Alterations of atrial electrophysiology induced by electrolyte variations: Combined computational and P-wave analysis. *Europace.* 2010;12:842–849.
100. Drighil A, Madias JE, Yazidi A, et al. P-wave and QRS complex measurements in patients undergoing hemodialysis. *J Electrocardiol.* 2008;41:60.e61–60.e67.
101. Ozmen N, Cebeci BS, Kardesoglu E, et al. Relationship between P-wave dispersion and effective hemodialysis in chronic hemodialysis patients. *Med Princ Pract.* 2007;16:147–150.
102. Drighil A, Madias JE, El Mosalami H, et al. Impact of hemodialysis on P-wave amplitude, duration, and dispersion. *Indian Pacing Electrophysiol J.* 2007;7:85–96.

103. Yavuzkir M, Ozturk A, Dagli N, et al. Effect of ongoing inflammation in rheumatoid arthritis on P-wave dispersion. *J Int Med Res.* 2007;35:796–802.
104. Guler H, Seyfeli E, Sahin G, et al. P wave dispersion in patients with rheumatoid arthritis: its relation with clinical and echocardiographic parameters. *Rheumatol Int.* 2007;27:813–818.
105. Akkaya H, Karakas MS, Sahin O, Borlu M, Oguzhan A. The effect of nebivolol on P wave duration and dispersion in patients with Behcet's disease; a prospective single-arm controlled study. *Anadolu Kardiyol Derg.* 2013;13:682–687.
106. Dogan SM, Aydin M, Gursurer M, et al. The increase in P-wave dispersion is associated with the duration of disease in patients with Behcet's disease. *Int J Cardiol.* 2008;124:407–410.
107. Bacaksiz A, Erdogan E, Tasal A, et al. Electrocardiographic P-wave characteristics in patients with psoriasis vulgaris. *Ups J Med Sci.* 2013;118:35–41.
108. Magnani JW, Williamson MA, Ellinor PT, Monahan KM, Benjamin EJ. P wave indices: current status and future directions in epidemiology, clinical, and research applications. *Circ Arrhythm Electrophysiol.* 2009;2:72–79.
109. Tsai WC, Lee KT, Wu MT, et al. Significant correlation of P-wave parameters with left atrial volume index and left ventricular diastolic function. *Am J Med Sci.* 2013;346:45–51.
110. Magnani JW, Johnson VM, Sullivan LM, et al. P wave duration and risk of longitudinal atrial fibrillation in persons ≥ 60 years old (from the Framingham heart study). *Am J Cardiol.* 2011;107:917–921.
111. Ishida K, Hayashi H, Miyamoto A, et al. P wave and the development of atrial fibrillation. *Heart Rhythm.* 2010;7:289–294.
112. Cheng S, Keyes MJ, Larson MG, et al. Long-term outcomes in individuals with prolonged PR interval or first-degree atrioventricular block. *JAMA.* 2009;301:2571–2577.
113. De Sisti A, Leclercq JF, Stiubei M, et al. P wave duration and morphology predict atrial fibrillation recurrence in patients with sinus node dysfunction and atrial-based pacemaker. *Pacing Clin Electrophysiol.* 2002;25:1546–1554.
114. Snoeck J, Decoster H, Vrints C, et al. Predictive value of the P wave at implantation for atrial fibrillation after VVI pacemaker implantation. *Pacing Clin Electrophysiol.* 1992;15:2077–2083.
115. Padeletti L, Santini M, Boriani G, et al. Duration of P-wave is associated with atrial fibrillation hospitalizations in patients with atrial fibrillation and paced for bradycardia. *Pacing Clin Electrophysiol.* 2007;30:961–969.
116. Healey JS, Israel CW, Connolly SJ, et al. Relevance of electrical remodeling in human atrial fibrillation: Results of the Asymptomatic Atrial Fibrillation and Stroke Evaluation in Pacemaker Patients and the Atrial Fibrillation Reduction Atrial Pacing Trial mechanisms of atrial fibrillation study. *Circ Arrhythm Electrophysiol.* 2012;5:626–631.
117. Dilaveris PE, Gialafos EJ, Sideris SK, et al. Simple electrocardiographic markers for the prediction of paroxysmal idiopathic atrial fibrillation. *Am Heart J.* 1998;135:733–738.
118. Dogan U, Dogan EA, Tekinalp M, et al. P-wave dispersion for predicting paroxysmal atrial fibrillation in acute ischemic stroke. *Int J Med Sci.* 2012;9:108–114.
119. Altunkeser BB, Ozdemir K, Gok H, et al. Can P wave parameters obtained from 12-lead surface electrocardiogram be a predictor for atrial fibrillation in patients who have structural heart disease? *Angiology.* 2003;54:475–479.
120. Girasis C, Vassilikos V, Efthimiadis GK, et al. Patients with hypertrophic cardiomyopathy at risk for paroxysmal atrial fibrillation: advanced echocardiographic evaluation of the left atrium combined with non-invasive P-wave analysis. *Eur Heart J Cardiovasc Imaging.* 2013;14:425–434.
121. Aytemir K, Amasyali B, Kose S, et al. Maximum P-wave duration and P-wave dispersion predict recurrence of paroxysmal atrial fibrillation in patients with Wolff-Parkinson-White syndrome after successful radiofrequency catheter ablation. *J Interv Card Electrophysiol.* 2004;11:21–27.
122. De Bacquer D, Willekens J, De Backer G. Long-term prognostic value of P-wave characteristics for the development of atrial fibrillation in subjects aged 55 to 74 years at baseline. *Am J Cardiol.* 2007;100:850–854.
123. Dogan A, Acar G, Gedikli O, et al. A comparison of P-wave duration and dispersion in patients with short-term and long-term atrial fibrillation. *J Electrocardiol.* 2003;36:251–255.
124. Ozdemir O, Soylu M, Demir AD, et al. P-wave durations in patients experiencing atrial fibrillation during exercise testing. *Angiology.* 2007;58:97–101.
125. le Polain de Waroux JB, Talajic M, Khairy P, et al. Pulmonary vein isolation for the treatment of atrial fibrillation: Past, present and future. *Future Cardiol.* 2010;6:51–66.
126. Zhao L, Jiang WF, Zhou L, Liu X. Early-phase changes of P-wave characteristics after circumferential pulmonary vein isolation. *Chin Med J (Engl).* 2013;126:2607–2612.
127. Janin S, Wojcik M, Kuniss M, et al. Pulmonary vein antrum isolation and terminal part of the P wave. *Pacing Clin Electrophysiol.* 2010;33:784–789.
128. Nassif M, Krul SP, Driessen AH, et al. Electrocardiographic P wave changes after thoracoscopic pulmonary vein isolation for atrial fibrillation. *J Interv Card Electrophysiol.* 2013;37:275–282.
129. Gonna H, Gallagher MM, Guo XH, et al. P-wave abnormality predicts recurrence of atrial fibrillation after electrical cardioversion: A prospective study. *Ann Noninvasive Electrocardiol.* 2014;19:57-62.
130. Gorenek B, Birdane A, Kudaiberdieva G, et al. P wave amplitude and duration may predict immediate recurrence of atrial fibrillation after internal cardioversion. *Ann Noninvasive Electrocardiol.* 2003;8:215–218.
131. Ozdemir O, Soylu M, Demir AD, et al. Does P-wave dispersion predict the atrial fibrillation occurrence after direct-current shock therapy? *Angiology.* 2006;57:93–98.

132. Salah A, Zhou S, Liu Q, Yan H. P wave indices to predict atrial fibrillation recurrences post pulmonary vein isolation. *Arq Bras Cardiol.* 2013;101:519-527.
133. Ogawa M, Kumagai K, Vakulenko M, et al. Reduction of P-wave duration and successful pulmonary vein isolation in patients with atrial fibrillation. *J Cardiovasc Electrophysiol.* 2007;18:931–938.
134. Caldwell J, Koppikar S, Barake W, et al. Prolonged P-wave duration is associated with atrial fibrillation recurrence after successful pulmonary vein isolation for paroxysmal atrial fibrillation. *J Interv Card Electrophysiol.* 2014;39:131-138.
135. Siebert J, Anisimowicz L, Lango R, et al. Atrial fibrillation after coronary artery bypass grafting: Does the type of procedure influence the early postoperative incidence? *Eur J Cardiothorac Surg.* 2001;19:455–459.
136. Buxton AE, Josephson ME. The role of P wave duration as a predictor of postoperative atrial arrhythmias. *Chest.* 1981;80:68–73.
137. Tsikouris JP, Kluger J, Song J, White CM. Changes in P-wave dispersion and P-wave duration after open heart surgery are associated with the peak incidence of atrial fibrillation. *Heart Lung.* 2001;30:466–471.
138. Chandy J, Nakai T, Lee RJ, et al. Increases in P-wave dispersion predict postoperative atrial fibrillation after coronary artery bypass graft surgery. *Anesth Analg.* 2004;98:303–310.
139. Chang CM, Lee SH, Lu MJ, et al. The role of P wave in prediction of atrial fibrillation after coronary artery surgery. *Int J Cardiol.* 1999;68:303–308.
140. Akutsu Y, Kaneko K, Kodama Y, et al. A combination of P wave electrocardiography and plasma brain natriuretic peptide level for predicting the progression to persistent atrial fibrillation: Comparisons of sympathetic activity and left atrial size. *J Interv Card Electrophysiol.* 2013;38:79–84.
141. Cotter PE, Martin PJ, Pugh PJ, et al. Increased incidence of interatrial block in younger adults with cryptogenic stroke and patent foramen ovale. *Cerebrovasc Dis Extra.* 2011;1:36–43.
142. Magnani JW, Gorodeski EZ, Johnson VM, et al. P wave duration is associated with cardiovascular and all-cause mortality outcomes: the National Health and Nutrition Examination Survey. *Heart Rhythm.* 2011;8:93–100.
143. Aro AL, Anttonen O, Kerola T, et al. Prognostic significance of prolonged PR interval in the general population. *Eur Heart J.* 2014;35:123–129.
144. Soliman EZ, Cammarata M, Li Y. Explaining the inconsistent associations of PR interval with mortality: the role of P-duration contribution to the length of PR interval. *Heart Rhythm.* 2014;11:93–98.
145. Liu G, Tamura A, Torigoe K, et al. Abnormal P-wave terminal force in lead V1 is associated with cardiac death or hospitalization for heart failure in prior myocardial infarction. *Heart Vessels.* 2013;28:690–695.
146. Li Y, Shah AJ, Soliman EZ. Effect of electrocardiographic P-wave axis on mortality. *Am J Cardiol.* 2014;113:372–376.
147. Gudbjartsson DF, Arnar DO, Helgadottir A, et al. Variants conferring risk of atrial fibrillation on chromosome 4q25. *Nature.* 2007;448:353–357.
148. Benjamin EJ, Rice KM, Arking DE, et al. Variants in ZFHX3 are associated with atrial fibrillation in individuals of European ancestry. *Nat Genet.* 2009;41:879–881.
149. Ellinor PT, Lunetta KL, Glazer NL, et al. Common variants in KCNN3 are associated with lone atrial fibrillation. *Nat Genet.* 2010;42:240–244.
150. Sinner MF, Pfeufer A, Akyol M, et al. The non-synonymous coding IKr-channel variant KCNH2-K897T is associated with atrial fibrillation: results from a systematic candidate gene-based analysis of KCNH2 (HERG). *Eur Heart J.* 2008;29:907–914.
151. Lubitz SA, Sinner MF, Lunetta KL, et al. Independent susceptibility markers for atrial fibrillation on chromosome 4q25. *Circulation.* 2010;122:976–984.
152. Lin H, Sinner MF, Brody JA, et al. Targeted sequencing in candidate genes for atrial fibrillation: The cohorts for heart and aging research in genomic epidemiology targeted sequencing study. *Heart Rhythm.* 2014;11:452-457.
153. Havlik RJ, Garrison RJ, Fabsitz R, Feinleib M. Variability of heart rate, P-R, QRS and Q-T durations in twins. *J Electrocardiol.* 1980;13:45–48.
154. Hanson B, Tuna N, Bouchard T, et al. Genetic factors in the electrocardiogram and heart rate of twins reared apart and together. *Am J Cardiol.* 1989;63:606–609.
155. Pilia G, Chen WM, Scuteri A, et al. Heritability of cardiovascular and personality traits in 6,148 sardinians. *PLoS Genet.* 2006;2:e132.
156. Newton-Cheh C, Guo CY, Wang TJ, et al. Genome-wide association study of electrocardiographic and heart rate variability traits: the Framingham heart study. *BMC Med Genet.* 2007;8(suppl 1):S7.
157. Pfeufer A, van Noord C, Marciante KD, et al. Genome-wide association study of PR interval. *Nat Genet.* 2010;42:153–159.
158. Rabert DK, Koch BD, Ilnicka M, et al. A tetrodotoxin-resistant voltage-gated sodium channel from human dorsal root ganglia, HPN3/SCN10A. *Pain.* 1998;78:107–114.
159. Remme CA, Wilde AA, Bezzina CR. Cardiac sodium channel overlap syndromes: Different faces of SCN5A mutations. *Trends Cardiovasc Med.* 2008;18:78–87.
160. Kristensen L, Nielsen JC, Mortensen PT, et al. Sinus and paced P wave duration and dispersion as predictors of atrial fibrillation after pacemaker implantation in patients with isolated sick sinus syndrome. *Pacing Clin Electrophysiol.* 2004;27:606–614.

CHAPTER

4

The Athlete's Electrocardiogram

Yousef Bader, MD, Mark S. Link, MD, and N.A. Mark Estes III, MD

INTRODUCTION

Changes in the ECG are common in the athlete due to physiological adaptations that occur in myocardial conduction, repolarization, and impulse formation in response to athletic conditioning and alterations in autonomic tone. The athlete's heart represents a largely benign increase in cardiac mass with circulatory and morphological alterations in response to athletic training. These structural and electric adaptations may mimic findings associated with cardiovascular disease (CVD). Structural findings include chamber enlargement and ventricular hypertrophy. Electric abnormalities include increased QRS voltage, abnormal Q waves, and T-wave inversions. ECG findings such as bradyarrhythmia, ventricular hypertrophy, or repolarization abnormalities are physiological rather than pathologic.[1–31] Less commonly, the athlete's ECG may manifest changes indicating the possibility of an underlying cardiovascular condition predisposing to sudden cardiac death.[1–31] Distinguishing physiologic ECG changes in the athlete from findings with a cardiovascular condition that may be life-threatening remains a clinical challenge.[1–31] It is particularly important for physicians interpreting ECGs to have both knowledge and understanding of changes that result from athletic conditioning and those that may be a marker of underlying structural heart disease or vulnerability to cardiac arrhythmias. Variation in the range of normal for an athlete's ECG occur based on age, gender, ethnicity, sport, position on a team, and level of conditioning.[1–31] Recent publications of consensus recommendations related to this issue provide a constructive framework for interpretation of the athlete's ECG.[32–47] However, some inconsistencies in the definition of ECG abnormalities, gray zones, and challenges in interpretation persist.[32–47]

The related, but separate, issue of ECG-inclusive preparticipation screening of athletes is beyond the scope of this chapter.[48–57] However, it is appropriate to recognize that some have recommended that the 12-lead ECG be included in preparticipation athletic screening.[48–57] The rationale is that the ECG has incremental value over standard screening with a history and physical examination to detect cardiovascular conditions that predisposed to sudden death during sports.[48–57] The clinical utility of the ECG for detecting cardiomyopathies, channelopathies, and other conditions that predispose to athletic sudden death is dependent on the sensitivity, specificity, and positive and negative predictive values of the ECG.[48–57] Based on the principle of Bayesian analysis, it is evident that a low prevalence of cardiovascular conditions predisposing to sudden death limits the predictive

The ECG Handbook of Contemporary Challenges © 2015 Mohammad Shenasa, Mark E. Josephson, N.A. Mark Estes III
Cardiotext Publishing, ISBN: 978-1-935395-88-1

accuracy of the ECG even with otherwise favorable sensitivity and specificity.[48–57] Uncertainty persists regarding the criteria for definitive diagnosis of many cardiovascular conditions with secondary testing such as echocardiograms and cardiac magnetic resonance imaging (MRI).[48–57] The unresolved controversies related to the inclusion of the ECG in preparticipation athletic screening are addressed in many recent publications.[48–57] The evaluation and management of the cardiovascular conditions that predispose to athletic sudden death are also the subject of many recent publications.[58–64] Detailed descriptions of the specific ECG abnormalities accompanying the multiple cardiovascular conditions predisposing to sudden athletic death are included in separate chapters in this book.[59–64] These include ECG changes in hypertrophic cardiomyopathy (HCM), arrhythmogenic right ventricular (RV) dysplasia, Brugada syndrome, early repolarization, long QT syndrome, and other conditions that predispose to sudden cardiac death of the athlete.[59–63] The purpose of this chapter is to provide the best available recommendations for distinguishing the physiological ECG changes that accompany the cardiovascular remodeling resulting from athletic training and ECG alterations that may serve as a marker of cardiovascular conditions predisposing to athletic sudden death. In addition, this chapter will serve to discuss the limitations of classification schemes that have been proposed to distinguish ECG changes attributable to the athlete's heart and those that may indicate an underlying cardiovascular condition predisposing to sudden death.

Multiple ECG changes attributed to cardiovascular remodeling in the conditioned athlete have been described as being within the spectrum of normal for a conditioned athlete (Table 4.1).[37–47] Recently, ECG changes in athletes have been classified into 2 distinct groups.[37–39] These are defined as: (1) common and training-related and (2) uncommon and not training-related (Table 4.2).[37–39] These classifications are based on prevalence, relation to exercise training, association with an increased cardiovascular risk, and need for further clinical investigation to confirm or exclude an underlying CVD.[37–39] This classification scheme for ECG changes in the athlete will serve as a useful, yet imperfect, framework for subsequent sections on ECG changes that are common and training-related or uncommon and not training-related.[37–39]

Table 4.1. **Common electrocardiographic findings in athletes.**

Sinus bradycardia (>30 bpm)
Sinus arrhythmia
Ectopic atrial rhythm
First-degree AV block (PR > 200 ms)
Mobitz type I/Wenckebach second-degree AV block
Incomplete RBBB
Notched P Waves
Isolated QRS voltage criteria for LVH • Except QRS voltage criteria for LVH occurring with any nonvoltage criteria for LVH, such as left atrial enlargement, left axis deviation, ST-segment depression, T-wave inversion, or pathological Q waves
Early repolarization
Repolarization abnormalities • Including ST segment elevation or depression (ST-elevation, J-point elevation, J waves, or terminal QRS slurring)
Convex ("domed") ST segment elevation • Combined with T-wave inversion in leads V_1–V_4 in black/African athletes.

Common training-related ECG alterations are physiological adaptations to regular exercise and as such are considered normal variants in athletes and do not require further evaluation in asymptomatic athletes. (Modified with permission.[37–39])
Abbreviations: AV, atrioventricular; bpm, beats per minute; LVH, left ventricular hypertrophy; ms, milliseconds; RBBB, right bundle branch block.

SINUS BRADYCARDIA, SINUS ARRHYTHMIA, JUNCTIONAL RHYTHM, AND ECTOPIC ATRIAL RHYTHM

There is a broad spectrum of normal bradyarrhythmias seen in the athlete due to high vagal tone and reduction of sympathetic tone that accompanies physical training. These changes are attributed to physiological, electrical, and structural remodeling and autonomic nervous system changes in response to substantial physical activity.[1,2,14] The sinus node, by mechanism of automaticity, sympathetic, and parasympathetic inputs, determines a person's necessary heart rate depending on the physiologic state.[1,2,14] Sinus bradycardia, defined as a heart rate less than 60 beats per minute (bpm), is among the most common finding in the athlete (Figure 4.1). Up to 91% of athletes have sinus bradycardia at rest, although this depends upon the type of athletic activity.[1,2,14] With endurance sports such as long-distance running, bicycling, and swimming, athlete's resting heart rates become lower with higher levels of conditioning.[1,2,14] Athletes may have resting heart rates in the 30s, which is a result of high vagal tone and is considered normal in asymptomatic individuals. Some authors have suggested that there are changes within the SA node independent of increased vagal tone, which

Table 4.2. **Uncommon, abnormal ECG findings in athletes.**

T-wave inversion
- >1 mm in depth in 2 or more leads V_2–V_6, II and aVF, or I and aVL (excludes III, aVR, and V_1)

ST-segment depression
- ≥0.5 mm in depth in 2 or more leads

Pathologic Q waves
- >3 mm in depth or >40 ms in duration in 2 or more leads (except for III and aVR)

Complete LBBB
- QRS ≥120 ms, predominantly negative QRS complex in lead V_1 (QS or rS), and upright, monophasic R wave in leads I and V_6

Intraventricular conduction delay
- Any QRS duration ≥140 ms

Left axis deviation
- −30° to −90°

Left atrial enlargement
- Prolonged P-wave duration of >120 ms in leads I or II with negative portion of the P wave ≥1 mm in depth and ≥40 ms in duration in lead V_1

Ventricular pre-excitation
- PR interval <120 ms with a delta wave (slurred upstroke in the QRS complex) and wide QRS (>120 ms)

Long QT interval
- QTc ≥ 470 ms (male)
- QTc ≥ 480 ms (female)
- QTc ≥ 500 ms (marked QT prolongation)

Short QT interval
- QTc ≤ 320 ms

Brugada-like ECG pattern
- High take-off and down-sloping ST segment elevation followed by a negative T wave in ≥2 leads in V_1 to V_3

Profound sinus bradycardia
- <30 bpm or sinus pauses ≥ 3 seconds

Ventricular arrhythmias
- Couplets, triplets, and nonsustained VT

These are not considered normal variants in athletes and require further evaluation in athletes. (Modified with permission.[37–39])

result in decreased automaticity of the SA node. However, with exercise, athletes with resting sinus bradycardia demonstrated a normal chronotropic response.[1,2,14]

Sinus arrhythmia, or the increase of heart rate related to inspiration is also seen more commonly in highly conditioned athletes reflecting heightened vagal tone (Figure 4.2).[1,2,14] This variability in heart rate with respiration is known as sinus arrhythmia and is commonly found in children. It is also reported in up to 69% of athletes.[1,2,14,38] The heart rate typically increases slightly during inspiration and slows slightly during expiration. This is also a benign finding in athletes and does not warrant further workup.[1,2,29]

In addition to ectopic atrial rhythms and wandering atrial pacemakers, athletes may have junctional rhythm. The sinus node lies in the posterior right atrium at the junction of the superior vena cava and right atrium.[1,2,14] Therefore, one would expect P waves to be upright in leads I, II, and usually V_1 on a 12-lead ECG. Due to suppression of the sinus node by the mechanisms described above, other automatic foci in the atria can occasionally drive the heart rate.[1,2,14] Athletes may have an ectopic atrial rhythm whereby the P-wave morphology would be different than that seen in normal sinus rhythm (NSR). Occasionally, greater than 2 atrial foci can be seen in a single lead, and this is known as multifocal atrial rhythm or wandering atrial pacemaker.[1,2,14] It is considered physiologic when the native junctional rate of a conditioned athlete is faster than the baseline or rest sinus rate.[1,2,14] A typical junctional escape rate is 40 to 60 bpm and sinus bradycardia in the athlete with rates less than this are common; thus, junctional escape beats are commonly seen (Figure 4.3).[1,2,14]

Distinguishing normal from abnormal arrhythmias in athletes always needs to be done in the context of symptoms documented to be due to the arrhythmia or cardiovascular abnormality.[1,2,37–39] Heart rates that normalize with exercise and bradycardias that reverse with reduction in athletic training are considered to be indicators of physiologic bradycardia rather than a manifestation of primary sinus node dysfunction.[1,2,37–39] Generally, only symptomatic bradycardia or profound sinus bradycardia or sinus arrhythmia with heart rates < 30 bpm or pauses > 3 seconds during the waking hours should be considered as possible manifestations of underlying sinus node dysfunction.[1,2,37–39]

RIGHT AND LEFT ATRIAL ABNORMALITIES

Historically, multiple studies noted that the P-wave amplitude is greater in athletes than nonathletes.[1,2,5,31] This was presumed to be due to atrial hypertrophy. In one report, 25% of elite runners had P-wave amplitude of 2.5 to 3 mm in any lead. In addition, it has been noted that there is a high frequency of notched P waves in athletes, with 18 of 26 runners having this finding in one series.[25] However, this finding was not noted in another series of Finnish athletes, where only 41 of 651 were noted to have notching of the P wave.[26] More recently, ECG evidence of right atrial enlargement has been classified as an

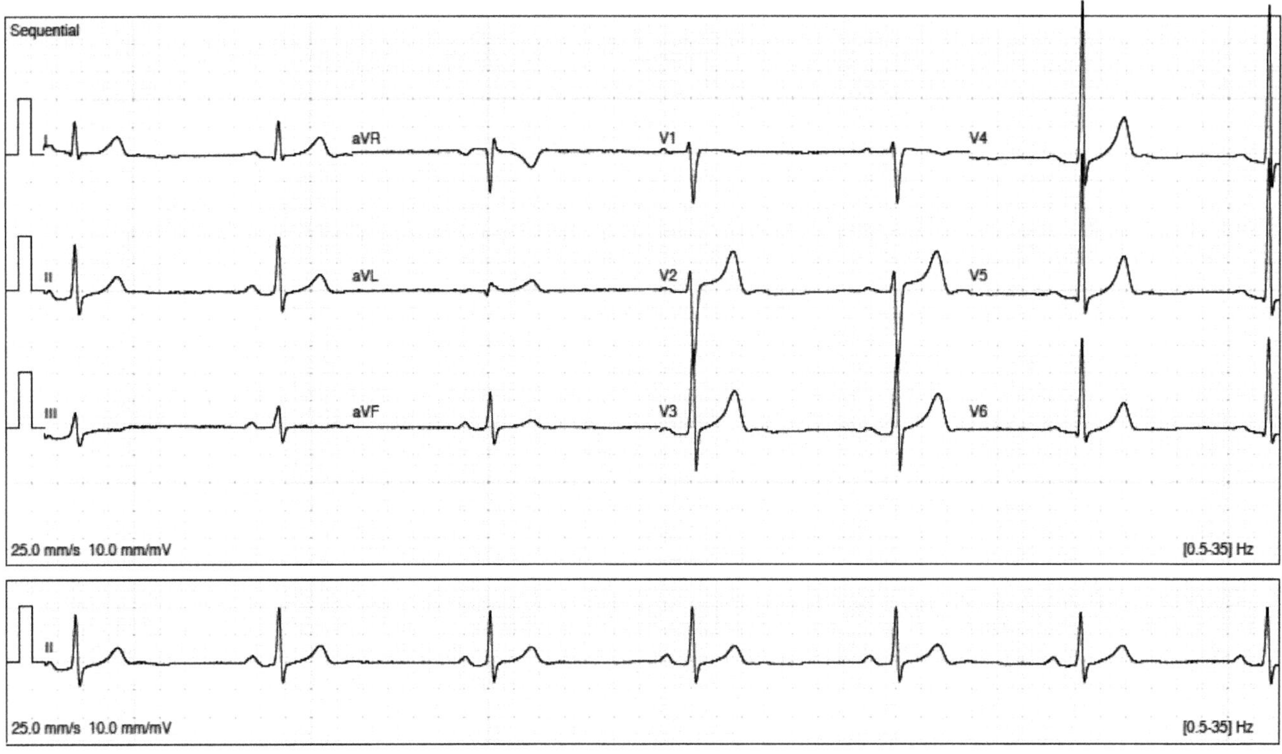

Figure 4.1. Sinus bradycardia in a asymptomatic 18-year-old female long distance runner.

uncommon finding in athletes.[38] In one series of 1108, it was reported that there was a prevalence of 0.08% for right atrial enlargement.[3] Based on this more recent data, the recent consensus recommendation note that, if present, the ECG pattern of right atrial enlargement should not be interpreted as a manifestation of exercise-induced cardiac remodeling. The presence of either congenital or acquired heart diseases associated with an increased right atrial size should be excluded.[38]

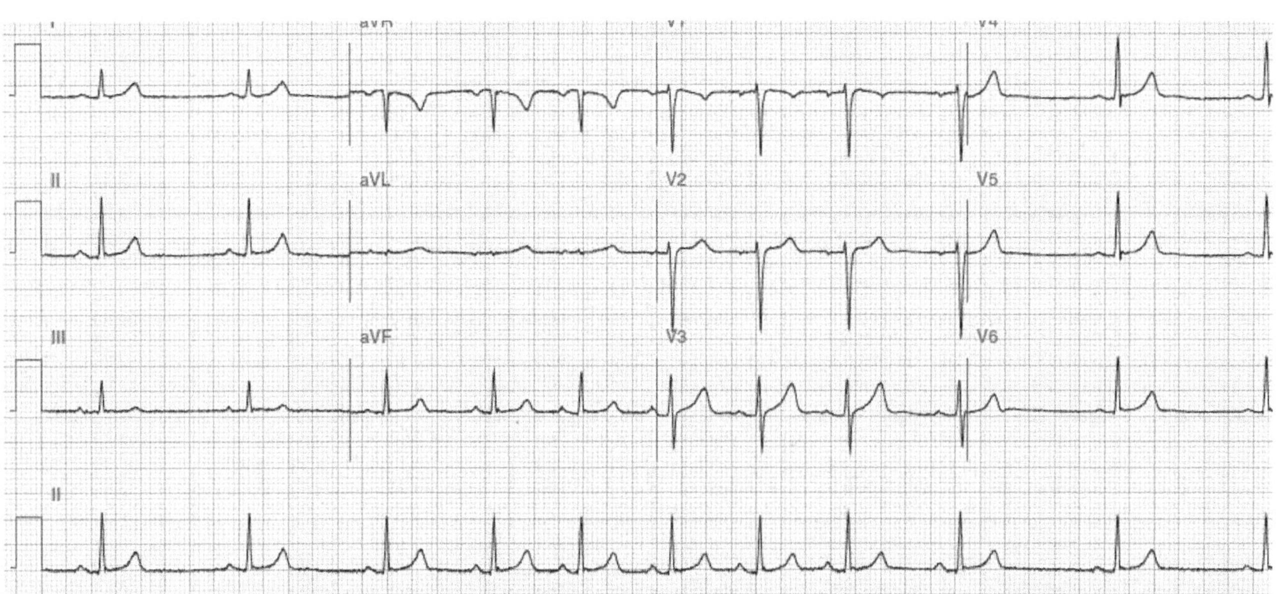

Figure 4.2. Sinus arrhythmia manifesting with an increase in heart rate with inspiration in a 20-year-old male hockey player.

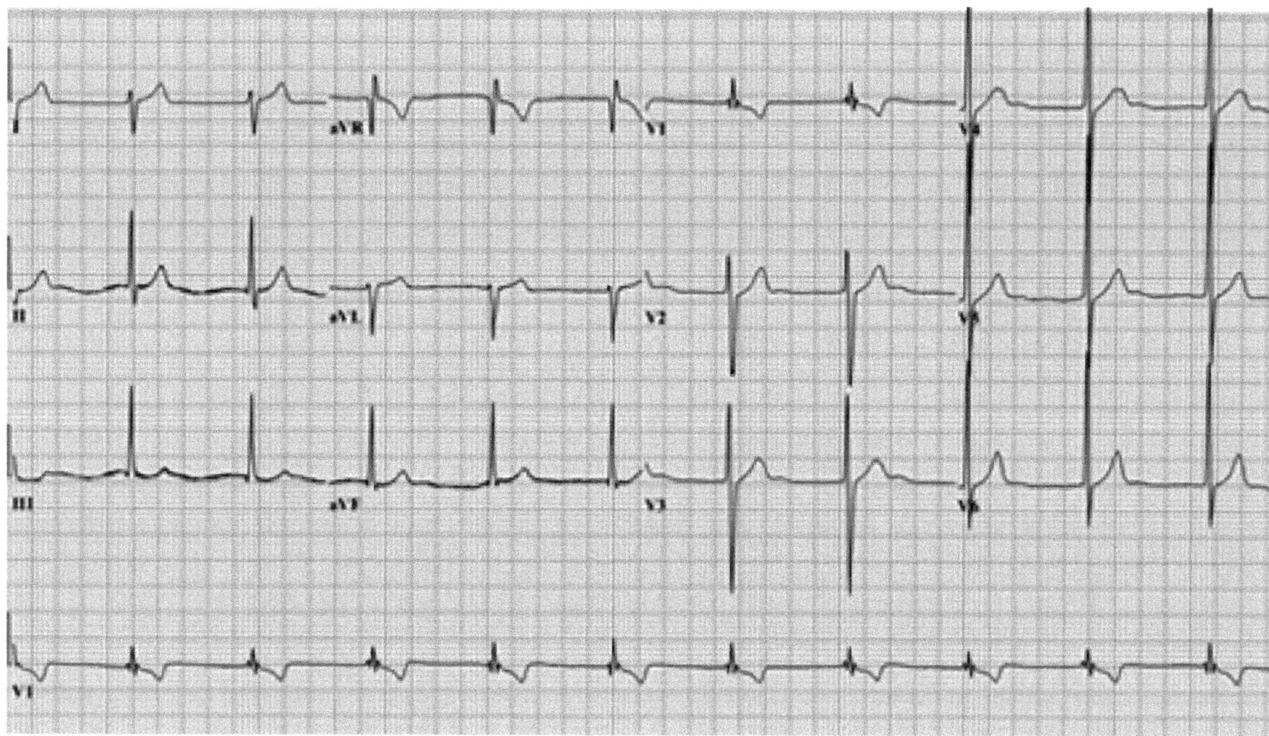

Figure 4.3. Junctional rhythm in an asymptomatic 19-year-old swimmer. Note the absence of P-waves prior to the QRS complexes.

The prevalence of left atrial abnormality is defined on the ECG based on a negative P wave in V_1 or V_2 of 40 ms duration and 1 mm in amplitude or total P-wave duration of 120 ms. Some studies have reported left atrial abnormalities in up to 18% of athletes, whereas others report a prevalence as low as 0.7%.[3,13,16] Current recommendations are that isolated atrial abnormalities in younger athletes who are asymptomatic and have an unremarkable personal and family history do not require further workup.[37–39] However, it is recommended that collegiate and adult athletes should have further workup with fulfilling criteria for atrial abnormalities.[37,38]

ATRIOVENTRICULAR CONDUCTION

The effects of high vagal tone in athletes are also evident by its effect on the atrioventricular (AV) node. First-degree AV block (PR interval > 200 ms) and Mobitz type I (Wenckebach) second-degree AV block are common and benign findings in trained athletes (Figure 4.4).[1,2,37–39] They are reported to be present in 35% and 10% of athletes' ECGs, respectively.[38] With exercise and acceleration of the sinus rate, conduction through the AV node should improve with physiological decrease in AV conduction in response to sympathetic activation.[1,2,38] In athletes with type II second-degree (Mobitz type II) and third-degree AV block, a careful diagnostic evaluation is indicated with the potential need for placement of a pacemaker.[1,2,37–39]

A 2:1 block is possible with both Mobitz I and II; if the QRS is not prolonged, then in all likelihood the block is in the AV node (Mobitz I). If the QRS is > 120 ms, then it is likely that the block is in the His-Purkinje system (Mobitz II).

CONDUCTION ABNORMALITIES: RBBB, LBBB, AND INTRAVENTRICULAR CONDUCTION DELAY

Infranodal and infra-Hisian conduction delays are also often seen in athletes. Incomplete right bundle branch block (RBBB) is a common finding seen in 12% to 32% of athletes and is due to RV enlargement, which is a normal response to regular training.[1–3,13,37–39] The cause of incomplete RBBB is thought to be a result of mild RV enlargement resulting in increased cavity size, which in turn leads to delayed conduction through the RV myocardium as opposed to delay within the His-Purkinje system.[18] This ECG finding is more often noted in athletes in endurance sports with a striking male predominance.[38]

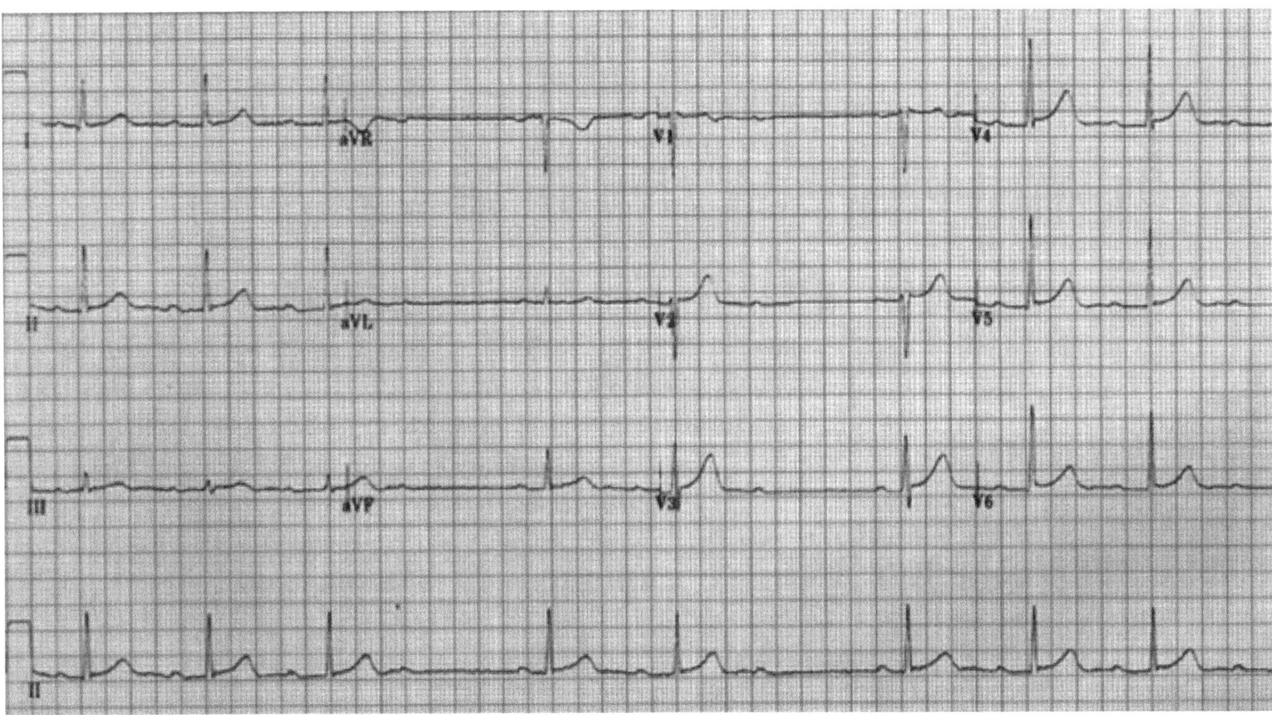

Figure 4.4. Progressive prolongation of the PR interval followed by a nonconducted P wave and subsequent shortening of the PR interval in a 4:3 P wave to QRS ratio demonstrating Mobitz type I (Wenckebach) conduction at the level of the AV node.

In general, an incomplete RBBB in an athlete does not require further evaluation in the absence of symptoms.[38] However, in the presence of fixed splitting of the second heart sound, an ostium secundum atrial septal defect (ASD) should be excluded.[38]

Intraventricular conduction delays > 110 ms, complete bundle branch block (BBB) with a QRS > 120 ms, and hemiblocks are uncommon in athletes and may represent underlying disease.[35] The prevalence of RBBB and left bundle branch block (LBBB) in athletes is similar to the general population and is approximately 0.4%.[3] A study done on football players found that linemen had a longer QRS duration (102 ± 10 ms) when compared to lighter players (96 ± 7 ms). Transthoracic echocardiograms of these athletes showed greater calculated left ventricular (LV) mass and LV end-diastolic diameter in linemen, whether adjusted for body surface area or not. This finding suggests that the type of sport has variable effects on an athlete's heart and QRS duration. Athletes with greater LV mass have slightly longer QRS durations.[7]

Complete RBBB is uncommon in healthy asymptomatic individuals but usually represents an isolated, benign conduction disturbance (Figure 4.5).[1,2,37–39] LBBB, on the other hand, is rare in healthy, asymptomatic individuals and is a predictor of underlying structural heart disease.[1,2,37–39] Even if imaging reveals a structurally normal heart, LBBB may be a marker of future cardiomyopathy. QRS duration of greater than 120 ms is uncommon in healthy individuals, warrants further evaluation, and is considered abnormal.[37–39]

QRS AXIS

The normal QRS axis is rightward at birth and shifts leftward in infancy and childhood. Right axis deviation >120° is common, particularly in younger athletes, with a prevalence reported as high as 20%.[1,2,37–39] Several cohort studies have correlated QRS axis with age and found that athletes <20 years of age had a QRS axis from 0° to 102° and athletes from 20 to 29 years of age had an axis between 10° and 95°.[15] In adults, right axis deviation is uncommon and is usually a result of significant pulmonary disease. Left axis deviation, however, is very common affecting 8% of adults.[15] Generally, asymptomatic athletes with a QRS axis between −30° and 120° do not require further evaluation. Those with mild right axis deviation and pulmonary disease or left axis deviation and systemic hypertension warrant further workup.[37–39]

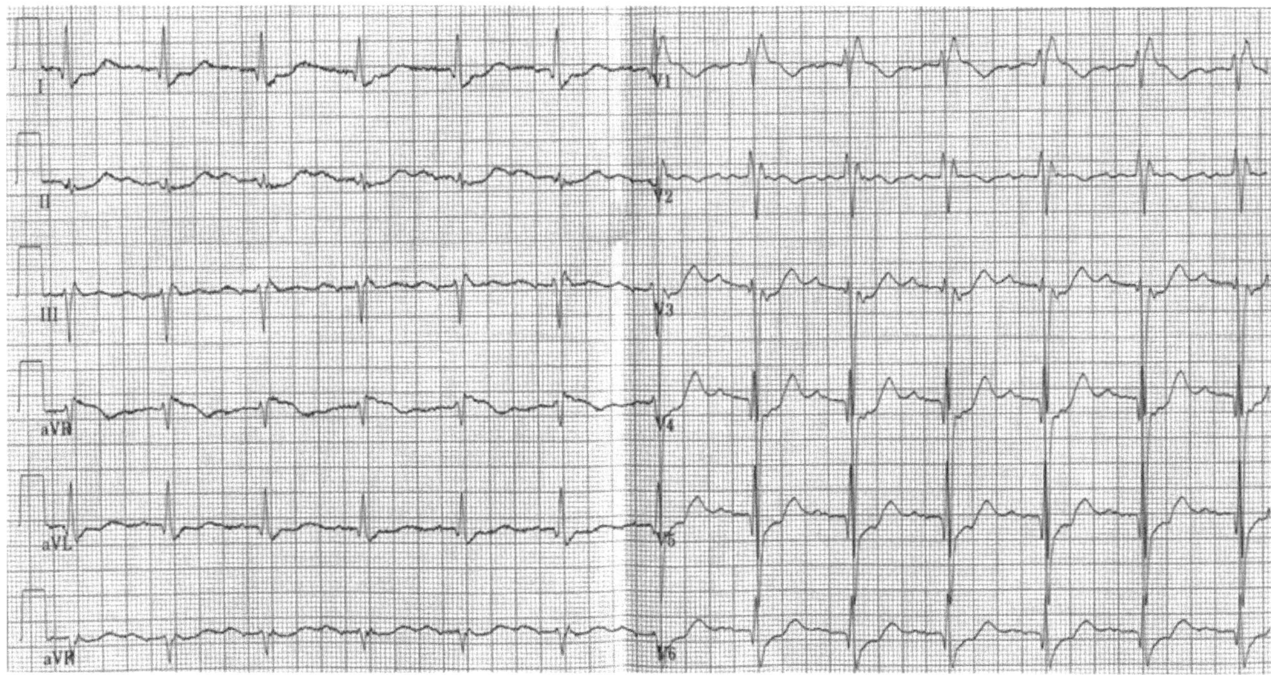

Figure 4.5. Complete RBBB with first-degree AV block in a 53-year-old athlete preparing for a marathon.

Q WAVES

Q waves are seen in ischemic heart disease, infiltrative cardiomyopathies, and HCM, but the pathophysiology underlying their presence in these conditions is different. In HCM, Q waves are likely a result of asymmetrical myocardial hypertrophy with electrical force moving away from the anterior precordial leads. By contrast, in ischemic heart disease, Q waves are a result of depolarization forces directed away from scar.[1,2,37–39] In ischemic heart disease, the World Health Organization's diagnostic criteria for pathologic Q waves are those ≥40 ms in duration with an amplitude of >24% of the R wave in 2 contiguous leads.[65] Ischemic heart disease is rare in individuals younger than 40 years of age, so HCM should be considered if Q waves are present on an ECG of an athlete younger than 40 years. Pathologic Q waves on any ECG are considered to be those that are >3 mm in depth or >40 ms in duration in 2 or more leads except for leads III and aVR.

RIGHT VENTRICULAR HYPERTROPHY (RVH)

The Sokolow–Lyon voltage criteria for RVH (R in V_1 + S in V_5 > 10.5 mm) have been applied to athletes in several studies. Younger athletes are more likely to fulfill the criteria for RVH. Sharma et al reported this finding in a study on young elite athletes, the majority of whom were less than 16 years of age. The prevalence of RVH was 12% in athletes compared to 10% in the control group.[16] Generally, if present, the ECG pattern of RV hypertrophy should not be interpreted as a manifestation of exercise-induced cardiac remodeling.[37–38] When voltage-only criteria are present for RVH in an athlete, it has been noted that this likely represents physiologic hypertrophy.[37] By contrast, further evaluation is warranted when additional findings, such as right atrial enlargement, T-wave inversion in V_2 or V_3 and/or right axis deviation, are present.[37] The presence of either congenital or acquired heart diseases associated with an increased right atrial size and/or pathological RV dilatation/hypertrophy should be excluded with further cardiac imaging.[38]

LEFT VENTRICULAR HYPERTROPHY (LVH)

Intensive athletic training and conditioning are associated with changes in the right and left ventricles, including increased ventricular mass, end diastolic dimensions, and wall thickness.[37–39] These changes are reflected on the surface ECG.[37–39] QRS voltage varies from individual to individual based on age, sex, race, and body habitus. There are a number of voltage criteria to aid in the diagnosis of LVH including the Sokolow–Lyon (S in V_1 + R in V_5 or V_6 ≥ 35 mm or R in aVL ≥ 11 mm) and Cornell criteria (S in V_3 + R in aVL > 28 mm or S in V_3 + R in aVL > 20 mm).

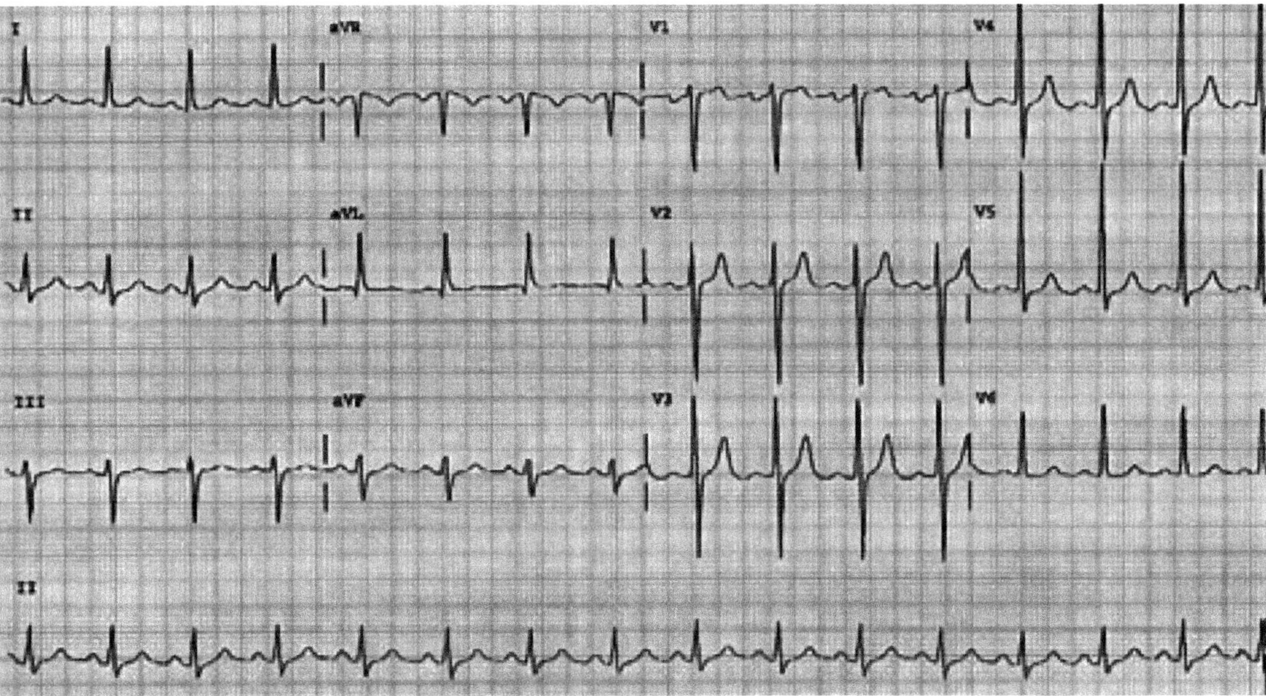

Figure 4.6. Voltage criteria for LVH without secondary changes in an asymptomatic 41-year-old runner.

In general, the commonly used QRS voltage criteria apply to adults older than 35 years. Standards for the 16- to 35-year age group are not as well established, and the diagnosis of LVH based on voltage alone has a low accuracy in this age group.[37–39]

The diagnosis of LVH in highly trained athletes is especially problematic because many athletes meet the standard voltage criteria.[1,2] It is more common in men and seen more frequently in athletes participating in endurance disciplines, such as rowing, cycling, and cross-country skiing (Figure 4.6).[1,2] Black athletes have more prevalent and pronounced ECG changes, and this may be a reflection of more dramatic myocardial changes. Approximately one in five black athletes exhibit LV wall thickness of >12 mm, and 3% of black athletes have LV thickness >15 mm. This is in comparison to white athletes, 4% of whom meet LVH criteria.[37–39] A study done on Stanford football players demonstrated differences in QRS voltage and LV mass index in white players versus black players. Black players had higher QRS vector magnitudes 3.2 ± 0.7 versus 2.7 ± 0.8, and this is likely a reflection of increased LV mass index seen in black players (77 ± 11 g/m^2 versus 71 ± 11g/m^2).[8]

In patients with mild or moderate hypertension, the Sokolow–Lyon criterion has a higher sensitivity and lower specificity in African Americans than in Euro-Americans, whereas the Cornell voltage criterion shows lower sensitivity and higher specificity in African Americans than in Euro-Americans.[37–39] Based on the best available data, the current recommendations regarding athletes who show pure QRS voltage criteria for LV hypertrophy on 12-lead ECG do not require systematic echocardiographic evaluation, unless they have relevant symptoms, a family history of CVDs and/or SCD, or nonvoltage ECG criteria suggesting pathological LV hypertrophy.[38] Therefore, in the absence of other ECG abnormalities such as left atrial enlargement, pathologic Q waves, ST changes, or left axis deviation, fulfilling LVH voltage criteria is considered a nonspecific finding in athletes.

Recent consensus documents stress the potential of the ECG to distinguish between pathological and physiological hypertrophy.[37–39] Based on their experience, they note that the ECG abnormalities of structural heart diseases manifesting with LV hypertrophy, such as cardiomyopathies including HCM, valve diseases, or hypertensive heart disease, overlap only marginally with training-related ECG changes.[37–39] An isolated QRS voltage criterion for LV hypertrophy (Sokolow–Lyon or Cornell criteria) is a very unusual pattern (1.9%) in HCM patients in whom pathological LV hypertrophy is characteristically associated with one or more additional nonvoltage criteria such as left atrial enlargement, left axis deviation, delayed intrinsicoid deflection, ST-segment and T-wave abnormalities, and pathological Q waves.[37–39] Based on this, it is recommended that all athletes with nonvoltage criteria for LV hypertrophy require an echocardiographic evaluation in order to exclude underlying structural heart disease and pathological LV hypertrophy.[37–39]

REPOLARIZATION CHANGES: ST-SEGMENT ELEVATION, ST-SEGMENT DEPRESSION, AND T-WAVE INVERSION

ST-segment elevation in the athlete can be due to benign exercise-related early repolarization or a manifestation of an increased risk of cardiac arrest due to an early repolarization syndrome or Brugada syndrome.[32–36] While it is evident that properly characterizing these repolarization changes is extremely important, the distinction between them can be challenging. Benign early repolarization is characterized by J-point elevation with concave upward ST-segment elevation in 2 contiguous leads with either slurring or notching of the terminal portion of the QRS complex (Figure 4.7).[32–36] The majority of early repolarization patterns are normal variants and benign. Early repolarization with ST-segment elevation in precordial and anterolateral leads is a common finding in athletes, occurring in 45% of white athletes and up to 90% of black athletes.[65,66] Inferior early repolarization is also a common finding seen in approximately 25% of athletes. This finding is more common in black athletes, those with increased QRS voltage and slower heart rates. There is no relationship between early repolarization and underlying structural heart disease. When ST elevation occurs in V_1 to V_2, the ECG needs to be reviewed carefully for the possibility of a Brugada pattern. When early repolarization occurs in conjunction with increased QRS voltage, patients should be followed serially, as this may be a precursor to developing phenotypic HCM, but not eliminated from sport.

Recently, the early repolarization syndrome has been described as a clinical entity distinct from benign early repolarization associated with an increased risk of sudden death.[32–36,65,66] This early repolarization syndrome is characterized by a slurring downstroke of the QRS complex or J waves in 2 contiguous inferior or lateral leads in the absence of ST elevation.[32–36,65,66] Early repolarization in inferior leads characterized by terminal slurring of the QRS or J waves was associated with a 2- to 4-fold increase in idiopathic ventricular tachycardia (VT) and ventricular fibrillation in a study published by Haïssaguerre et al.[66] The ESC's diagnostic criteria recommendations for early repolarization are in line with these findings.[38]

While ST-segment elevation due to benign early repolarization is a common finding in the ECG of trained athletes, ST-segment depression is

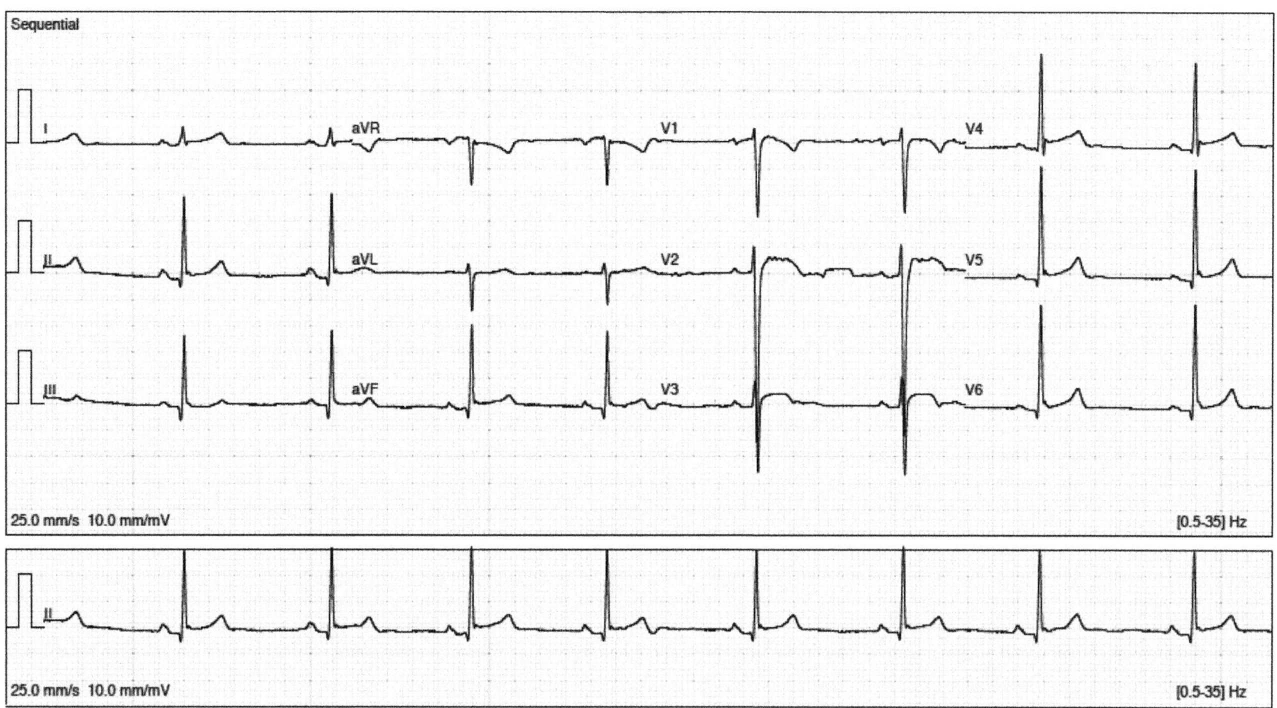

Figure 4.7. Pattern of benign early repolarization in an asymptomatic 22-year-old football player.

uncommon.[37–39] Visually apparent ST-segment depression >0.5 mm below a line isoelectric with the PR interval on resting ECG in any of the lateral leads (I, aVL, V_5, V_6) or one >1 mm in any lead or associated with T-wave inversion should be further evaluated to exclude underlying heart disease.[37–39]

The prevalence of T-wave inversions is similar in athletes and sedentary individuals affecting about 2% to 4% of people.[16,37] T-wave abnormalities are more common in black athletes, particularly in women. In non-black athletes with T-wave inversions >1 mm in leads other than III, aVR, V_1, and V_2, a diagnostic evaluation is necessary to rule out underlying disease. Black female athletes demonstrated a higher prevalence of T-wave inversion compared with matched nonblack athletes (14% vs. 2%).[16] However, because T-wave inversions are also seen in cardiomyopathies, the presence of T-wave inversions ≥ 2 mm in 2 or more adjacent leads in an athlete is considered a potential marker of CVD and merits further evaluation.[37] It is recommended that a secondary evaluation be performed with minor and significant T-wave inversions.

QT ABNORMALITIES

It is well accepted that a QTc >500 ms is associated with a higher risk of sudden cardiac death in males and females; however, applying the traditional criteria of >440 ms in men and in women >460 ms results in a high false-positive rate for true long QT syndrome.[1,2,37–39] Consensus recommendation in both athletes and nonathletes indicate that a QTc interval >500 ms is sufficient for a definitive diagnosis of the long QT syndrome in the absence of drugs or metabolic abnormalities that would prolong the QT interval.[37–39,58] QTc intervals between 440 to 500 ms in men and 460 to 500 ms in women are considered an indeterminate zone that requires further evaluation.[37–39,58] The short QT syndrome is an extremely rare ECG finding, defined as a QTc as <330 ms. Further evaluation is recommended for a QTc interval less than 330 ms.[38]

VALIDATION OF CRITERIA FOR NORMAL VERSUS ABNORMAL ECG CRITERIA IN THE ATHLETE

While the proposed criteria for differentiating normal from abnormal ECGs in athletes provide a useful framework, clinicians with the responsibility of interpreting the ECG should be mindful of the limitations of all proposed classification schemes. The ESC criteria were developed in 2010, when an international group of experts published new recommendations for interpreting ECGs in athletes in the *European Heart Journal*.[38] The authors applied their recommendations to a group of 1005 Olympic-level athletes who were previously studied by Pelliccia et al. Using their new recommendations, they decreased the number of ECGs reported with abnormal findings from 40% to 11%. Uberoi et al applied the ESC recommendations to Stanford college athletes and had similar findings with a reduction in abnormal ECGs warranting further work-up from 10% to 4%.[37] The ESC criteria and the recommendations by Uberoi et al led to a significant increase in specificity with much fewer false positives. These criteria, however, have yet to be tested prospectively.[37]

Recent studies have been noted that the 2010 ESC guidelines for interpreting the ECG have been associated with a relatively high false-positive rate related to atrial abnormalities.[67] A prospective evaluation of the criteria for abnormal atrial enlargement or axis deviation in isolation as proposed by the ESC was found to be 13% among 2533 athletes. Echocardiographic evaluation of these athletes failed to show any major structural or functional abnormalities.[67] Exclusion of atrial enlargement or axis deviation reduced the false-positive rate from 13% to 7.5% and improved specificity from 90% to 94% with a minimum reduction in sensitivity (91%–89.5%). It is evident that the European and other proposed criteria for ECG interpretation merit further validation and refinement.[67]

Insights into some of the diagnostic challenges in distinguishing normal from abnormal ECG and secondary tests are gained from another recent investigation.[68] Comparison of the ECGs and RV echocardiographic data of 300 consecutive black athletes with data from 375 white athletes and 153 control subjects was performed.[68,69] The control group consisted of a similar proportion of blacks who were not athletes.[68,69] Anterior T-wave inversion (leads V_1–V_4) was more common in black athletes (14.3%; P = 0.001) compared with either White athletes or control subjects of either race.[68,69] Both black and white athletes had greater RV dimensions compared with control subjects of the same ethnicity, including RV outflow tract dimensions.[68,69] Compared with white athletes, black athletes had significantly lower values for all the 3 measures of RV outflow tract dimensions and RV longitudinal dimensions.[68,69] On echocardiogram, 4 white and 4 black athletes had RV apical wall motion abnormalities on the apical 4-chamber view.[68,69] The combination of T-wave inversion in V_1 through V_3 and RV dilation meeting the modified ARVC diagnostic criteria occurred in 3% of black athletes and only 0.3% of white athletes.[68,69] To meet the revised criteria for a diagnosis of ARVC, RV wall motion abnormalities need to accompany dilatation.[70]

Only 2 of the 4 black athletes with RV wall motion abnormalities on echocardiogram had the combination of all 3 findings (wall motion abnormalities, RV dilatation, and T-wave inversion).[68] Cardiac MRI of those athletes revealed normal RV wall motion, thereby excluding the diagnosis of ARVC. The authors conclude that highly trained athletes, regardless of ethnicity, exhibit RV enlargement, but because of the higher incidence of T-wave inversion in V_1 through V_3 in black athletes, the potential for erroneous diagnosis of ARVC exists.[68,69] The Multiethnic Study of Atherosclerosis-Right Ventricle (MESA-RV) evaluated 4062 noncardiac patients with cardiac MRI and manually contoured the RV margins in diastole and systole. The authors applied the RVH ECG criteria from the 2009 American Heart Association recommendations for standardization and interpretation of the ECG to their patient population. Of these, 6% had MRI findings consistent with mild RVH. They found the criteria to be specific (>95%), but had a low sensitivity and low positive predictive value (12%).[70]

These and multiple other studies have demonstrated a high prevalence of ECG abnormalities, in particular voltage criteria for LVH, when applying the ESC sports cardiology consensus criteria to young, nonathletic individuals.[71–82] Many of these abnormalities are nonspecific in isolation and may warrant further investigations to exclude quiescent cardiac disease.[71–82] Such a high burden of ECG abnormalities has significant implications on the feasibility and cost-effectiveness of a national cardiovascular screening program in young individuals and questions the suitability of such guidelines in the nonathletic population.[71–83]

ECG MARKERS CARDIOVASCULAR CONDITIONS PREDISPOSING TO SUDDEN CARDIAC DEATH

The cardiovascular conditions that predispose athletes to the risk of sudden death and the abnormalities, which may manifest on their ECGs, are well characterized.[56,58–63,65,83–85] These include HCM, arrhythmogenic RV dysplasia, long QT syndrome, short QT syndrome, and catecholaminergic polymorphic VT.[56,58–63,65,71,72] Brugada syndrome can also be diagnosed on the standard ECG, but there is no recommendation for restricting patients with this condition from athletic activities (Table 4.3).[73] Anomalous origin of a coronary artery also is a cause of sudden death in athletes.[56,58–63,65,71,72] However, this condition does not manifest with any abnormalities on the surface ECG. The diagnostic criteria for these conditions, ECG changes, recommendations for athletic restriction, and disease management are reviewed in detail in many recent consensus documents, reviews, manuscripts, and multiple chapters in this book (Table 4.4).[56,58–63,65,83–85]

Table 4.3. **Cardiovascular conditions predisposing to sudden cardiac death in the athlete and ECG abnormalities.**

HCM Voltage criteria for LVH, septal Q waves, secondary repolarization changes including ST segment depression and T-wave inversion.
Arrhythmogenic RV dysplasia Major: Repolarization abnormalities: Inverted T waves in right precordial leads (V_1, V_2, and V_3) or beyond in individuals >14 years of age (in the absence of complete right bundle-branch block QRS >120 ms): Epsilon wave (reproducible low-amplitude signals between end of QRS complex to onset of the T wave) in the right precordial leads (V_1–V_3). Minor: Inverted T waves in leads V_1 and V_2 in individuals >14 years of age (in the absence of complete right bundle-branch block) or in V_4, V_5, or V_6 inverted T waves in leads V_1, V_2, V_3, and V_4 in individuals >14 years of age in the presence of complete right bundle-branch block.
Brugada syndrome Presence of Type 1 pattern with coved ST segment in V_1 and V_2 gradually descending into the T wave. High take-off and downsloping ST segment elevation followed by a negative T wave in ≥2 leads in V_1–V_3.
Long Q-T syndrome QTc > 470 ms in males, > 480 ms in females.
Short QT syndrome QTc < 340 ms.
Arrhythmogenic RV dysplasia T-wave inversions in V_1 to V_3, Epsilon waves.
Ventricular Preexcitation Delta wave and PR < 120 ms.

Table 4.4. **Recommendations for interpretation of the ECG in athletes.**

ECG Abnormality	Criteria for further evaluation	Example
Q waves	>3 mm in depth or >40 ms duration in any lead except III, aVR, aVL and V_1.	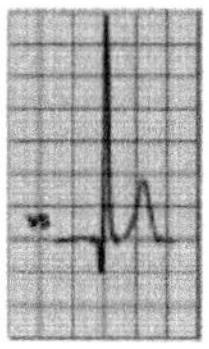
ST depression	>0.5 mm below PR isoelectric line between J-junction and beginning of T waves in V_4, V_5, V_6, I, aVL. >1 mm in any lead.	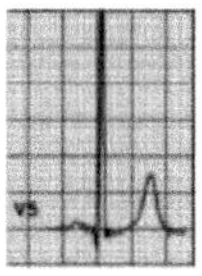
T-wave inversion	>1 mm in leads other than III, aVR and V_1 (except V_2 and V_3 in women <25 years).	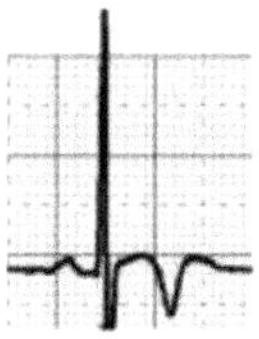
Atrial abnormalities	Right: P wave amplitude >2.5 mm Left: 1) Negative portion of P wave in V_1, V_2 of >40 ms duration and 1 mm in depth; or 2) total P wave duration >120 ms	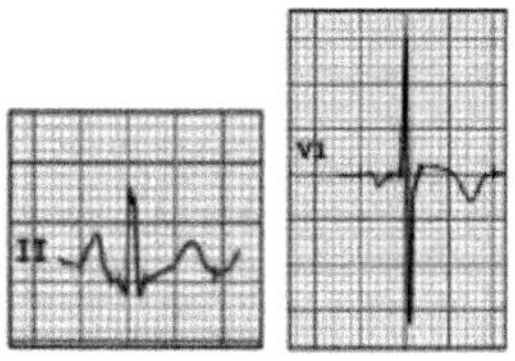
Right ventricular hypertrophy	>30 years: 1) R wave >7 mm in V_1; or 2) R/S ratio >1 in V_1; or 3) sum of R wave in V_1 and S wave in V_5 or V_6 >10.5 mm <30 years: above plus right atrial enlargement, T-wave inversion in V_2, V_3, or right axis deviation >115°	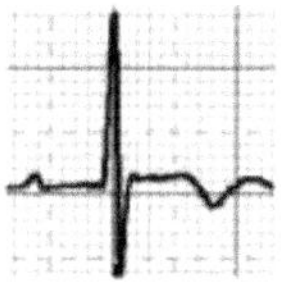
LBBB RBBB IVCD	Any QRS >120 ms	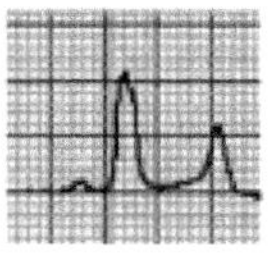
QRS axis deviation	More leftward than −30° More rightward than 115°	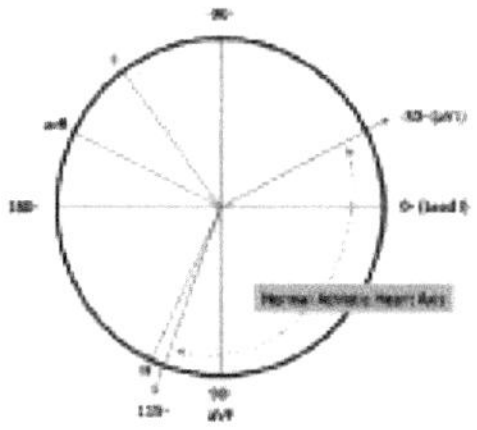

RAA, right atrial abnormality; LAA, left atrial abnormality; RVH, right ventricular hypertrophy; RAD, right axis deviation; RBBB, right bundle branch block; TWI, T-wave inversion; and QTc, heart-rate correction of the QT interval. (Modified with permission.[38])

CONCLUSION

Considerable progress has been made in defining the ECG changes that commonly occur in the athlete based on physiologic adaptations to exercise. Nonetheless, distinguishing physiologic ECG changes in the athlete from findings that may represent underlying CVD predisposing to sudden cardiac death remains a clinical challenge. Recent publications of consensus recommendations related to interpretation of the athlete's ECG have considerably advanced the field. However, inconsistencies in the definition of ECG abnormalities remain. Prospective evaluation of the proposed criteria to establish their validity in a heterogenous population of athletes has not yet been performed. Despite the limitations of the ECG criteria and the absence of validation, the recommendations represent the best available guidance for clinicians interpreting the ECGs of athletes. It is evident that while considerable progress has been made allowing clinicians to differentiate physiologic changes in the athlete's ECG from pathologic, many fundamental gaps in knowledge remain.

REFERENCES

1. Foote C, Michaud G. The athlete's electrocardiogram: Distinguishing normal from abnormal. In: Estes NAM III, Salem D, Wang PJ, eds. *Sudden Cardiac Death in the Athlete.* New York, NY: Futura; 1998:101–115.
2. Estes NAM, Link MS, Homoud MH, Wang PJ. Electrocardiographic variants and cardiac rhythm disturbances in the athlete. In: Thompson PD, ed. *Exercise and Sports Cardiology.* New York, NY: McGraw Hill; 2001:211–232.
3. Pelliccia A, Maron BJ, Culasso F, et al. Clinical significance of abnormal electrocardiographic patterns in trained athletes. *Circulation.* 2000;102:278–284.
4. Pelliccia A, Culasso F, Di Paolo FM, et al. Prevalence of abnormal electrocardiograms in a large, unselected population undergoing pre-participation cardiovascular screening. *Eur Heart J.* 2007;28(16):2006–2010.
5. Venerando A, Rully V. Frequency, morphology and meaning of the electrocardiographic anomalies found in Olympic marathon runners. *Sports Med Phys Fitness.* 1964;50:135–141.
6. Hanne-Paparo N, Drory Y, Schoenfeld Y, Shapira Y, Kellermann JJ. Common ECG changes in athletes. *Cardiology.* 1976;61(4):267–278.
7. Uberoi A, Sadik J, Lipinski MJ, Van Le V, Froelicher V. Association between cardiac dimensions and athlete lineup position: Analysis using echocardiography in NCAA football team players. *Phys Sportsmed.* 2013;41(3):58–66.
8. Haddad F, Peter S, Hulme O, et al. Race differences in ventricular remodeling and function among college football players. *Am J Cardiol.* 2013;112(1):128–134.
9. Talan DA, Bauernfeind RA, Ashley WW, Kanakis C Jr, Rosen KM. Twenty-four hour continuous ECG recordings in long-distance runners. *Chest.* 1982;82:19–24.
10. Boraita A, Serratosa L. "El corazón del deportista": hallazgos electrocardiográficos más frecuentes. *Rev Esp Cardiol.* 1998;51:356–368.
11. Tintoré S. Electrocardiografía del deportista. In: Bayés de Luna A, Furlanello F, Maron BJ, Serra Grima JR, eds. *Cardiología Deportiva.* Barcelona: Mosby/Doyma Libros; 1994:42-61.
12. Zehender M, Meinertz T, Keul J, Just H. ECG variants and cardiac arrhythmias in athletes: Clinical and prognostic importance. *Am Heart J.* 1990;119:1378–1391.
13. Sharma S. Athlete's heart—effect of age, sex, ethnicity and sporting discipline. *Exp Physiol.* 2003;88:665–669.
14. Stein R, Medeiros CM, Rosito GA, et al. Intrinsic sinus and atrioventricular node electrophysiologic adaptations in endurance athletes. *J Am Coll Cardiol.* 2002;39:1033–1038.
15. Mason JW, Ramseth DJ, Chanter DO, et al. Electrocardiographic reference ranges derived from 79,743 ambulatory subjects. *J Electrocardiol.* 2007;40:228–234.
16. Sharma S, Whyte G, Elliott P, et al. Electrocardiographic changes in 1000 highly trained junior elite athletes. *Br J Sports Med.* 1999;33:319–324.
17. Di Paolo FM, Schmied C, Zerguini YA, et al. The athlete's heart in adolescent Africans: an electrocardiographic and echocardiographic study. *J Am Coll Cardiol.* 2012;59:1029–1036.
18. Langdeau JB, Blier L, Turcotte H, et al. Electrocardiographic findings in athletes: the prevalence of left ventricular hypertrophy and conduction defects. *Can J Cardiol.* 2001;17:655–659.
19. Douglas P, O'Toole M, Hiller D, Hackney K, Reichek N. Electrocardiographic diagnosis of exercise-induced left ventricular hypertrophy. *Am Heart J.* 1988;116:784.
20. Bjornstad H, Smith G, Storstein L, Meen H, Hals O. Electrocardiographic and echocardiographic findings in top athletes, athletic students and sedentary controls. *Cardiology.* 1993;82:66–74.
21. Wu J, Stork TL, Perron AD, Brady WJ. The athlete's electrocardiogram. *Am J Emerg Med.* 2006;24:77–86.
22. Serra-Grima R, Estorch M, Carrio I, et al. Marked ventricular repolarization abnormalities in highly trained athletes electrocardiograms: clinical and prognostic implications. *J Am Coll Cardiol.* 2000;36:1310–1316.
23. Kasikcioglu E. QT dispersion: Is it a screening parameter for athletes who have high cardiovascular risk? *Ann Noninvasive Electrocardiol.* 2005;10:391.
24. Lonati LM, Magnaghi G, Bizzi C, Leonetti G. Patterns of QT dispersion in athletic and hypertensive left ventricular hypertrophy. *Ann. Noninvasive Electrocardiol.* 2004;9:252–256.
25. Nakamato K. Electrocardiograms of 25 marathon runners before and after 100 meter dash. *Jpn Circ J.* 1969;33:105–126.
26. Klemola E. Electrocariographic observations on 650 Finnish athletes. *Ann Med Finn.* 1951;40:121–132.
27. Myetes I, Kaplinsky E, Yahini J, Hanne-Paparo N, Neufeld HN. Wenckenbach AV block: A frequent feature following heavy physical training. *Am Heart J.* 1975;990:426–430.
28. Van Ganse W, Versee L, Eylenbosch W, Vuylsteek K. The electrocardiogram of athletes. Comparison with untrained subjects. *Br Heart J.* 1970;32(2):160–164.
29. Balady GJ, Cadigan JB, Ryan TJ. Electrocardiogram of the athlete: an analysis of 289 professional football players. *Am J Cardiol.* 1984;53(9):1339–1343.
30. Northcote RJ, Canning GP, Ballantyne D. Electrocardiographic findings in male veteran endurance athletes. *Br Heart J.* 1989;61(2):155–160.
31. Ikäheimo MJ, Palatsi IJ, Takkunen JT. Noninvasive evaluation of the athletic heart: Sprinters versus endurance runners. *Am J Cardiol.* 1979;44(1):24–30.

32. Gibbons LW, Cooper KH, Martin RP, Pollock ML. Medical examination and electrocardiographic analysis of elite distance runners. *Ann NY Acad Sci.* 1977;301:283–296.
33. Kligfield P, Gettes LS, Bailey JJ, et al. Recommendations for the standardization and interpretation of the electrocardiogram: part I: The electrocardiogram and its technology: A scientific statement from the American Heart Association Electrocardiography and Arrhythmias Committee, Council on Clinical Cardiology; the American College of Cardiology Foundation; and the Heart Rhythm Society. Endorsed by the International Society for Computerized Electrocardiology. *J Am Coll Cardiol.* 2007;49:1109–1127.
34. Wagner GS, Macfarlane P, Wellens H, et al. AHA/ACCF/HRS recommendations for the standardization and interpretation of the electrocardiogram: part VI: Acute ischemia/infarction: a scientific statement from the American Heart Association Electrocardiography and Arrhythmias Committee, Council on Clinical Cardiology; the American College of Cardiology Foundation; and the Heart Rhythm Society. Endorsed by the International Society for Computerized Electrocardiology. *J Am Coll Cardiol.* 2009;53:1003–1011.
35. Hancock EW, Deal BJ, Mirvis DM, et al. AHA/ACCF/HRS recommendations for the standardization and interpretation of the electrocardiogram: part V: electrocardiogram changes associated with cardiac chamber hypertrophy: a scientific statement from the American Heart Association Electrocardiography and Arrhythmias Committee, Council on Clinical Cardiology; the American College of Cardiology Foundation; and the Heart Rhythm Society. Endorsed by the International Society for Computerized Electrocardiology. *J Am Coll Cardiol.* 2009;53:992–1002.
36. Surawicz B, Childers R, Deal BJ, et al. AHA/ACCF/HRS recommendations for the standardization and interpretation of the electrocardiogram: part III: intraventricular conduction disturbances: A scientific statement from the American Heart Association electrocardiography and arrhythmias committee, council on clinical cardiology; the American College of Cardiology Foundation; and the Heart Rhythm Society. Endorsed by the International Society for Computerized Electrocardiology. *J Am Coll Cardiol.* 2009;53:976–981.
37. Rautaharju PM, Surawicz B, Gettes LS, et al. AHA/ACCF/HRS recommendations for the standardization and interpretation of the electrocardiogram: part IV: The ST segment, T and U waves, and the QT interval: A scientific statement from the American Heart Association Electrocardiography and Arrhythmias Committee, Council on Clinical Cardiology; the American College of Cardiology Foundation; and the Heart Rhythm Society: Endorsed by the International Society for Computerized Electrocardiology. *Circulation.* 2009;119:e241–e250.
38. Uberoi A, Stein R, Perez MV, et al. Interpretation of the electrocardiogram of young athletes. *Circulation.* 2011;124:746–757.
39. Corrado D, Pelliccia A, Heidbuchel H, et al. Recommendations for interpretation of 12-lead electrocardiogram in the athlete. *Eur Heart J.* 2010;31(2):243–259.
40. Drezner JA, Ackerman MJ, Anderson J, et al. Electrocardiographic interpretation in athletes: The 'Seattle Criteria'. *Br J Sports Med.* 2013;47:122–124.
41. Drezner JA, Asif IM, Owens DS, et al. Accuracy of ECG interpretation in competitive athletes: The impact of using standised ECG criteria. *Br J Sports Med.* 2012;46:335–340.
42. Drezner JA, Ashley E, Baggish AL, et al. Abnormal electrocardiographic findings in athletes: recognizing changes suggestive of cardiomyopathy. *Br J Sports Med.* 2013;47:137-52.
43. Pelliccia A, Fagard R, Bjornstad HH, et al. Recommendations for competitive sports participation in athletes with cardiovascular disease: a consensus document from the Study Group of Sports Cardiology of the Working Group of Cardiac Rehabilitation and Exercise Physiology and the Working Group of Myocardial and Pericardial Diseases of the European Society of Cardiology. *Eur Heart J.* 2005;26:1422–1445.
44. Corrado D, Basso C, Schiavon M, Thiene G. Screening for hypertrophic cardiomyopathy in young athletes. *N Engl J Med.* 1998;339:364–369.
45. Corrado D, Pelliccia A, Bjørnstad HH, et al. Cardiovascular pre-participation screening of young competitive athletes for prevention of sudden death: proposal for a common European protocol. Consensus statement of the study group of sport cardiology of the working group of cardiac rehabilitation and exercise physiology and the working group of myocardial and pericardial diseases of the European Society of Cardiology. *Eur Heart J.* 2005;26:516–524.
46. Marek JC. Electrocardiography and preparticipation screening of competitive high school athletes. *Ann Intern Med.* 2010;153:131–132.
47. Weiner RB, Hutter AM, Wang F, et al. Performance of the 2010 European Society of Cardiology criteria for ECG interpretation in athletes. *Heart.* 2011;97:1573–1577.
48. Drezner JA. ECG screening in athletes: Time to develop infrastructure. *Heart Rhythm.* 2011;8:1560–1561.
49. Steinvil A, Chundadze T, Zeltser D, et al. Mandatory electrocardiographic screening of athletes to reduce their risk for sudden death proven fact or wishful thinking? *J Am Coll Cardiol.* 2011;57:1291–1296.
50. Corrado D, Basso C, Schiavon M, Pelliccia A, Thiene G. Pre-participation screening of young competitive athletes for prevention of sudden cardiac death. *J Am Coll Cardiol.* 2008;52:1981–1989.
51. Asif IM, Drezner JA. Sudden cardiac death and preparticipation screening: The debate continues in support of electrocardiogram-inclusive preparticipation screening. *Prog Cardiovasc Dis.* 2012;54:445–450.
52. Corrado D, Migliore F, Zorzi A, et al. Preparticipation electrocardiographic screening for the prevention of sudden death in sports medicine. *G Ital Cardiol.* 2011;12:697–706.
53. Maron BJ, Thompson PD, Ackerman MJ, et al. Recommendations and considerations related

to preparticipation screening for cardiovascular abnormalities in competitive athletes: 2007 update: A scientific statement from the American Heart Association Council on Nutrition, Physical Activity, and Metabolism: Endorsed by the American College of Cardiology Foundation. *Circulation.* 2007;115:1643–1455.

54. Estes NAM III, Link MS. Preparticipation athletic screening including an electrocardiogram: An unproven strategy for prevention of sudden cardiac death in the athlete. *Prog Cardiovasc Dis.* 2012;54:451–454.
55. Corrado D, Basso C, Schiavon M, Thiene G. Screening for hypertrophic cardiomyopathy in young athletes. *N Engl J Med.* 1998;339:364–369.
56. Link MS, Estes NAM. Sudden cardiac death in the athlete: bridging the gaps between evidence, policy, and practice. *Circulation.* 2012;125:2511–2516.
57. Maron BJ, Haas, TS, Doerer JJ, Thompson PD, Hodges JS. Comparison of U.S. and Italian experiences with sudden cardiac deaths in young competitive athletes and implications for preparticipation screening strategies. *Am J Cardiol.* 2009;104:276–280.
58. Dougherty KR, Friedman RA, Link MS, Estes NAM III. Prediction and prevention of sudden death in young populations: the role of ECG screening. *J Interv Card Electrophysiol.* 2013;36(2):167–175.
59. Priori SG, Wilde AA, Horie M, et al. HRS/EHRA/APHRS expert consensus statement on the diagnosis and management of patients with inherited primary arrhythmia syndromes: document endorsed by HRS, EHRA, and APHRS in May 2013 and by ACCF, AHA, PACES, and AEPC. *Heart Rhythm.* 2013;10(12):1932–1963.
60. Walsh E, Abrams DJ. Electrocardiographic markers of arrhythmic risk and sudden cardiac death in pediatric and adolescent populations. In: Shenasa M, Josephson MD, Estes NAM III, eds. *The Electrocardiogram: Contemporary Challenges.* Minneapolis, MN: Cardiotext Publishing; 2015.
61. Shenasa M, Shenasa H. Electrocardiographic markers of sudden death in different substrates. In: Shenasa, M, Josephson MD, Estes NAM III, eds. *The Electrocardiogram: Contemporary Challenges.* Minneapolis, MN: Cardiotext Publishing; 2015.
62. Richter S, Brugada J, Brugada R, Brugada P. Electrocardiographic markers of arrhythmic events and sudden death in channelopathies. In: Shenasa M, Josephson MD, Estes NAM III, eds. *The Electrocardiogram: Contemporary Challenges.* Minneapolis, MN: Cardiotext Publishing; 2015.
63. Hocini M, Shah AJ, Jaïs P, Haïssaguerre M. Diagnostic electrocardiographic criteria for early repolarization and idiopathic ventricular fibrillation. In: Shenasa M, Josephson MD, Estes NAM III, eds. *The Electrocardiogram: Contemporary Challenges.* Minneapolis, MN: Cardiotext Publishing; 2015.
64. Probst V, Le Marec H. Electrocardiographic markers of progressive cardiac conduction disease. In: Shenasa M, Josephson MD, Estes NAM III, eds. *The Electrocardiogram: Contemporary Challenges.* Minneapolis, MN: Cardiotext Publishing; 2015.
65. Ammar KA, Kors JA, Yawn BP, Rodeheffer RJ. Defining unrecognized myocardial infarction: a call for standardized electrocardiographic diagnostic criteria. *Am Heart J.* 2004;148:277–284.
66. Cappato R, Furlanello F, Giovinazzo V, et al. J wave, QRS slurring, and ST elevation in athletes with cardiac arrest in the absence of heart disease: marker of risk or innocent bystander? *Circ Arrhythm Electrophysiol.* 2010;3:305–311.
67. Haïssaguerre M, Derval N, Sacher F, et al. Sudden cardiac arrest associated with early repolarization. *N Engl J Med.* 2008;358:2016–2023.
68. Gati S, Sheikh N, Ghani S, et al. Should axis deviation or atrial enlargement be categorized as abnormal in young athletes? The athlete's electrocardiogram: A time for re-appraisal of markers of pathology. *Eur Heart J.* 2013;34:3641–3648.
69. Zaidi A, Ghani S, Sharma R, et al. Physiological right ventricular adaptation in elite athletes of African and Afro-Caribbean origin *Circulation.* 2013;127(17):1783–1792.
70. Weinstock J, Estes NAM III. The heart of an athlete: black, white, and shades of grey with no gold standard. *Circulation.* 2013;127(17):1757–1759.
71. Whitman I, Patel V, Soliman E, et al. Validity of the surface electrocardiogram criteria for right ventricular hypertrophy: The MESA-RV study (multi-ethnic study of atherosclerosis-right ventricle). *J Am Coll Cardiol.* 2014;63(7):672–681.
72. Chandra N, Papadakis M, Duschl J, et al. Comparing the prevalence of ECG abnormalities between young athletes and non-athletes: the implications for a nationwide screening program. *Circulation.* 2010;A16692.
73. Zaidi A, Ghani S, Sheikh N, et al. Clinical significance of electrocardiographic right ventricular hypertrophy in athletes: Comparison with arrhythmogenic right ventricular cardiomyopathy and pulmonary hypertension. *Eur Heart J.* 2013;34(47):3649–3656.
74. Papadakis M, Sharma S. Sudden cardiac death in young athletes: Practical challenges and diagnostic dilemmas. *J Am Coll Cardiol.* 2013;61(10):1027–1040.
75. Gati S, Chandra N, Bennett RL, et al. Increased left ventricular trabeculation in highly trained athletes: do we need more stringent criteria for the diagnosis of left ventricular non-compaction in athletes? *Heart.* 2013;99(6):401–408.
76. Sheikh N, Papadakis M, Carre F, et al. Cardiac adaptation to exercise in adolescent athletes of African ethnicity: an emergent elite athletic population. *Br J Sports Med.* 2013;47(9):585–592.
77. Bastiaenen R, Raju H, Sharma S, et al. Characterization of early repolarization during ajmaline provocation and exercise tolerance testing. *Heart Rhythm.* 2013;10(2):247–254.
78. Papadakis M, Wilson MG, Ghani S, et al. Impact of ethnicity upon cardiovascular adaptation in competitive athletes: relevance to preparticipation screening. *Br J Sports Med.* 2012;46(suppl 1):i22–i28.

79. Chandra N, Papadakis M, Sharma S. Cardiac adaptation in athletes of black ethnicity: differentiating pathology from physiology. *Heart.* 2012;98(16):1194–1200.
80. Sharma S, Ghani S, Papadakis M. ESC criteria for ECG interpretation in athletes: better but not perfect. *Heart.* 2011;97(19):1540–1541.
81. Raju H, Papadakis M, Govindan M, et al. Low prevalence of risk markers in cases of sudden death due to Brugada syndrome relevance to risk stratification in Brugada syndrome. *J Am Coll Cardiol.* 2011;57(23):2340–2345.
82. Papadakis M, Carre F, Kervio G, et al. The prevalence, distribution, and clinical outcomes of electrocardiographic repolarization patterns in male athletes of African/Afro-Caribbean origin. *Eur Heart J.* 2011;32(18):2304–2313.
83. Rawlins J, Carre F, Kervio G, et al. Ethnic differences in physiological cardiac adaptation to intense physical exercise in highly trained female athletes. *Circulation.* 2010;121(9):1078–1085.
84. Marcus FI, McKenna WJ, Sherrill D, et al. Diagnosis of arrhythmogenic right ventricular cardiomyopathy/dysplasia: proposed modification of the task force criteria. *Circulation.* 2010;121:1533–1541.
85. Gersh BJ, Maron BJ, Bonow RO, et al. American College of Cardiology Foundation/American Heart Association Task Force on Practice Guidelines; 2011 ACCF/AHA guideline for the diagnosis and treatment of hypertrophic cardiomyopathy: executive summary: A report of the American College of Cardiology Foundation/American Heart Association Task Force on Practice Guidelines. *Circulation.* 2011;124(24):2761–2796.
86. Zipes DP, Ackerman MJ, Estes NAM 3rd, et al. Task Force 7: Bethesda 36th recommendations for evaluation and management of cardiovascular disease in the arrhythmias. *J Am Coll Cardiol.* 2005;45(8):1354–1363.

CHAPTER

5

Electrocardiographic Markers of Arrhythmic Risk and Sudden Cardiac Death in Pediatric and Adolescent Patients

Edward P. Walsh, MD and Dominic J. Abrams, MD

INTRODUCTION

This chapter will review aspects of the ECG that are most relevant to the identification of serious arrhythmias in young patients. Readers will certainly be aware that the ECG is imperfect as a stand-alone tool for this purpose owing to normal variants, false-negatives, maturational changes, and the confusing patterns that can accompany congenital heart defects (CHDs) in children and adolescents. Electrocardiography can only be viewed as one part of the diagnostic exercise that includes patient history, physical examination, family history, and supportive tests.[1] But, despite its limitations, the ECG remains the quickest, safest, and least expensive diagnostic technique at our disposal. With proper interpretation, it is often capable of providing potentially life-saving information.[2,3]

NORMAL ECG VARIANTS IN YOUNG PATIENTS

Accurate analysis of the ECG for children and adolescents first requires an understanding of certain age-specific patterns that can differ from normal adult tracings.

Changes in Right-Precordial T-wave Pattern with Age

The normal right-precordial T-wave pattern in young patients changes with age.[4] Normal newborns tend to register an upright T wave over the right chest immediately after birth, which then switches to a negative T-wave after the first week of life. Throughout the remaining childhood, the normal T-wave remains negative in leads V_1, V_2, and sometimes as far out as V_3 (Figure 5.1). Transition to a mature precordial T-wave pattern begins during adolescence, sometime between ages 12 and 18 years. Knowledge of this evolving T-wave pattern in youngsters becomes important during evaluation for familial disorders such as arrhythmogenic right ventricular cardiomyopathy.

Difficulties with QTc Measurements in Newborns

The QT interval is notoriously difficult to interpret in the first few days after birth. Mild to moderate prolongation (QTc up to 480 ms when corrected by Bazzet's formula) can be seen as a transient phenomenon in many normal newborns, likely due to some

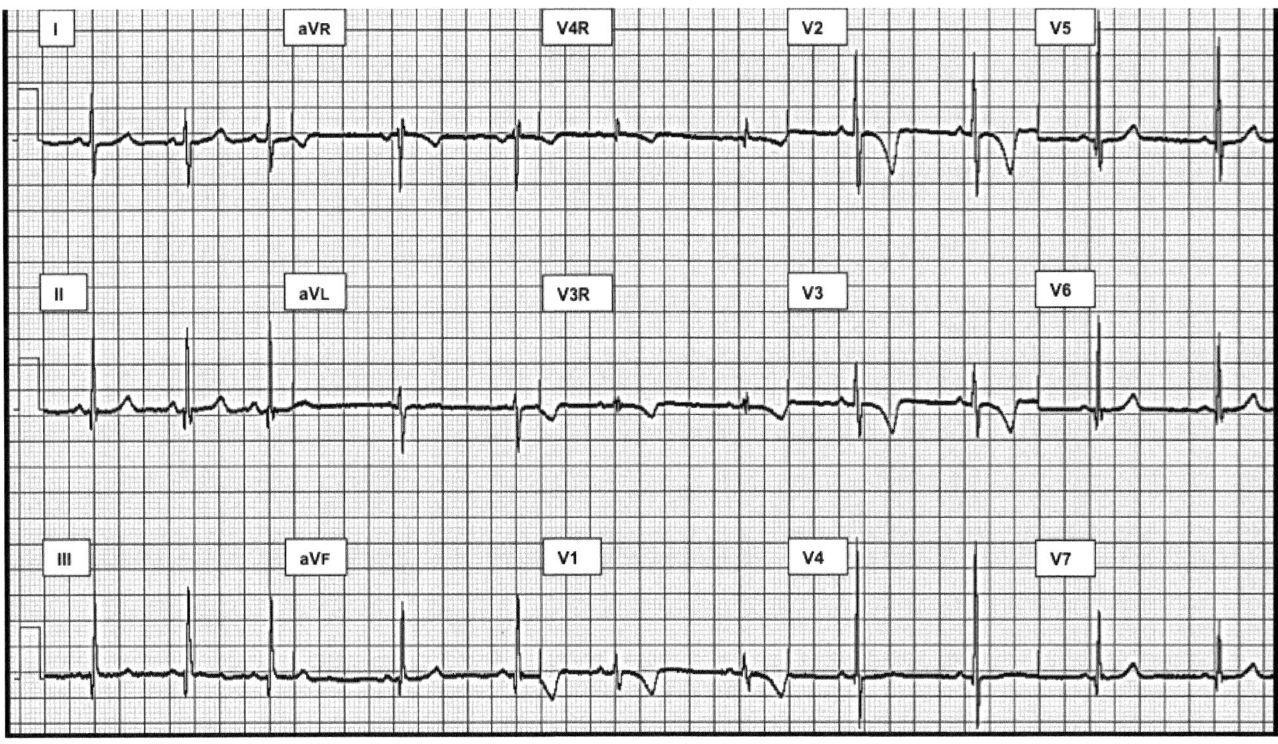

Figure 5.1. Normal variant in the precordial T-wave pattern seen in a 9-year-old with a structurally and functionally normal heart. The T wave can be negative in leads V_1 and V_2 (sometimes out as far as V_3 as in this case). The T wave will assume the normal "mature" pattern during adolescence.

combination of fluctuating calcium/magnesium levels and the changes in autonomic tone that accompany adaptation to extrauterine life. By the age of 7 days, the QTc stabilizes and can be interpreted by the same criteria used for adults. Inaccuracy of newborn QTc data is important to bear in mind when evaluating offspring in the setting of a positive family history of long QT syndrome. It is generally recommended that phenotypic evaluation by ECG be delayed until age > 7 days.[5]

Interpreting RSR′ Pattern in V_1

An RSR′ pattern in lead V_1 is a common normal variant on a pediatric ECG, and should not be confused with a true right-ventricular conduction disturbance. The benign RSR′ pattern has a normal QRS duration with a high frequency R′ deflection, an amplitude for the R′ component that is similar to the initial R wave, and an isoelectric ST segment. A RSR′ pattern with a very tall R′ component can be seen in patients with an atrial septal defect (ASD). In young patients with proven conditions, such as Brugada's syndrome and right-ventricular cardiomyopathy, the R′ component tends to have a noticeably lower slew rate than the initial R wave, consistent with actual conduction delay (Figure 5.2).

Normal Precordial Voltages According to Age

Diagnosing ventricular hypertrophy based on voltage criteria can be difficult at any age, but is particularly challenging in children. The normal ranges for precordial QRS amplitudes vary widely, and it is not uncommon to encounter healthy pediatric patients with R-wave voltages in V_5 and V_6 that far exceed the upper limit of normal for an adult. It is important that tables of age-adjusted normal voltages be consulted when interpreting the ECG in children and adolescents for hypertrophic conditions.[6]

The 15-lead ECG Format Used in Young Patients

Many of the ECGs displayed in this chapter use a 15-lead format that has become customary for pediatric recordings. This modification adds 2 precordial leads over the right chest (V_4R and V_3R) along with a far leftward chest lead (V_7). The primary purpose of the expanded lead system is to assist in recognition of dextrocardia and other complex malpositions. However, for purposes of rhythmic analysis, a standard 12-lead recording is entirely satisfactory across all age groups.

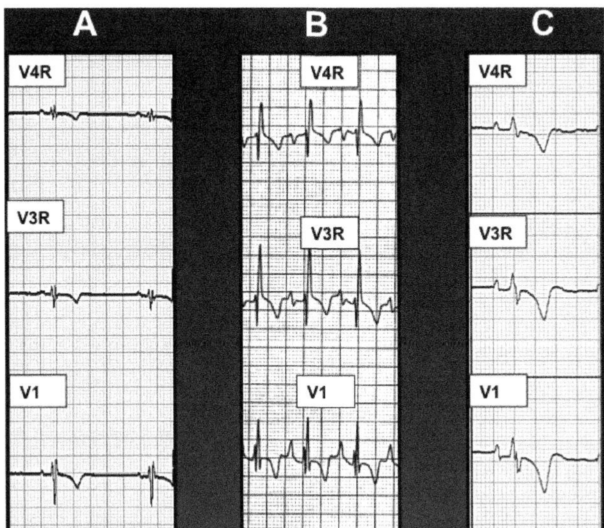

Figure 5.2. The RSR′ pattern in lead V_1 under 3 different conditions. A. Normal variant in a healthy 11-year-old with a small R′ wave. B. Tall R′ wave in a child with a large ASD. C. More complex pattern with true right ventricular conduction delay in a 15-year-old with documented right ventricular dysplasia and VT.

ECG PATTERNS FOR SERIOUS RHYTHMIC DISORDERS IN YOUNG PATIENTS

This section will avoid detailed discussion of specific arrhythmias and syndromes that are reviewed, more thoroughly, elsewhere in this textbook, and will instead focus on clinical presentations and electrocardiographic patterns that are somewhat unique to the pediatric and young adult populations.

Pediatric Presentations of Ion Channel Disease

The ion channel diseases show both age-related and variable penetrance even within families harboring the same mutations. Ion channel diseases that manifest in early childhood often display a severe phenotype with associated ECG abnormalities, and frequently relate to *de novo* mutations, although subsequent genotypic diagnoses in asymptomatic parents with lowly penetrant disease is well recognized.

Long QT Syndrome

The most common forms of long QT syndrome result from either reduced potassium conductance in the slow (I_{Ks}) or rapid (I_{Kr}) delayed rectifier currents or persistent, late activation of sodium channels (I_{Na}), leading to long QT1 (*KCNQ1*), 2 (*KCNH2*), and 3 (*SCN5A*), respectively. In children and adolescents, the prevalence of the 3 common types of long QT syndrome mirrors that seen in adults, with long QT1 (~45%–50%) more commonly seen in boys prepuberty and long QT2 (~40%–45%) in girls postpuberty, with long QT3 the rarest variant (~5%). In such cases, the ECG features are similar to older patients. However, presentation of long QT syndrome in infancy is often associated with severe prolongation of the QT interval and specific ECG features that may point to the clinical and genetic disease type. Phenotypic expression in LQTS relate to numerous genetic, epigenetic, and environmental factors, with the risk of cardiac events correlating with the degree of QT prolongation.

In the fetus and neonate, long QT1 is classically associated with sinus bradycardia often detected incidentally in an otherwise asymptomatic child. Conversely, long QT2 may manifest with 2:1 atrioventricular conduction (Figure 5.3), where functional atrioventricular block occurs due to prolonged ventricular refractoriness and QT intervals, and may be associated with refractory ventricular arrhythmias.[7] In infancy, the incidence of long QT3 related to SCN5A mutations is markedly increased compared to other types, with severe QT prolongation with the typical late-rising T wave after a prolonged isoelectric interval seen on the ECG, and as in long QT2, functional conduction disease is common. This reversed ratio of genotype weighted towards SCN5A is also seen in sudden infant death syndrome, where approximately 10% of all cases are associated with functionally deleterious mutations in the sodium channel gene.[8]

More complex genotypes frequently lead to clinical presentation in childhood, including compound heterozygote and digenic inheritance, and the autosomal recessive Jervell Lange-Nielsen (JLN) syndrome associated with sensorineural deafness and related to homozygous variants most commonly in *KCNQ1.* The ECG in JLN syndrome therefore displays the broad-based T wave associated with *KCNQ1* mutations and QT prolongation frequently greater than 550 ms, which is reflected in the high rate of cardiac events during childhood.[9]

Whilst long QT syndrome is an isolated cardiac condition, 2 conditions previously considered variants of long QT syndrome are recognized as distinct multisystem disorders. Andersen-Tawil syndrome is associated with mutations in the gene *KCNJ2* encoding the inward rectifier potassium channel Kir2.1, and is characterized by recurrent arrhythmias, abnormal facial features, and periodic paralysis. The ECG features typically display a normal QT interval, but prolonged QU interval with a wide T-U junction and dominant biphasic U waves (Figure 5.4). Other electrocardiographic features seen in Andersen-Tawil syndrome but not in classical LQTS include frequent ventricular premature beats, often bigeminal, and nonsustained ventricular tachycardia (VT) that frequently displays

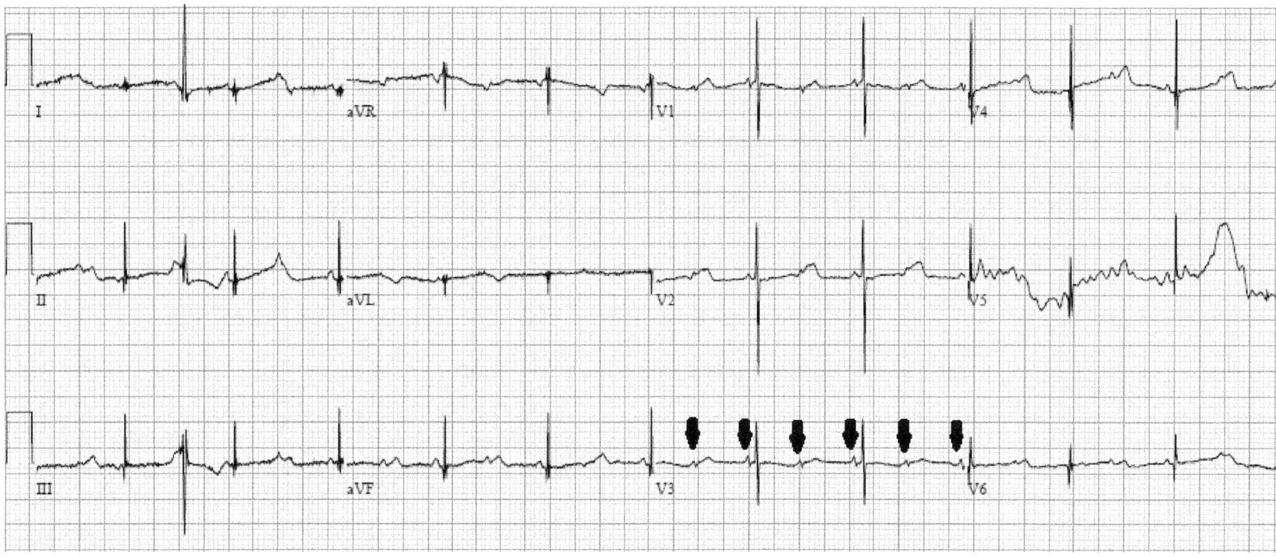

Figure 5.3. ECG from a 1-day-old girl with a severe phenotype of long QT syndrome. The atrial rate (P waves marked by arrows) is about 145 beats/min. Atrioventricular conduction (mostly 2:1) is limited by prolonged refractoriness in His-Purkinje and ventricular tissue.

a bidirectional pattern and conduction disorders. Conversely, torsade de pointes, the hallmark polymorphic VT of LQTS is rare in Andersen-Tawil syndrome.[10] Timothy syndrome relates to gain of function missense mutations in the calcium channel gene *CACNA1c* leading to loss of voltage-gated inactivation of the calcium channel CaV1.2. The ECG features of Timothy syndrome include severe QT prolongation (Figure 5.5), although as other cardiac manifestations including structural defects and pulmonary hypertension may occur, features of these may also be seen. Extracardiac manifestations include syndactyly, immune deficiency, endocrine disorders (hypoglycemia), and autism.[11]

Catecholaminergic Polymorphic VT (CPVT)

This arrhythmia most frequently presents during childhood with symptoms secondary to ventricular arrhythmias at times of catecholaminergic stress, typically exercise or emotion. Mutations in the ryanodine receptor gene (*RyR2*) cause cellular calcium overload leading to afterdepolarizations and triggered VT when the receptor is phosphorylated via the adrenergically stimulated cyclic AMP-protein kinase A pathway. At rest, the ECG is normal, although the characteristic appearance of ventricular ectopy, nonsustained, and bidirectional VT appear during exercise in a warm-up/cool-down pattern (Figure 5.6). Animal models have demonstrated the bidirectional pattern and are caused by alternating focal activation from Purkinje fibers in the right ventricle (RV) and left ventricle (LV),[12] and although exertional bidirectional VT is almost pathognomonic of CPVT, only about 35% to 40% of patients will display this characteristic ECG pattern.[13] Atrial arrhythmias, including focal atrial tachycardias and atrial fibrillation with rapid AV nodal conduction that may trigger ventricular arrhythmias, are increasingly recognized in CPVT.

Brugada Syndrome

Although the initial description of Brugada syndrome was in 2 young, highly symptomatic children, due to age-related penetrance the incidence is exceedingly low in the pediatric population. Although a proportion (25%–30%) of Brugada syndrome relates to mutations in the sodium channel gene (*SCN5A*), debate continues as to whether this is a disease of depolarization or repolarization and no single unifying mechanism has been proven. The ECG appearance is similar to that of adults with J-point elevation (>2 mm) and a coved or saddleback ST-segment in the anterior precordial leads (V_1–V_3). Perhaps the most powerful environmental modifier of the ECG appearance (and hence arrhythmic risk) in children is fever (Figure 5.7), which frequently precedes symptomatic cardiac events.[14]

Short QT Syndrome

Short QT syndrome may present in infancy or childhood with a peaked T-wave and a short QT interval. Early repolarization is commonly seen in association with short QT syndrome.[15]

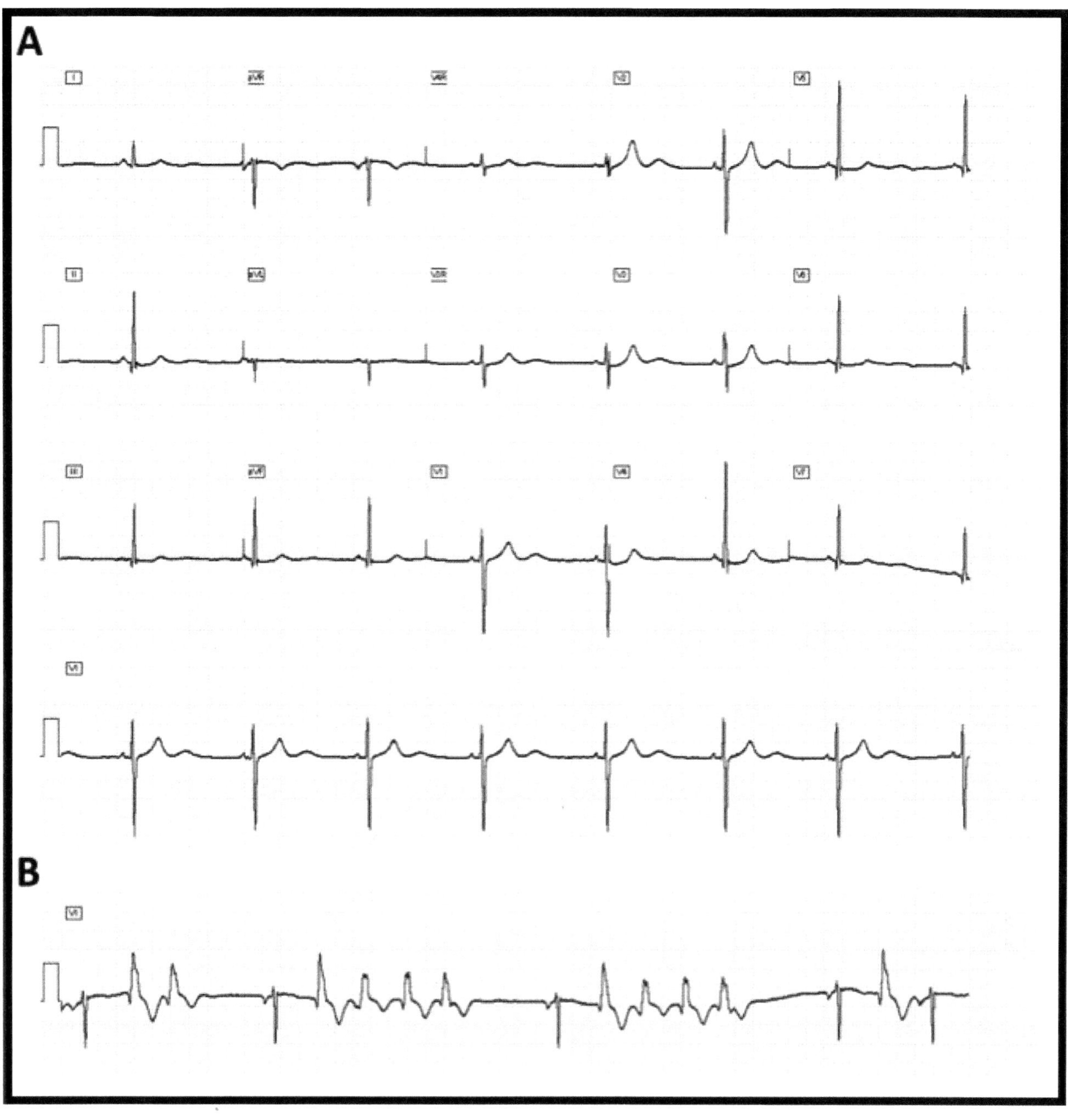

Figure 5.4. A. Teenager with Andersen-Tawil syndrome demonstrating a normal QT interval, but prominent, broad U-waves in several leads resulting in a markedly prolonged QU interval. B. A rhythm strip from lead V_1 recorded at a different time demonstrates a high burden of ventricular ectopy with variable right bundle branch morphology. Familial evaluation identified a variant in *KCNJ2.*

Cardiomyopathies in Children and Young Adults

Hypertrophic and Restrictive Cardiomyopathy

Sarcomeric mutations account for the majority of pediatric cases of hypertrophic cardiomyopathy (HCM), both sporadic and familial,[16] and although phenotypic expression typically occurs in adolescence, this can be seen at any stage during childhood. The ECG features seen in manifest HCM include Q waves (>1/3 the subsequent R wave or >0.3 mV, and >30 ms duration in at least 2 contiguous leads); T-wave inversion (>0.1 mV) or other nonspecific ST segment-T wave morphological abnormalities, typically seen in the anterolateral leads; and ST-segment depression (>0.1 mV if upsloping or >0.05 mV if downsloping or horizontal in at least contiguous leads) typically seen at higher heart rates and during exercise. Left ventricular hypertrophy may be defined by one of

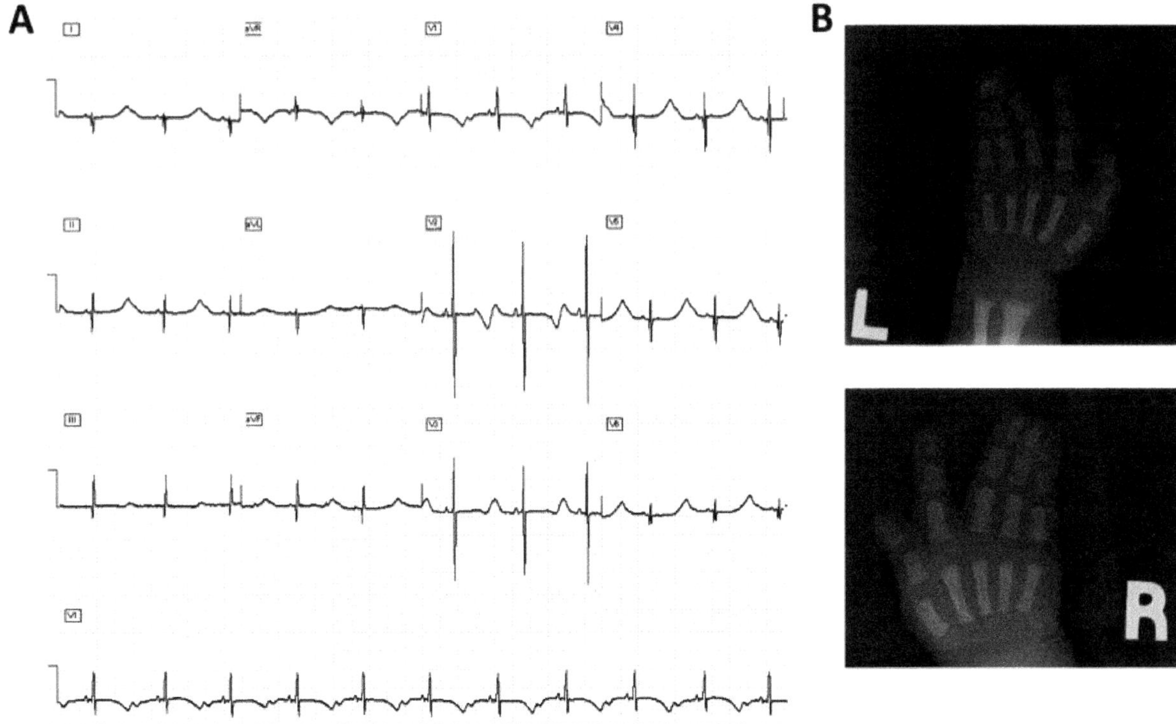

Figure 5.5. **A.** ECG from a neonate with Timothy syndrome demonstrating marked QT prolongation (QTc 640 ms) who presented with symptomatic hypoglycemia. **B.** Left and right hand x-rays from the same patient with syndactyly involving the 3 medial digits bilaterally. A mutation was found in *CACNA1c*.

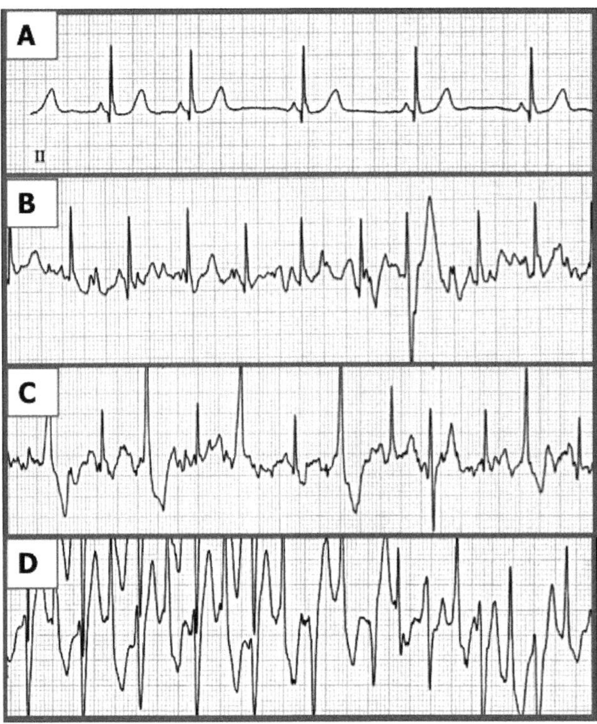

Figure 5.6. Rhythmic strips recorded from lead II demonstrating ventricular arrhythmia with increasing heart rates in CPVT. Sinus rhythm with normal QRS morphology is seen at lower heart rates during rest **(A)**. As the heart rate increases, ventricular ectopy **(B)** and then ventricular bigeminy **(C)** become evident, culminating in sustained bidirectional VT **(D)**.

many classifications, although increased precordial QRS amplitude is frequently seen in childhood and adolescence and overall the sensitivity of ECG criteria for left ventricular hypertrophy is low in children.[17] Q waves and nonspecific ST changes are highly specific findings in sarcomeric gene carriers prior to the development of overt ventricular hypertrophy, and therefore may act as early disease features in at-risk individuals.[18] QT prolongation (> 480 ms) relating to the mechanical effects of increased ventricular mass on repolarization have been reported in 13% of patients with HCM, more commonly in those who are symptomatic and/or those with left ventricular outflow tract (LVOT) obstruction.[19]

Restrictive cardiomyopathy often shows significant genotypic and phenotypic overlap with HCM and may display many of the ECG changes defined earlier (Figure 5.8). Given the marked increases in diastolic dysfunction, changes in P-wave morphology consistent with atrial dilatation and hypertrophy may be present. In adults, left atrial abnormalities are defined as either a widely notched (> 40 ms) P wave or prolongation of overall activation (>120 ms), and right atrial abnormalities by a tall, upright P wave (>2.5 mm) in lead 2.[20] Although marked differences in P-wave parameters exist throughout childhood, these values are consistent with the 98th percentile (P-wave amplitude 2.4 mm and duration 118 ms) seen in adolescents.

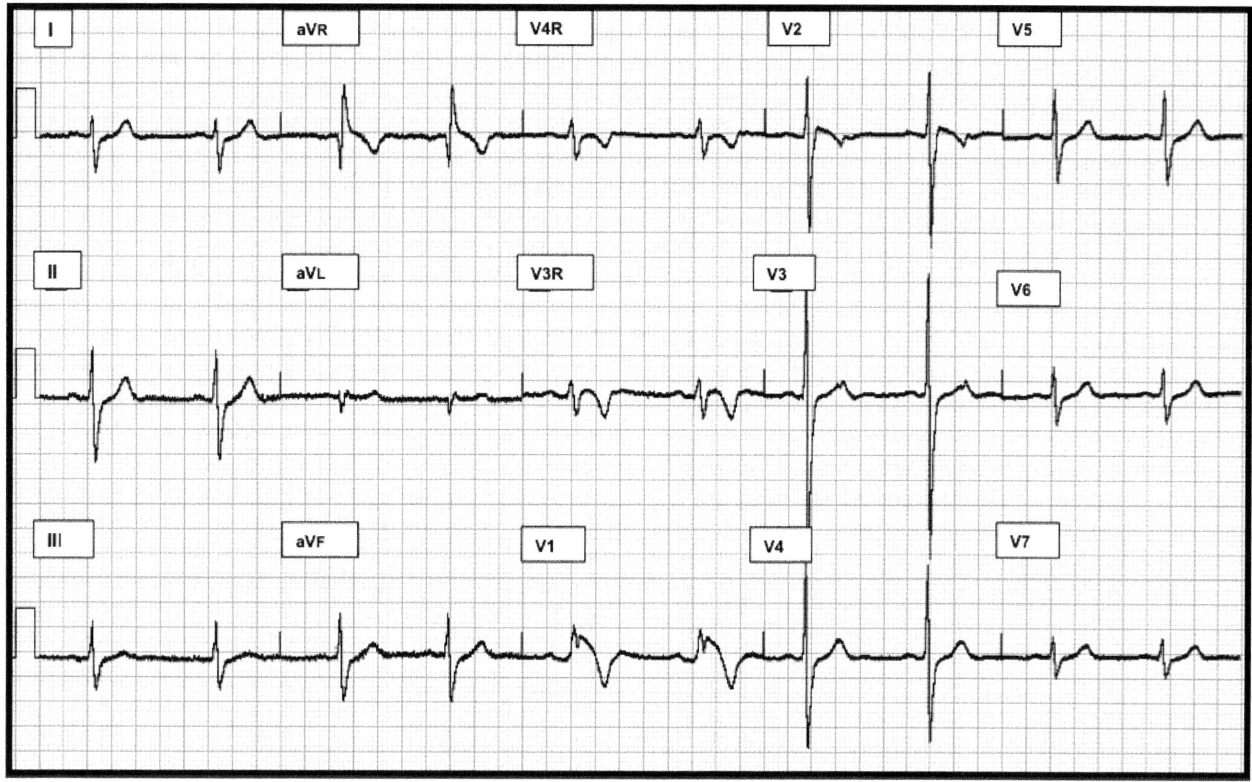

Figure 5.7. ECG from a 6-year-old with Brugada syndrome and recurrent VT. The abnormal precordial pattern was most dramatic during febrile illnesses.

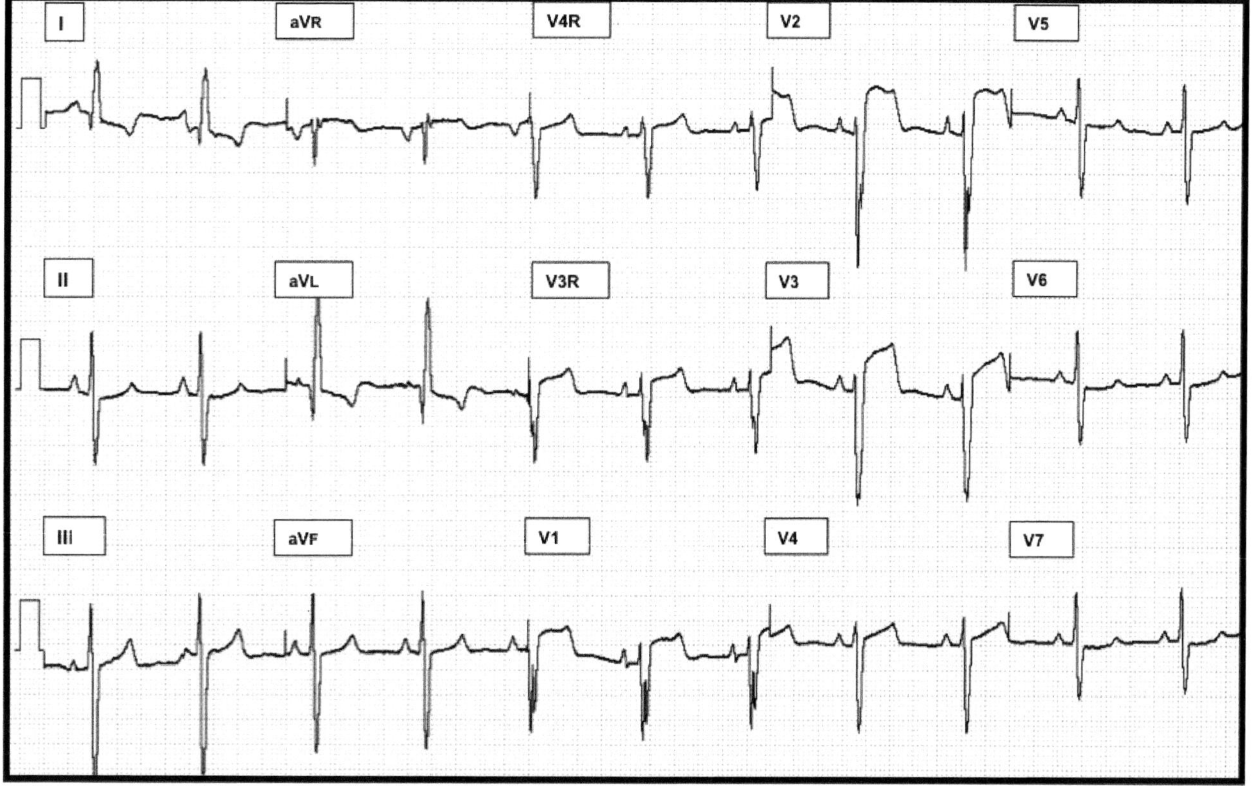

Figure 5.8. ECG from a 13-year-old girl investigated following a diagnosis of restrictive cardiomyopathy, conduction disease, and ventricular fibrillation in her mother. Widespread ST-segment abnormalities are seen with an RSR′ pattern in V_1. Note P-wave amplitude suggesting atrial enlargement secondary to restrictive ventricular physiology. Both mother and daughter carry a variant in the *DES* gene.

Children with restrictive cardiomyopathy may also show features of conduction disease, including PR and QRS prolongation progressing to complete heart block, features associated with a poor outcome.

Phenocopies of sarcomeric HCM typically manifest in the pediatric population and have specific ECG features that, along with the age of onset, may point to the underlying diagnosis. Pompe's disease is a glycogen storage disease resulting from deficiency of the alpha-glucosidase enzyme associated with sequence variants in the *GAA* gene. The condition typically presents in infancy, and although milder variants may be seen in older childhood and adults, only infantile-onset Pompe's is associated with the cardiac manifestations.[21] Electrocardiographic features characteristic of Pompe's disease include a short PR interval and marked increase in QRS amplitude (Figure 5.9), features believed to result from glycogen deposition within the atrioventricular node and myocardium, respectively,[22] which may regress with successful enzyme replacement therapy.[23]

Danon's disease is an aggressive X-linked storage disorder resulting from mutations in the lysosome-associated membrane protein gene (*LAMP2*), which typically presents in early adolescence with cardiac and extracardiac (skeletal myopathy and mental retardation) features. The ECG shows significant increases in QRS amplitude, reflecting the marked degree of left ventricular hypertrophy, and deep, inverted T-waves. Ventricular preexcitation is also frequently present, and the disease is typified by the rapid development of ventricular dilatation and systolic failure. Paroxysms of either atrial flutter or fibrillation are both common, reported in 6 of 7 patients in one study.[24]

Ventricular preexcitation is also seen in association with left ventricular hypertrophy in patients with mutations in the γ2 regulatory subunit of AMP-activated protein kinase (*PRKAG2*), where vacuolar glycogen storage leads to myocellular hypertrophy but myocyte disarray or fibrosis are not seen. Similar to patients with *LAMP2* mutations atrial flutter and fibrillation are both commonly seen, although the age of disease onset is typically older (third to fourth decade) and is frequently associated with both sinoatrial and atrioventricular node dysfunction requiring pacemaker implantation.[25] ECG findings include sinus bradycardia, a short PR interval and a wide QRS complex with a right bundle morphology. Although preexcitation typically relates to fasciculoventricular (FV) fibers, the properties of the AV node in these patients are atypical and despite the association with AV nodal conduction disease, rapid AV conduction of atrial arrhythmias with fatal outcomes has been documented.[26]

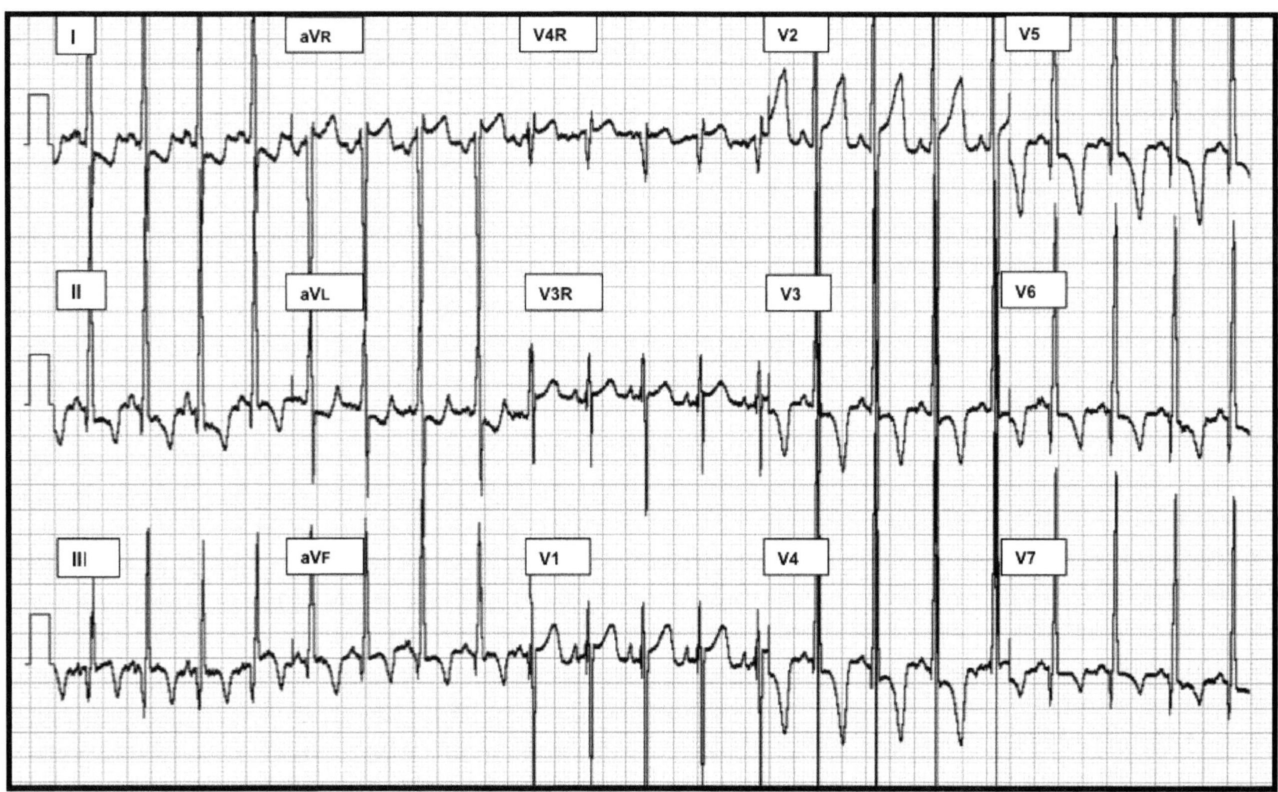

Figure 5.9. ECG from an 8-month-old infant with Pompe's disease demonstrating the typical short PR interval and marked increase in QRS amplitude secondary to severe ventricular hypertrophy.

Left ventricular hypertrophy is seen in 20% to 30% of Noonan's syndrome, although the ECG findings may be compounded by the electrocardiographic features typical of the condition, including left-axis deviation, poor precordial R-wave progression, and Q waves,[27] which may be seen in the absence of overt cardiac disease. Additional electrocardiographic features of other congenital cardiac lesions such as pulmonary valve stenosis, ASD, and aortic coarctation may be superimposed.[28]

Dilated Cardiomyopathy

Electrocardiographic findings in idiopathic or familial DCM are generally nonspecific and may include sinus tachycardia, anterolateral T-wave inversion, and septal Q waves, although even in cases of severe left ventricular dilation and dysfunction the ECG findings may be subtle, and rarely point to a specific diagnosis or etiology. In the young patient presenting with DCM, exclusion of potentially treatable causes (e.g., incessant arrhythmias, coronary abnormalities, and left heart obstructive lesions) is essential. Compared to the adult population, left bundle branch block is rare in pediatric DCM, although in adolescents and young adults it may be an early finding of lamin A/C cardiomyopathy, an autosomal dominant condition caused by mutations in the *LMNA* gene with cardiac features including left ventricular dilatation and dysfunction, conduction disease, atrial, and ventricular arrhythmias.[29]

Due to the high myocardial metabolic requirements and fundamental role of the mitochondria in energy utilization, DCM is a frequent manifestation of many maternally inherited mitochondrial disorders. Specific examples with childhood presentations include Barth syndrome (DCM and cyclical neutropenia), Leigh syndrome, mitochondrial encephalopathy, lactic acidosis, and stroke-like episodes (MELAS), and myoclonic epilepsy and red-ragged fibers (MERRF).

Arrhythmogenic Cardiomyopathy

Arrhythmogenic cardiomyopathy encompasses a range of myocardial disorders including classical arrhythmogenic right ventricular cardiomyopathy (ARVC), where right ventricular features predominate but progression to biventricular involvement may occur in later life, and left-sided variants with a spectrum from mild left ventricular involvement to phenocopies of DCM. Although numerous genes have been implicated in arrhythmogenic cardiomyopathy, including those encoding the desmosomal proteins (*PKP2, DSP, DSC-2, DSG-2,* and *JUP*), the intermediate filament desmin (*DES*), and the cytoskeletal protein titin (*TTN*), interpreting the true etiology is hindered by the high number of rare variants in these genes.

Arrhythmogenic cardiomyopathy shows age-related and highly variable penetrance, and disease expression is rare in childhood outside of the autosomal recessive cardiocutaneous Naxos disease and Cavajal syndrome, and those with compound heterozygosity.[30] A well-recognized concealed phase may be manifest in adolescence, where a high arrhythmic burden precedes any electrocardiographic or structural changes and potentially relates to an early inflammatory process,[31] so a normal ECG in a patient with malignant ventricular arrhythmias does not exclude the diagnosis. In right-sided disease, subsequent ECG changes include abnormal repolarization (T-wave inversion) and depolarization (terminal activation delay >55 ms defined as the time from the nadir of the S wave to the end of the QRS complex, and epsilon waves) in the anterior precordial leads.[32] Other findings include poor anterior R-wave progression and reduced QRS amplitude with notching in the inferior leads, which may be indicative of higher arrhythmic risk.[33] Ventricular ectopy may be seen on the 12-lead ECG with a left bundle morphology and either inferior or superior axis indicating origin within the outflow tract or body of the right ventricle. Left-sided variants may display only anterolateral T-wave inversion and left axis deviation, with an arrhythmic burden exceeding the degree of ventricular dysfunction.[34]

Incessant Tachycardias Causing Secondary Cardiomyopathy in Young Patients

Incessant tachycardias in young patients can occasionally lead to severe degrees of left ventricular dysfunction. It is critical to make the proper rhythm diagnosis promptly and treat accordingly, since this is one of the rare forms of cardiomyopathy that is entirely reversible.

Ectopic Atrial Tachycardia (EAT)

Atrial tachycardia involving a focus of abnormal automaticity can cause cardiomyopathy if sufficiently rapid and persistent. Although these foci can arise from anywhere in the right or left atrium, there is a tendency in young patients for EAT to cluster towards the atrial appendages, the pulmonary vein (PV) orifices, and the crista terminalis. The ECG pattern of an abnormal P-wave morphology is easily recognizable when the focus is located in the left appendage or the left PVs (Figure 5.10). However, foci located near the right PVs, the right appendage, or along the crista will sometimes generate a P-wave morphology that is difficult to differentiate from sinus tachycardia, in which

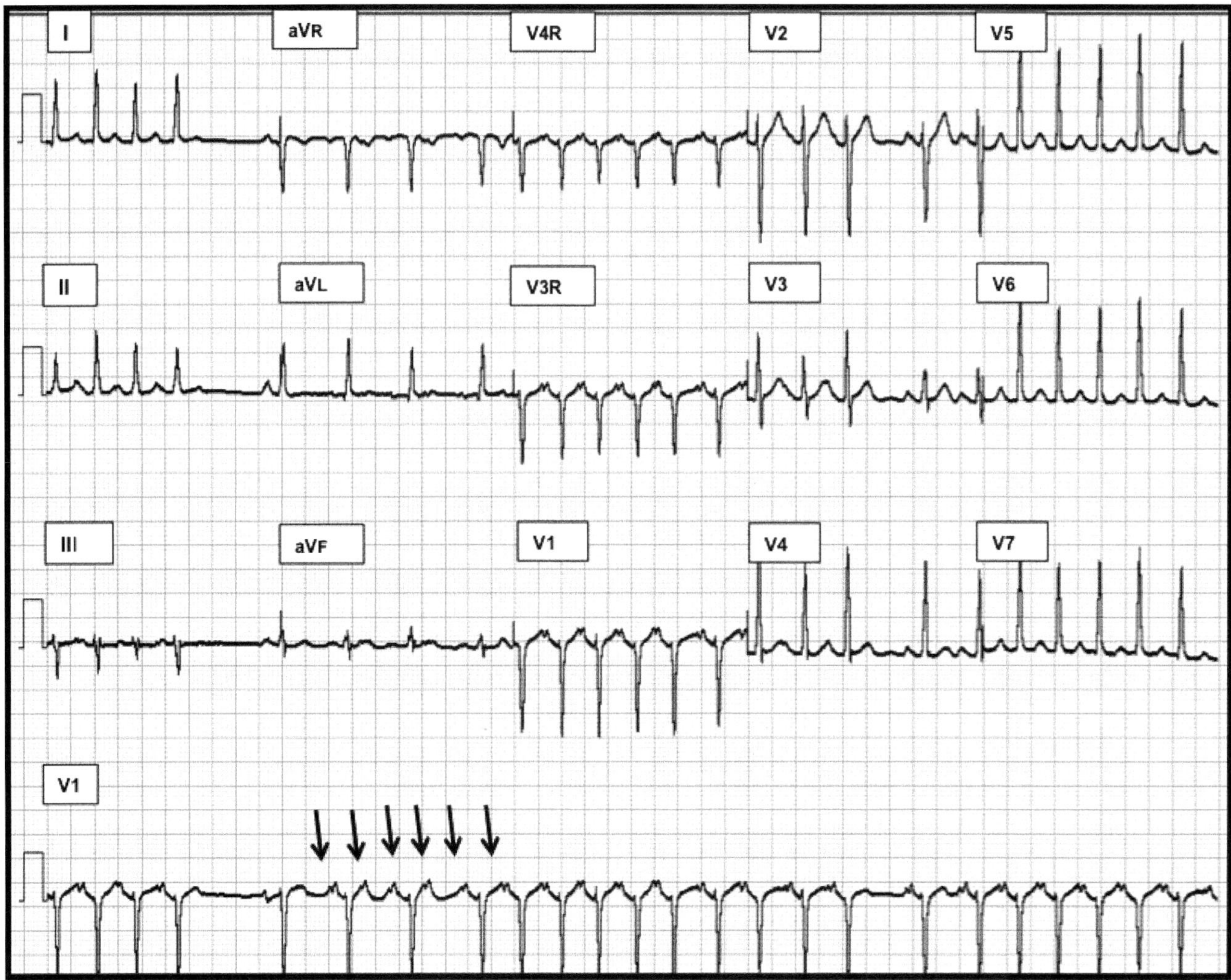

Figure 5.10. EAT (left atrial origin) in a teenager with secondary cardiomyopathy. Note instances of nonconducted P waves (arrows) without interruption of tachycardia, supporting atrial origin rather than a reciprocating mechanism.

case formal intracardiac mapping may be required to make a firm diagnosis.[35]

Permanent Form of Junctional Reciprocating Tachycardia (PJRT)

The ECG appearance of PJRT is distinctive (Figure 5.11), with deeply negative P waves in leads II, III, and aVF. The ventriculo-atrial interval is quite long due to slow conduction through a decremental concealed accessory pathway, with a relatively normal PR interval time.[36] A definitive diagnosis can be made by the observation of brief termination for a beat or two in response to vagal maneuvers or adenosine, with immediate resumption of tachycardia.

Focal VT

Although focal outflow VT is a generally benign condition, myopathy will develop occasionally in young patients with relatively fast rates and a high burden of ventricular beats. The ECG pattern for outflow VT in children is identical to that seen in adults.[37]

Complex Preexcitation

Accessory pathways are a source of high morbidity (and occasional mortality) in young patients, especially when the clinical picture is complicated by coexistent structural heart disease. It is unnecessary to review the basic ECG features of Wolff-Parkinson-White (WPW) and related disorders here, but it is worth highlighting some complex pediatric presentations.

WPW and Atriofascicular Fibers in Structural Heart Disease

A number of young patients presenting with preexcitation have associated structural disease in the form

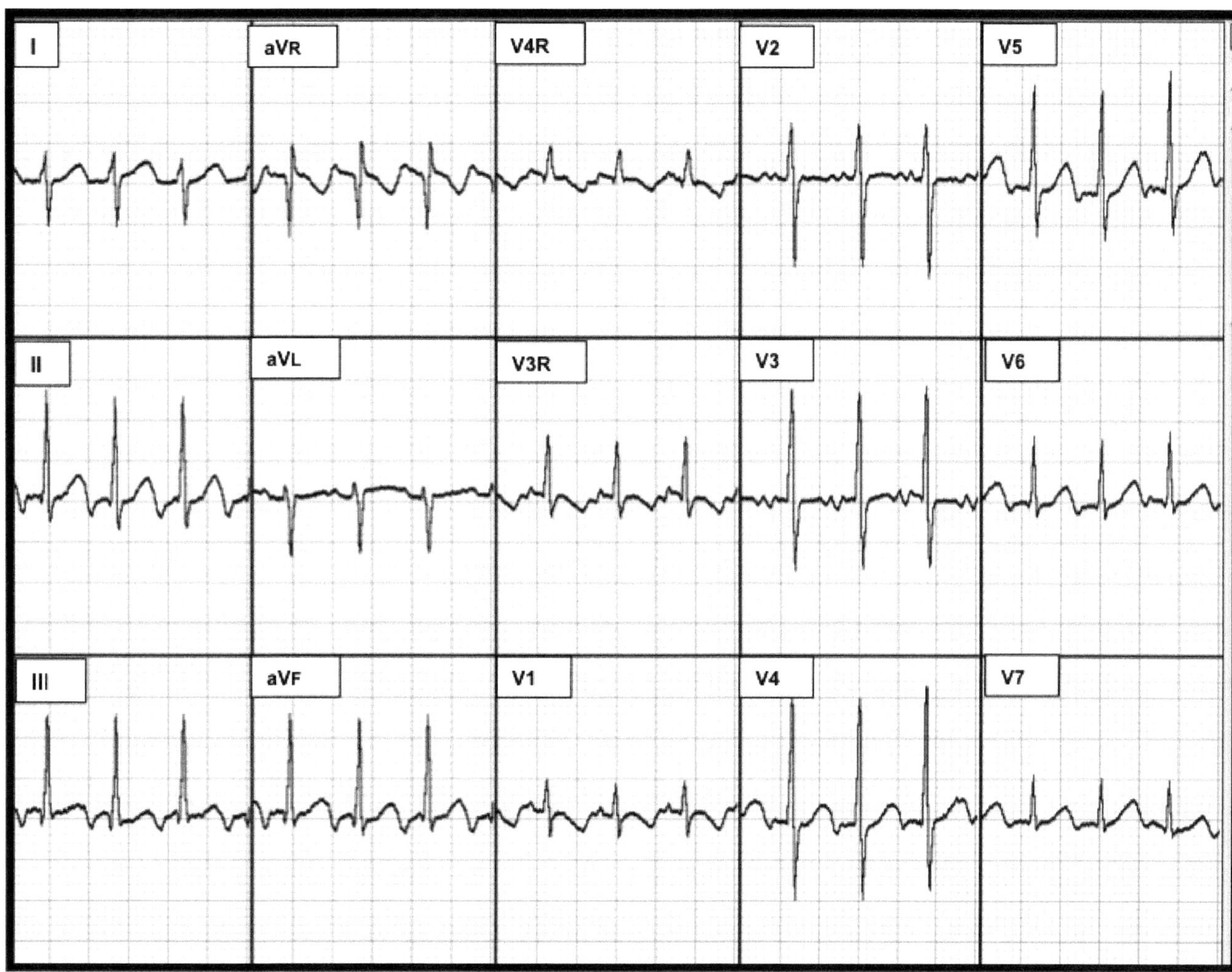

Figure 5.11. The PJRT showing classic timing and morphology for the retrograde P wave (standard calibration).

of cardiomyopathy or CHDs. Aside from the obvious disadvantages of reentrant tachycardia under conditions of suboptimal hemodynamics, risks are further increased by the fact that more than a quarter of patients with preexcitation in the setting of structural disease are likely to have multiple accessory pathways.[38] Preexcitation is known to be associated with several forms of cardiomyopathy in young patients, especially the hypertrophic and noncompaction varieties. The CHD associated with the highest incidence of accessory pathways is Ebstein's anomaly of the tricuspid valve (TV). These patients have a remarkably high incidence of both WPW pathways and atriofascicular fibers that are localized along the tricuspid ring where valve leaflets are most displaced down into the right ventricle.[39] The ECG pattern in Ebstein's patients with preexcitation can sometimes be confusing. Because the accessory pathway typically inserts into very abnormal right ventricular muscle, the delta wave is often low frequency and low amplitude (Figure 5.12). Additionally, since most Ebstein's patients have an underlying right bundle branch block (RBBB), fusion with sluggish preexcitation from a right-sided accessory pathway or atriofascicular fiber can result in artifactual normalization of the QRS. There should be a high index of suspicion for accessory pathways in any Ebstein's patient without a normal PR interval and RBBB.

Pseudo-preexcitation

An ECG appearance of relatively short PR interval and slurred QRS onset can be seen in select forms of pediatric heart disease that do not involve actual preexcitation. The most common condition is single ventricle (e.g., tricuspid atresia or hypoplastic left heart) where absence of normal septal depolarization distorts the initial QRS contour. When coupled with the atrial enlargement that is so common in single-ventricle patients, a remarkably good mimic of a WPW

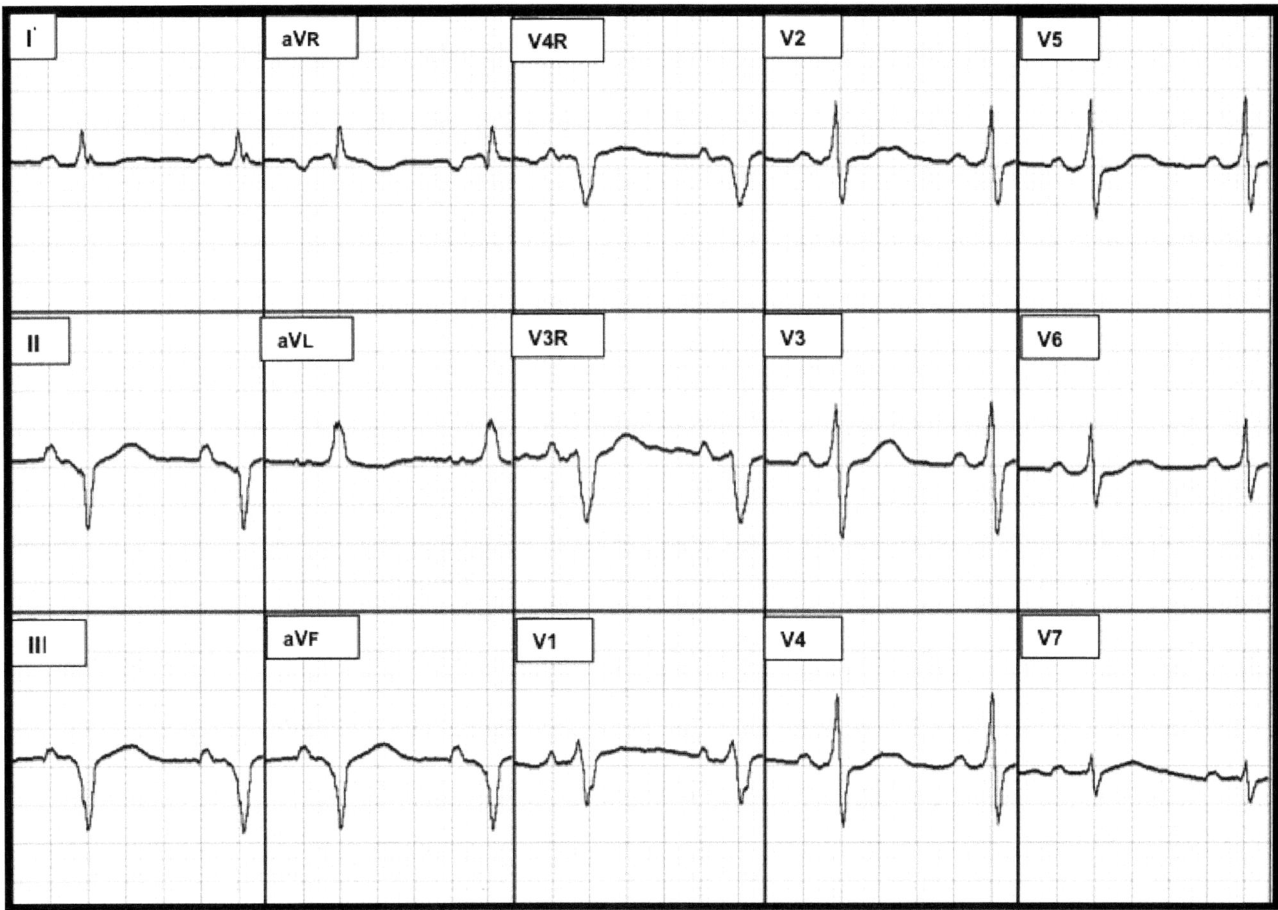

Figure 5.12. WPW in a child with Ebstein's anomaly. This was a conventional atrioventricular connection rather than an atriofascicular connection, even though the PR interval appears longer than expected due to slow conduction of the preexcitation wavefront through the abnormal tissue along the TV ring. The patient's ECG had the expected pattern of complete RBBB following successful catheter ablation of this right-posterior accessory pathway (standard calibration).

pattern is produced. Formal electrophysiologic testing may be required to differentiate this finding from the true preexcitation. Similar confusion can occur when interpreting the ECG in some young patients with HCM (Figure 5.13) or glycogen storage disease.

Conduction Defects

Congenital heart block due in utero exposure to maternal autoantibodies and acquired heart block from surgical trauma during congenital heart repairs are the most common causes of permanent AV conduction disturbances in young patients. These 2 entities have a fairly predictable natural history and treatment approach, and do not require a review here. There are, however, some less common conduction diseases that are more insidious in their presentation, have implications for cardiac structure and function, and may pose serious risk to young patients if unrecognized.

Abnormalities of TBX5 gene (Holt-Oram syndrome) or Nkx2-5 gene 3

Mutations of either of these 2 genes are associated with varied degrees of AV block[40,41] and septal defects (usually at the atrial level). In the case of Holt-Oram syndrome, deformities of the forelimbs are also present. In extreme cases, the cardiac involvement can progress to include complete AV block, atrial arrhythmias, and cardiomyopathy (Figure 5.14).

Kearns-Sayre Syndrome

This rare syndrome is caused by a deletion in mitochondrial DNA and is characterized by external ophthalmoplegia and diffuses conduction system disease that can be rapidly progressive in young patients (Figure 5.15). Occasional patients also may develop severe cardiomyopathy.[42]

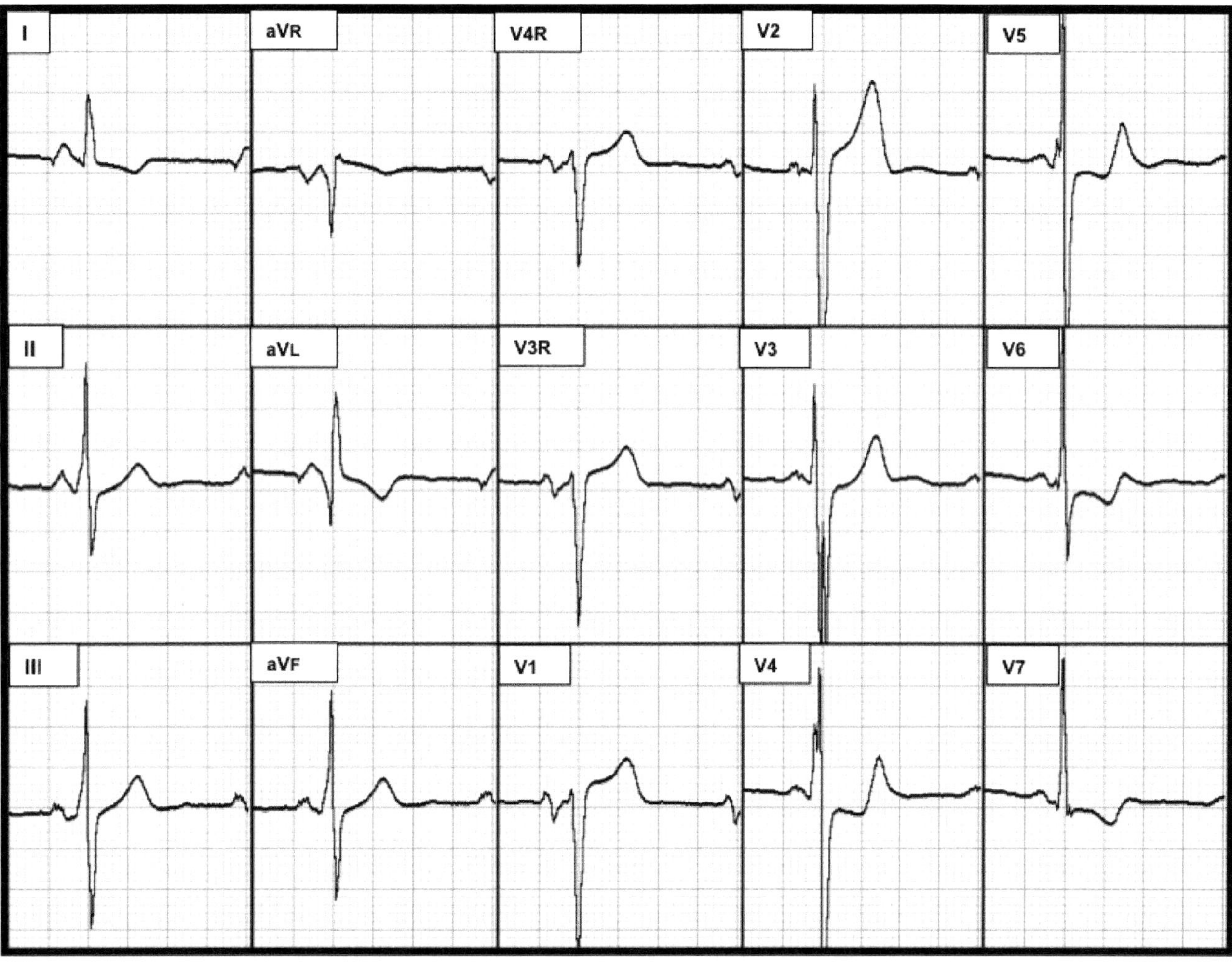

Figure 5.13. Pseudo-preexcitation in a teenager with HCM. The QRS onset has a pattern suggestive of a delta wave in leads V_5 and V_6. Preexcitation was ruled out with formal electrophysiology (EP) study (standard calibration).

Intrinsically Abnormal AV Conduction in CHDs

Certain forms of congenital heart disease (CHD) are associated with developmental abnormalities of the AV conduction tissues and complete heart block that may develop at any time from fetal life through adulthood. The best known of these conditions is L-transposition of the great arteries (also referred to as "congenitally corrected" transposition) which involves inversion of the RVs and LVs while the atria and great vessels remain in their normal positions. The conduction tissues are abnormally located and relatively fragile, resulting in an incidence of AV block as high as 30% by adulthood.[43] The ECG in these patients will show varied degrees of AV block, and a peculiar QRS contour that reflects the fact that early septal activation is occurring right-to-left owing to the reversed ventricular orientation (Figure 5.16). The AV conduction tissues can also be marginal in patients born with septal defects in the AV canal region.

Tachyarrhythmias in Patients with CHD

Arrhythmias remain a major late complication of CHD. Atrial and VTs may develop over time related to the unique myocardial substrate created by surgical scars and patches in conjunction with cyanosis and abnormal pressure/volume loads.[44,45] The ECG provides several markers that can be used as part of the risk-stratification process for these patients.

Atrial Tachycardias

The most common mechanism for tachycardia in the CHD population is macro-reentry within atrial muscle. The term intra-atrial reentrant tachycardia (IART) has become the customary label for this arrhythmia in order to distinguish it from typical atrial flutter that occurs in structurally normal hearts. In the setting of a healthy AV node, IART will conduct rapidly and can cause significant hemodynamic compromise. Patients prone to IART often have concomitant sinus

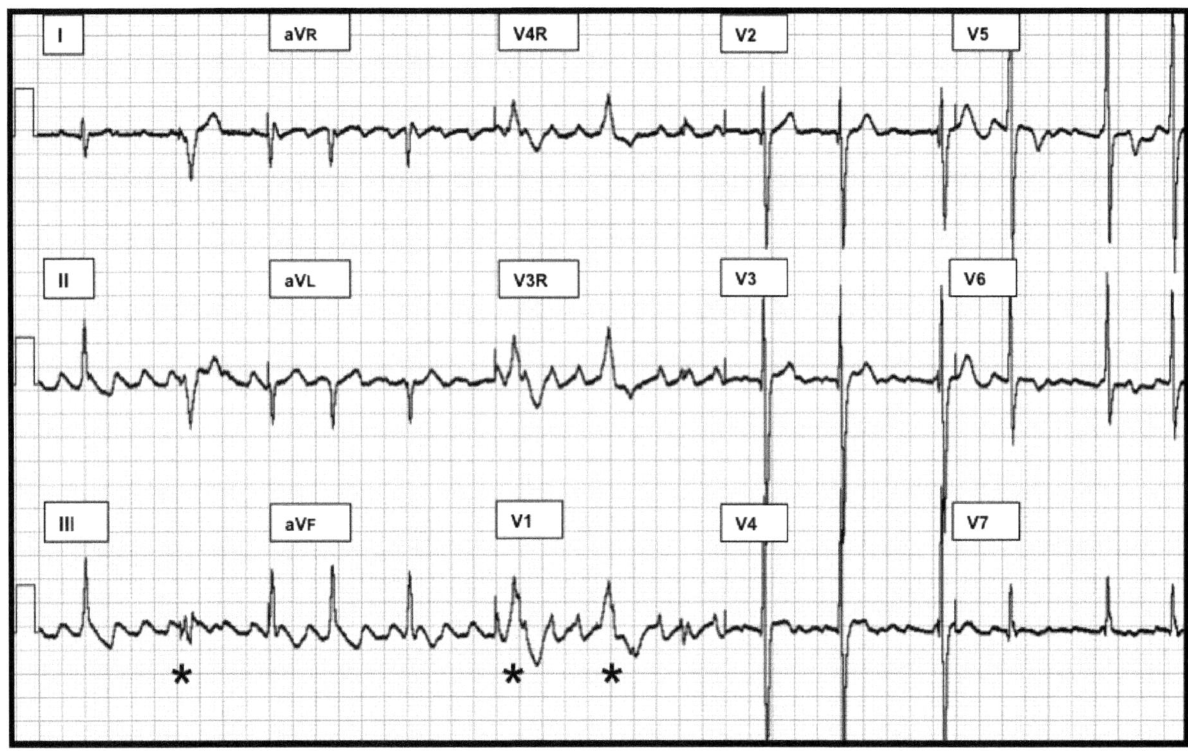

Figure 5.14. A 16-year-old with Holt-Oram syndrome who underwent successful closure of an ASD at 4 years. He developed recurrent atrial flutter and progressive delay in atrioventricular conduction that ultimately required permanent pacemaker implant. The ventricular response to atrial flutter on this tracing is relatively slow, at times defaulting (stars) to VVI pacing.

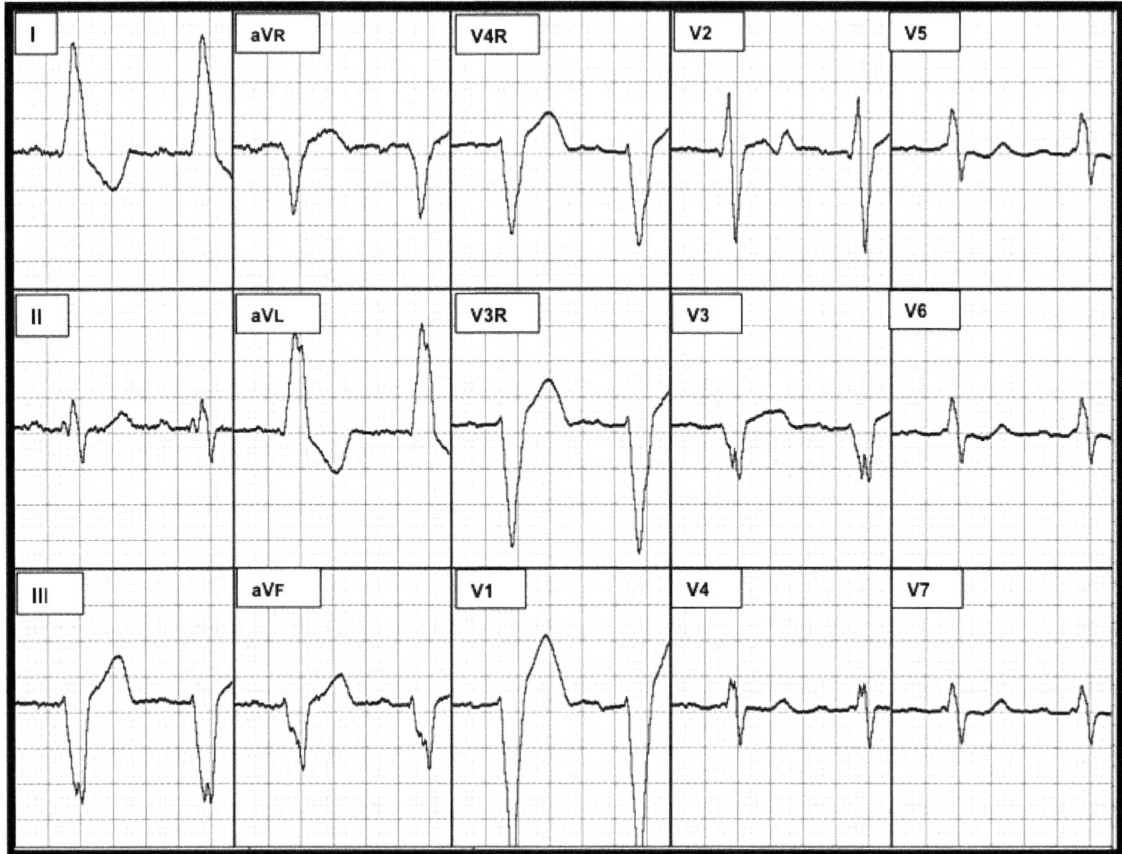

Figure 5.15. First-degree atrioventricular block and complete left bundle branch block in an 11-year-old with a rapidly progressive form of Kearns-Sayre syndrome (standard calibration).

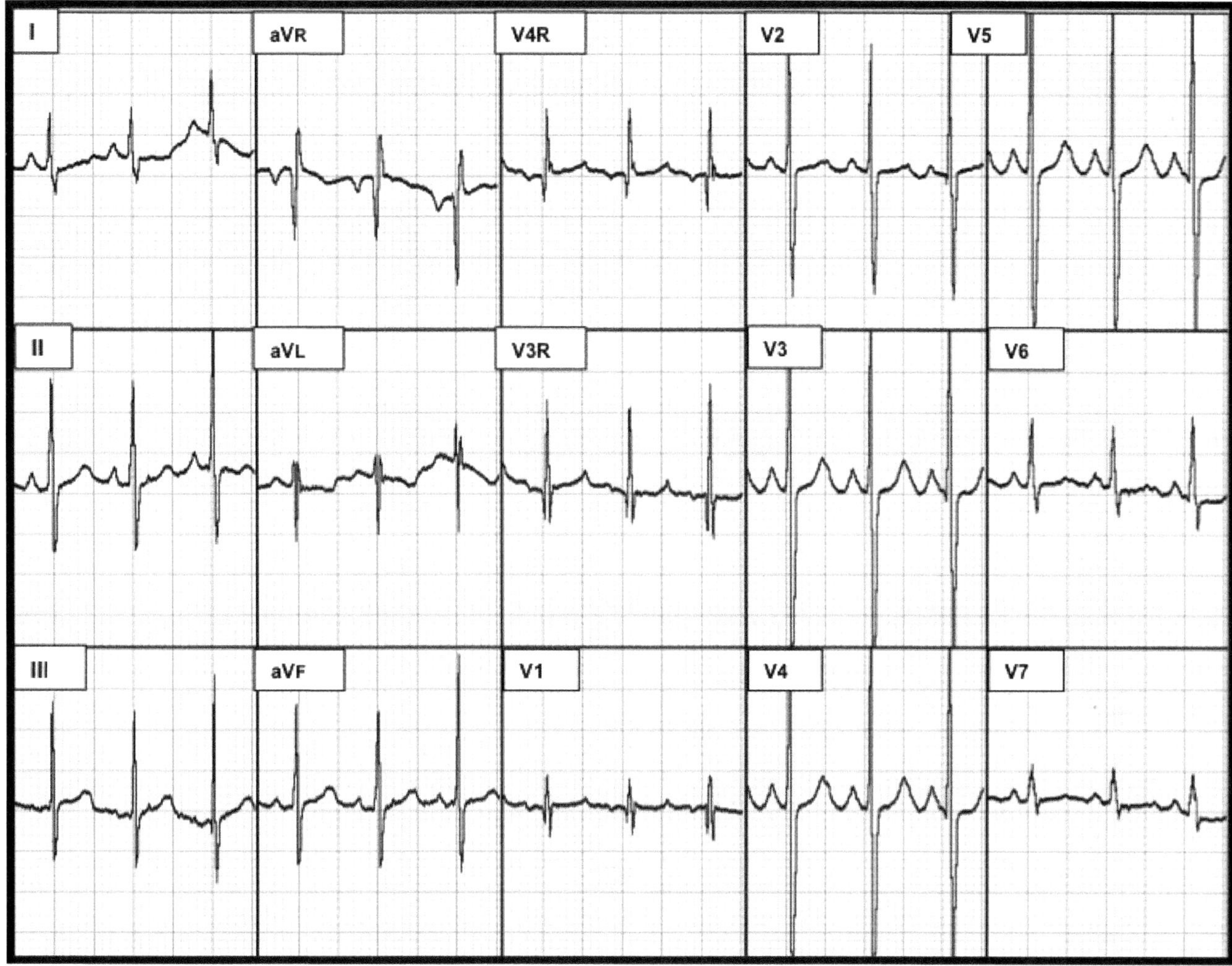

Figure 5.16. ECG from an infant with L-TGA (so-called "congenitally corrected" transposition). Atrioventricular conduction was intact at this point. The conducted QRS shows features suggesting septal activation occurs in a right-to-left direction due to the inverted ventricles, with sharp Q wave in the right precordium, absent Q wave in V_5 and V_6, and an RSR pattern in aVL (standard calibration).

node dysfunction and atrial enlargement. Consequently, the ECG in baseline rhythm can demonstrate an assortment of slow atrial and junctional escape rhythms (Figure 5.17A). The route of propagation for an IART circuit is modulated by regions of fibrosis from suture lines or patches, which function in combination with natural conduction barriers to channel the wavefront along its macro-reentrant loop. If a TV is present, the isthmus between the valve ring and the inferior vena cava is commonly involved, but atypical paths along the lateral atrial wall and the septum are also seen.[46] Multiple IART circuits are frequently encountered in the same patient.[47] The ECG pattern during an IART episode resembles classic atrial flutter in most respects, although the rates are generally slower (150–250 per minute) due to delayed conduction through scarred atrial muscle. Some circuits involving zones of exceptionally slow conduction through a well-protected corridor will register isoelectric times between P waves rather than the more continuous saw-tooth appearance of classic flutter (Figure 5.17B). It is important to emphasize that IART will occasionally conduct in a fixed 2:1 pattern on ECG that is occasionally misinterpreted as sinus rhythm when atrial activity is obscured by the QRS and T-wave. The index of suspicion for IART should always be high in CHD patients, particularly those who have undergone extensive atrial baffling operations such as the Mustard, Senning, or older-style Fontan operations.

VT

VT remains an uncommon but serious complication of CHD. It is useful to distinguish 2 categories of VT in this population. The first involves anatomical and surgical abnormalities in ventricular muscle that create discrete conduction corridors capable of supporting one or more monomorphic reentrant VT circuits. The lesion that best exemplifies this anatomic

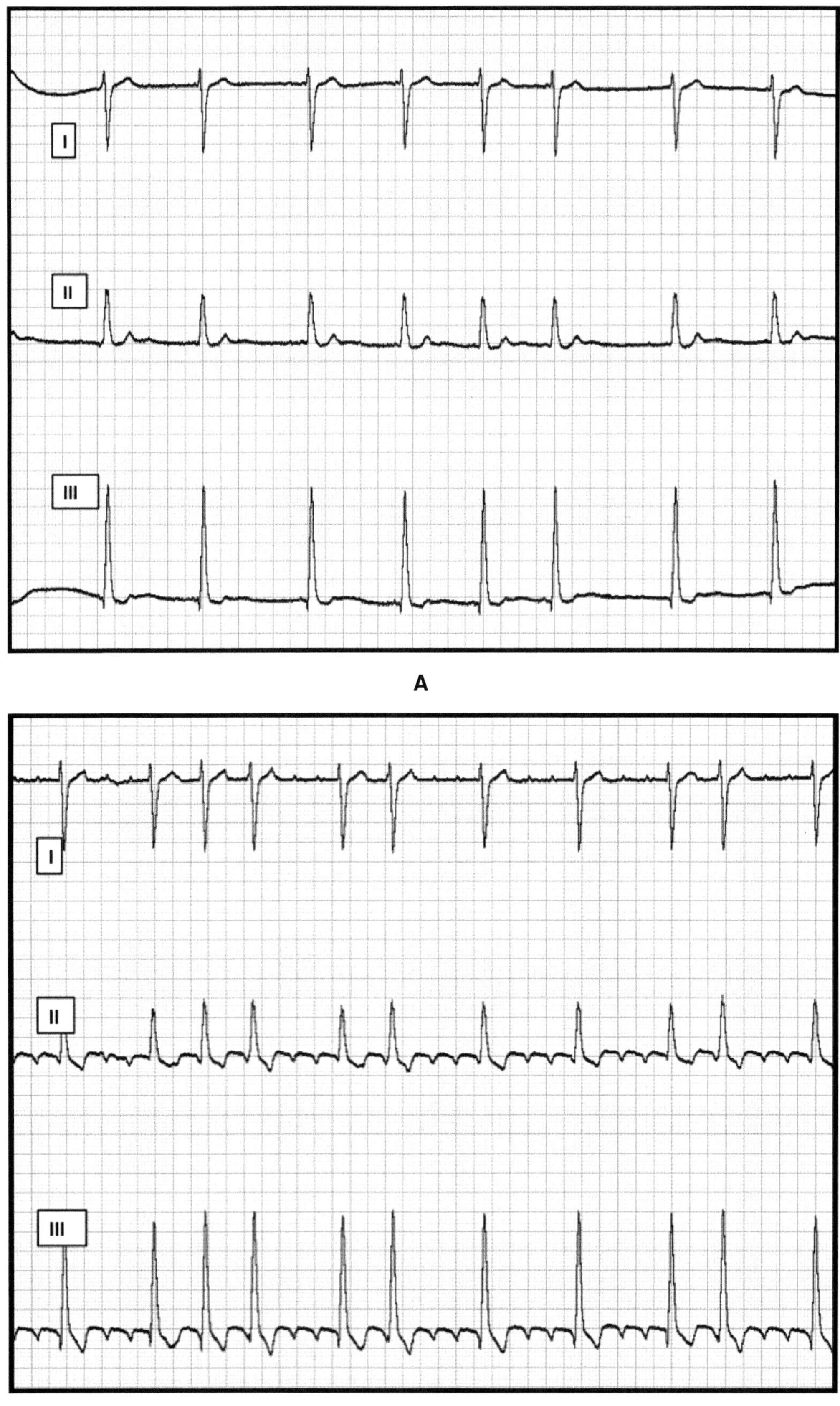

Figure 5.17. Rhythm strips demonstrating "tachy-brady" syndrome in a 25-year-old with single ventricle who has undergone a Fontan operation. A. Baseline rhythm with atrial and junctional escape beats. B. Same patient during IART.

predisposition to macro-reentrant VT is tetralogy of Fallot (TOF), where an organized circuit develops within the abnormal tissues of the right ventricular outflow tract (RVOT).[48] A second category involves nonspecific polymorphic VT and/or ventricular fibrillation from diffusely abnormal myocardium, similar to arrhythmias seen in other forms of hypertrophic or DCM. The myopathic substrate in CHD patients is caused by long-standing pressure and volume loads complicated by periods of cyanosis that ultimately results in advanced degrees of hypertrophy and fibrosis. Lesions associated with VT of the myopathic variety can include congenital aortic outflow obstruction and surgical corrections such as the Mustard

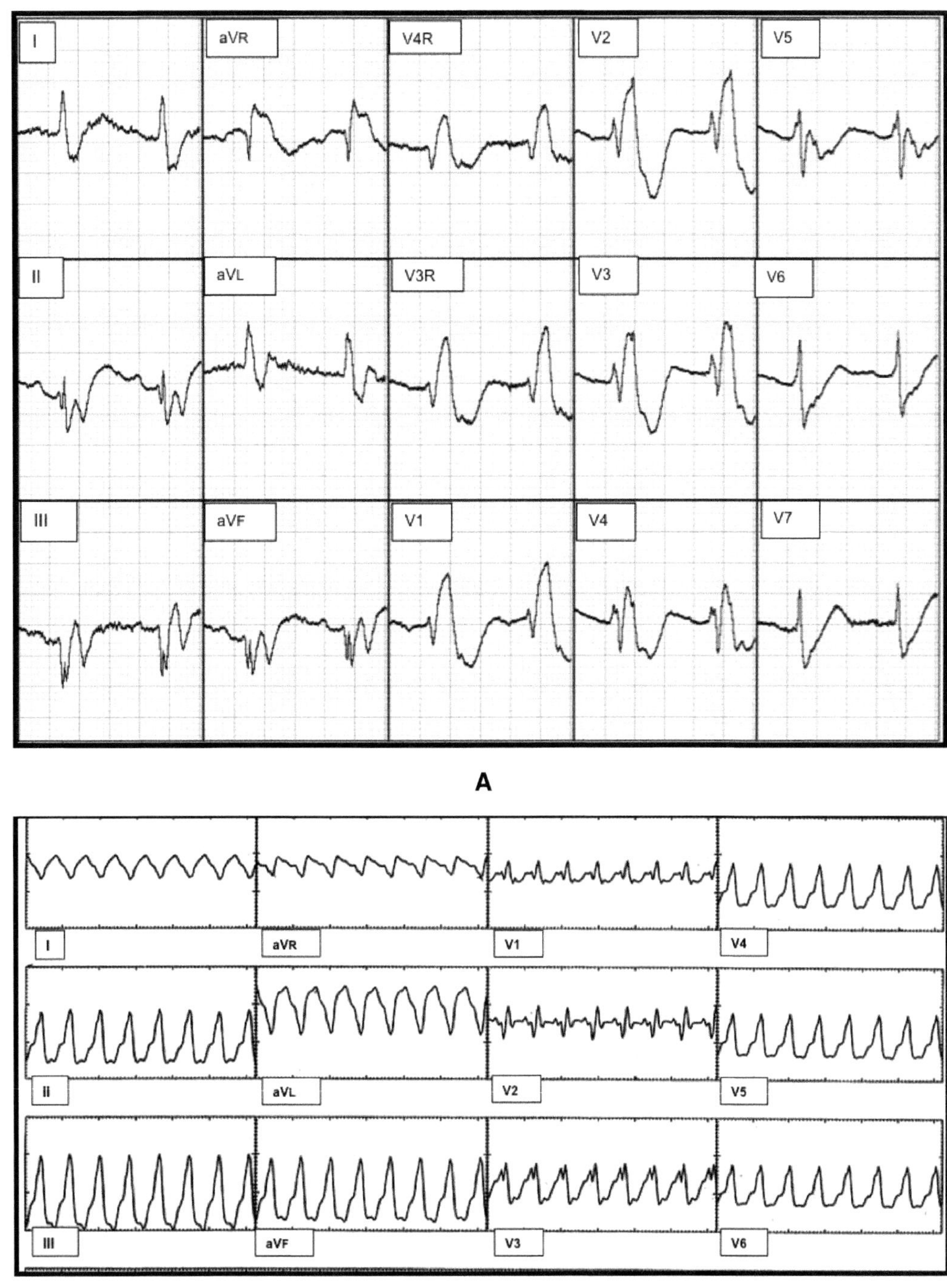

Figure 5.18. Recordings from patients with repaired of TOF. **A.** Sinus rhythm with RBBB and left anterior hemiblock in a 28-year-old who has a prolonged QRS duration of over 200 ms and recurrent VT (standard calibration). **B.** Sustained monomorphic VT in a 34-year-old with a morphology suggesting a tachycardia origin the right ventricular outflow region where successful catheter ablation was carried out.

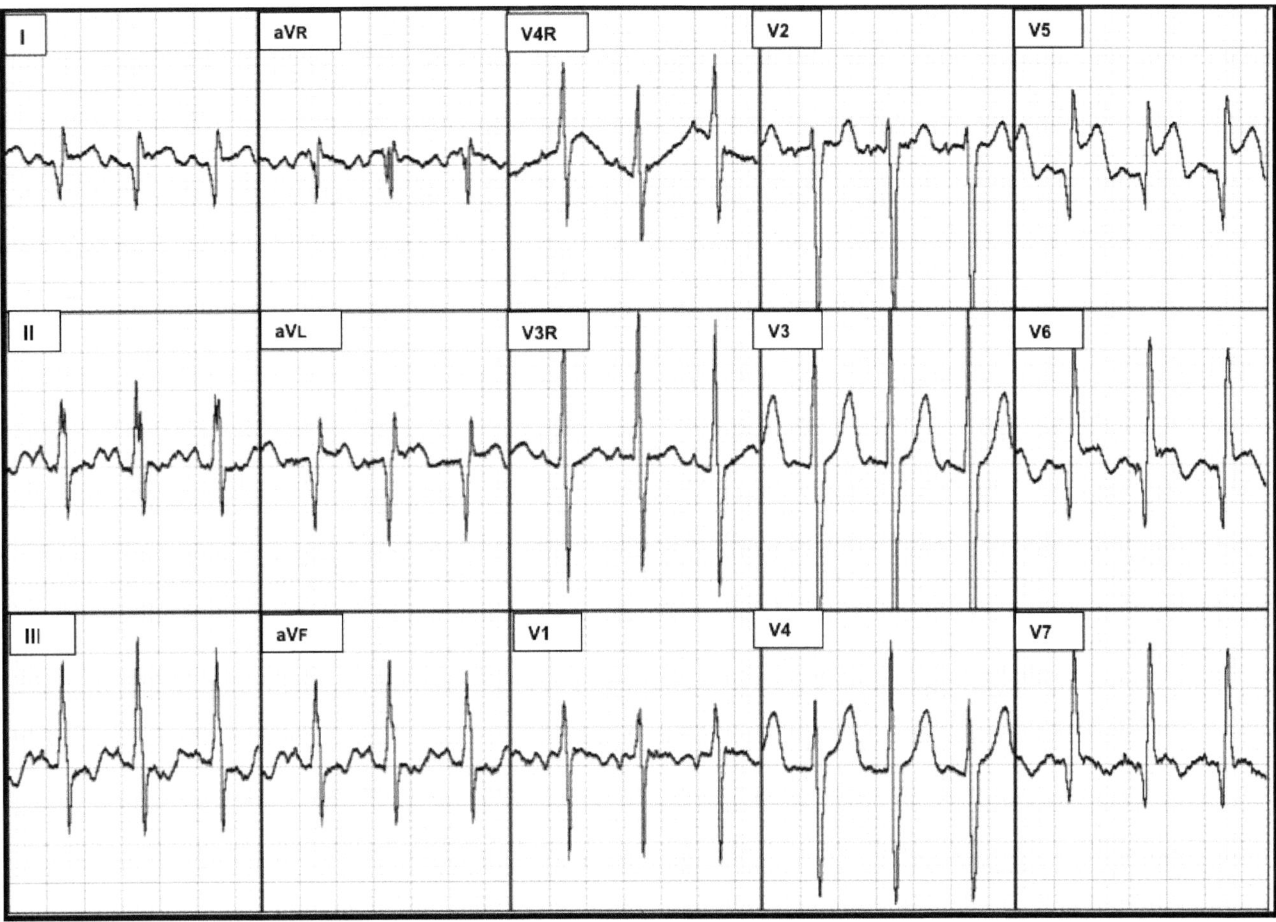

Figure 5.19. A 6-month-old with ALCAPA. The ECG suggests ischemia/infarct over the left-anterior precordium (standard calibration).

operation where the right ventricle has been recruited as the systemic ventricle. Most of the literature regarding VT in CHD has centered on the monomorphic type of VT seen in TOF. Sustained VT is relatively uncommon in children and adolescents with TOF, but the risk then accelerates in adulthood to reach as high as 1% per year by the fourth or fifth decades of life. Risk stratification for VT and sudden death in TOF patients has long been a topic of intense investigation, and numerous studies have identified clinical variables with modest prognostic value, including the ECG. More than 90% of postoperative TOF patients will exhibit a pattern of RBBB on their baseline ECG,[49] with a QRS duration ranging from 120 ms to over 200 ms. The QRS duration for a given patient appears to have reasonable correlation with right ventricular size and function,[50] and status of the right ventricle in turn correlates reasonably well with the risk of VT and sudden death. A very prolonged QRS duration exceeding 180 ms has therefore been suggested as a marker for TOF patients at highest risk (Figure 5.18A and B). Although the predictive accuracy of QRS duration is far from perfect,[51] it is nonetheless a practical, noninvasive tool for monitoring the long-term status of these patients.

Congenital Coronary Artery Anomalies

Anomalous origin of the left coronary artery from the pulmonary artery (ALCAPA) is a rare but serious disorder that can contribute to sudden death in pediatric patients. The presentation can vary, but most often the initial symptom is acute cardiovascular collapse in an infant.[52] The ECG for the distressed infant usually shows a clear infarct pattern with deep Q waves and loss of R wave in leads V_3 to V_6, along with left-axis deviation (Figure 5.19). What is truly remarkable about the ECG in this condition is that ventricular function can recover and the ECG fully normalize within just a few months of surgical correction when it is performed early in life.

REFERENCES

1. Walsh EP, Alexander ME, Cecchin F. Electrocardiography and introduction to electrophysiologic techniques. In: Keane JF, Lock JE, Fyler DC, ed(s). *Nadas' Pediatric Cardiology*. 2nd ed. Philadelphia, PA: Saunders/Elsevier; 2006:145–182.
2. Singh HR. The asymptomatic teenager with an abnormal electrocardiogram. *Pediatr Clin North Am.* 2014;61:45–61.
3. Fish FA, Kannankeril PJ. Diagnosis and management of sudden death in children. *Curr Opin Pediatr.* 2012;24:592–602.
4. Garson A Jr., ed. *The Electrocardiogram in Infants and Children*. Philadelphia, PA: Lea and Febiger, 1983.
5. Schwartz PJ, Stramba-Badiale M. Repolarization abnormalities in the newborn. *J Cardiovasc Pharmacol.* 2010;55:539–543.
6. Davignon A, Rautaharju P, Boisselle E, et al. Normal ECG standards for infants and children. *Pediatr Cardiol.* 1979;1:123–131.
7. Lupoglazoff JM, Denjoy I, Villain E, et al. Long QT syndrome in neonates: conduction disorders associated with HERG mutations and sinus bradycardia with KCNQ1 mutations. *J Am Coll Cardiol.* 2004;43:826–830.
8. Wang DW, Desai RR, Crotti L, et al. Cardiac sodium channel dysfunction in sudden infant death syndrome. *Circulation.* 2007;115:368–376.
9. Schwartz PJ, Spazzolini C, Crotti L, Bathen J, et al. The Jervell and Lange-Nielsen syndrome: Natural history, molecular basis and clinical outcome. *Circulation.* 2006;113:783–790.
10. Zhang L, Benson DW, Tristani-Firouzi M, et al. Electrocardiographic features in Andersen-Tawil syndrome patients with KCNJ2 mutations: Characteristic T-U-wave patterns predict the KCNJ2 genotype. *Circulation.* 2005;111:2720–2726.
11. Splawski I, Timothy KW, Sharpe LM, et al. Ca(V)1.2 calcium channel dysfunction causes a multisystem disorder including arrhythmia and autism. *Cell.* 2004;119:19–31.
12. Cerrone M, Noujaim SF, Tolkacheva EG, et al. Arrhythmogenic mechanisms in a mouse model of catecholaminergic polymorphic ventricular tachycardia. *Circ Res.* 2007;101:1039–1048.
13. Priori SG, Napolitano C, Memmi M, et al. Clinical and molecular characterization of patients with catecholaminergic polymorphic ventricular tachycardia. *Circulation.* 2002;106:69–74.
14. Probst V, Denjoy I, Meregalli PG, et al. Clinical aspects and prognosis of Brugada syndrome in children. *Circulation.* 2007;115:2042–2048.
15. Villafañe J, Atallah J, Gollob MH, et al. Long-term follow-up of a pediatric cohort with short QT syndrome. *J Am Coll Cardiol.* 2013;61:1183–1191.
16. Morita H, Rehm HL, Menesses A, et al. Shared genetic causes of cardiac hypertrophy in children and adults. *N Engl J Med.* 2008;358:1899–1908.
17. Hancock EW, Deal BJ, Mirvis DM, et al. American Heart Association Electrocardiography and Arrhythmias Committee, Council on Clinical Cardiology; American College of Cardiology Foundation; Heart Rhythm Society. AHA/ACCF/HRS recommendations for the standardization and interpretation of the electrocardiogram: Part V: electrocardiogram changes associated with cardiac chamber hypertrophy. *Circulation.* 2009;119:e251–e261.
18. Lakdawala NK, Thune JJ, Maron BJ, et al. Electrocardiographic features of sarcomere mutation carriers with and without clinically overt hypertrophic cardiomyopathy. *Am J Cardiol.* 2011;108:1606–1613.
19. Rijnbeek PR, Witsenburg M, Schrama E, Hess J, Kors JA. New normal limits for the paediatric electrocardiogram. *Eur Heart J.* 2001;22:702–711.
20. Walsh MA, Grenier MA, Jefferies JL, et al. Conduction abnormalities in pediatric patients with restrictive cardiomyopathy. *Circ Heart Failure.* 2012;5:267–273.
21. Gillette PC, Nihill MR, Singer DB. Electrophysiological mechanism of the short PR interval in Pompe's disease. *Am J Dis Child.* 1974;128:622–626.
22. Kroos M, Hoogeveen-Westerveld M, van der Ploeg A, Reuser AJ. The genotype-phenotype correlation in Pompe disease. *Am J Med Genet C Semin Med Genet.* 2012;160C:59–68.
23. Kishnani PS, Corzo D, Nicolino M, et al. Recombinant human acid α-glucosidase: Major clinical benefits in infantile-onset Pompe disease. *Neurology.* 2007;68:99–109.
24. Maron BJ, Roberts WC, Arad M, et al. Clinical outcome and phenotypic expression in LAMP2 cardiomyopathy. *JAMA.* 2009;301:1253–1259.
25. Gollob MH, Green MS, Tang AS, et al. Identification of a gene responsible for familial Wolff-Parkinson-White syndrome. *N Engl J Med.* 2001;344:1823–1831.
26. Sternick EB, Oliva A, Gerken LM, et al. Clinical, electrocardiographic, and electrophysiologic characteristics of patients with a fasciculoventricular pathway: The role of PRKAG2 mutation. *Heart Rhythm.* 2011;8:58–64.
27. Raaijmakers R, Noordam C, Noonan JA, et al. Are ECG abnormalities in Noonan syndrome characteristic for the syndrome? *Eur J Pediatr.* 2008;167:1363–1367.
28. Wilkinson JD, Lowe AM, Salbert BA, et al. Outcomes in children with Noonan syndrome and hypertrophic cardiomyopathy: a study from the Pediatric Cardiomyopathy Registry. *Am Heart J.* 2012;164:442–448.
29. Fatkin D, MacRae C, Sasaki T, et al. Missense mutations in the rod domain of the lamin A/C gene as causes of dilated cardiomyopathy and conduction-system disease. *N Engl J Med.* 1999;341:1715–17124.
30. Xu T, Yang Z, Vatta M, et al. Multidisciplinary study of right ventricular dysplasia investigators. compound and digenic heterozygosity contributes to arrhythmogenic right ventricular cardiomyopathy. *J Am Coll Cardiol.* 2010;55:587–597.
31. Asimaki A, Saffitz J. Gap junctions and arrhythmogenic cardiomyopathy. *Heart Rhythm.* 2012;9:992–995.
32. Marcus FI, McKenna WJ, Sherrill D, et al. Diagnosis of arrhythmogenic right ventricular cardiomyopathy/dysplasia: Proposed modification of the task force criteria. *Circulation.* 2010;121:1533–1541.

33. Peters S, Truemmel M, Koehler B. Prognostic value of QRS fragmentation in patients with arrhythmogenic right ventricular cardiomyopathy/dysplasia. *J Cardiovasc Med (Hagerstown).* 2012;13:295–298.
34. Sen-Chowdhry S, Syrris P, Prasad SK, et al. Left-dominant arrhythmogenic cardiomyopathy: An under-recognized clinical entity. *J Am Coll Cardiol.* 2008;52:2175–2187.
35. Walsh EP, Saul JP, Hulse JE, et al. Transcatheter ablation of ectopic atrial tachycardia in young patients using radiofrequency current. *Circulation.* 1992;86:1138–1146.
36. Critelli G. Recognizing and managing permanent junctional reciprocating tachycardia in the catheter ablation era. *J Cardiovasc Electrophysiol.* 1997;8:226–236.
37. Hoffmayer KS, Bhave PD, Marcus GM, et al. An electrocardiographic scoring system for distinguishing right ventricular outflow tract arrhythmias in patients with arrhythmogenic right ventricular cardiomyopathy from idiopathic ventricular tachycardia. *Heart Rhythm.* 2013;10:477–482.
38. Zachariah JP, Walsh EP, Triedman JK, et al. Multiple accessory pathways in the young: The impact of structural heart disease. *Am Heart J.* 2012;165:87–92.
39. Shivapour JKL, Sherwin ED, Alexander ME, et al. Utility of preoperative electrophysiology studies in patients with Ebstein's anomaly undergoing the Cone procedure. *Heart Rhythm.* 2014:11;182–186.
40. Huang T. Review of current advances in the Holt-Oram syndrome. *Curr Opin Pediatr.* 2002;14:691–695.
41. Pashmforoush M, Lu JT, Chen H, et al. Nkx2-5 pathways and congenital heart disease; loss of ventricular myocyte lineage specification leads to progressive cardiomyopathy and complete heart block. *Cell.* 2004;117:373–386.
42. Young TJ, Shah AK, Lee MH, Hayes DL. Kearns-Sayre syndrome: A case report and review of cardiovascular complications. *Pacing Clin Electrophysiol.* 2005;28:454–457.
43. Huhta JC, Maloney JD, Ritter DG, Ilstrup DM, Feldt RH. Complete atrioventricular block in patients with atrioventricular discordance. *Circulation.* 1983;67:1374–1377.
44. Sherwin ED, Triedman JK, Walsh EP. Update on interventional electrophysiology in patients with congenital heart disease: Evolving solutions for complex hearts. *Circ Arrhythm Electrophysiol.* 2013;6:1032–1040.
45. Walsh EP, Cecchin F. Arrhythmias in adult patients with congenital heart disease. *Circulation.* 2007;115:534–545.
46. Collins KK, Love BA, Walsh EP, et al. Location of acutely successful radiofrequency catheter ablation of intraatrial reentrant tachycardia in patients with congenital heart disease. *Am J Cardiol.* 2000;86:969–974.
47. Mah DY, Alexander ME, Cecchin F, Walsh EP, Triedman JK. The electroanatomic mechanisms of atrial tachycardia in patients with tetralogy of Fallot and double outlet right ventricle. *J Cardiovasc Electrophysiol.* 2011;10:1540–8167.
48. Zeppenfeld K, Schalij MJ, Bartelings MM, et al. Catheter ablation of ventricular tachycardia after repair of congenital heart disease: electroanatomic identification of the critical right ventricular isthmus. *Circulation.* 2007;116:2241–2252.
49. Walsh EP, Rockenmacher S, Keane JF, et al. Late results in patients with tetralogy of Fallot repaired during infancy. *Circulation.* 1988;77:1062–1067.
50. Gatzoulis MA, Till JA, Somerville J, Redington AN. Mechanoelectrical interaction in tetralogy of Fallot. QRS prolongation relates to right ventricular size and predicts malignant ventricular arrhythmias and sudden death. *Circulation.* 1995;92:231–237.
51. Gatzoulis MA, Balaji S, Webber SA, et al. Risk factors for arrhythmia and sudden cardiac death late after repair of tetralogy of Fallot: a multicentre study. *Lancet.* 2000;356:975–981.
52. Hoffman JI. Electrocardiogram of anomalous left coronary artery from the pulmonary artery in infants. *Pediatr Cardiol.* 2013;34:489–491.

CHAPTER

6

Electrocardiographic Markers of Sudden Cardiac Death in Different Substrates

Mohammad Shenasa, MD and Hossein Shenasa, MD

INTRODUCTION

The resting electrocardiogram (ECG) is widely used and can provide valuable information on a variety of cardiac and noncardiac diseases. Besides rate and rhythm, the ECG contains significant information when applied and used appropriately. This chapter will focus on the role of recent advances of the ECG as a risk marker/predictor for sudden cardiac death (SCD) in patients with hypertension, left ventricular hypertrophy (LVH), coronary artery disease (CAD), heart failure (HF), hypertrophic cardiomyopathy (HCM), dilated cardiomyopathy (DCM), arrhythmogenic right ventricular dysplasia/cardiomyopathy (ARVD/C), cardiac sarcoidosis, and other infiltrative cardiomyopathies. We will not discuss the specific pathophysiology and management of these individual diseases mentioned above. These markers are applied into different groups:

1. Patients without apparent structural heart disease.
2. Patients with mild to overt cardiac disease.
3. Patients with genetically inherited diseases.

The latter has been less explored until recently and is well described in other chapters of this book. It is hoped that better identification and analysis of these variables and their application to populations at risk can provide an ECG-based risk-stratification algorithm. It should always be kept in mind that risk predictors are not necessarily efficacy predictors.

The last 2 decades have provided important applications of the ECG in inherited channelopathies, screening for SCD in the young and athletes, and in patients with cardiac resynchronization therapy. The use of ECG, a simple and widely applicable technique, will teach us new and important data and will be used more and more extensively into the future.

Other advanced methods of ECG analysis such as T-wave alternans, heart rate turbulence (HRT), and signal-averaged ECG are discussed elsewhere in this book.

Electrocardiographic Markers of SCD

There are several ECG markers that predict SCD in a variety of different substrates that will be discussed under their specific titles. The following markers are important to note:

1. Abnormal rest or exercise ECG.[1]
2. LVH.

The ECG Handbook of Contemporary Challenges © 2015 Mohammad Shenasa, Mark E. Josephson, N.A. Mark Estes III
Cardiotext Publishing, ISBN: 978-1-935395-88-1

3. QRS prolongation.
4. Prolonged QTc and QT dispersion.
5. Wide QRS/T angle of ≥105 degrees (as an index of abnormal depolarization–repolarization relationship).[2]
6. Fragmented QRS (fQRS).
7. T-wave alternans (see Chapter 9 by Hohnloser).[3]
8. ST-T wave abnormalities.
9. Evidence of myocardial scar and ischemia.
10. Heart rate variability (HRV) and heart rate turbulence(HRT).

QRS Duration

Increased QRS duration is a predictor of all-cause mortality as well as SCD. Previous studies have demonstrated that prolonged QRS duration is associated with increased mortality in patients with CAD, cardiomyopathies, and congestive heart failure (CHF).[4]

Kurl et al reported on the relation of QRS complex duration in resting ECG to SCD in men. The study was comprised of 2049 men aged 42 to 60 years old, with a 19-year follow-up. During this time, 156 SCDs occurred, and each 10-ms increase in QRS duration was associated with 27% higher risk for SCD.[5] Multivariable analysis showed that QRS duration was an independent predictor of the risk of SCD. Therefore, this measurement may be of value for estimating SCD risk in a large population cohort.[6–8]

The LIFE study examined the predictive value of QRS duration as a marker for SCD in patients with hypertension and LVH and reported that after aggressive control of hypertension, prolonged QRS duration was an independent marker for risk of SCD.[9] Badheka et al reported on the relationship of QRS duration on ECG and cardiovascular mortality in a large cohort of 8527 patients from the National Health and Nutrition Examination Survey data set. Using a multivariable analysis, the addition of QRS duration by 10 ms increments resulted in 4.4% increase in cardiovascular mortality ($P = 0.00006$).[10]

QRS-T Angle

Recent data from screening a large ECG database of 15,000 to 20,000 patients revealed that patients with wide QRS-T angle of ≥105 degrees chosen as a surrogate for abnormal depolarization–repolarization relationship showed a 1-year mortality and risk of SCD of 8.8% to 13.9% compared to 3.8% to 5.5% of patients with normal QRS-T wave.[2] Patients with presence of myocardial scar by QRS scoring have significantly higher risk of SCD and appropriate implantable cardioverter-defibrillator (ICD) shocks, whereas the patients with no scar have significantly lower risk of SCD and less ICD shocks.[11]

fQRS Complex

fQRS is defined by complex notching in the QRS with various multiphasic RSR′ patterns or with the presence of numerous high-frequency deflections in the presence or absence of Q waves on a 12-lead resting ECG. The QRS duration may be normal, <120 ms, or may be prolonged >120 ms. fQRS has been identified as a risk for SCD in many diseases, such as CAD,[12–14] HF,[15] HCM,[16] ARVD/C,[17] DCM,[18,19] congenital heart disease (CHD),[20] and in many types of inhered channelopathies, such as Brugada syndrome and LQT syndrome.[21] Electrophysiologically, fQRS probably represents inhomogeneous activation of the ventricles due to conduction delays and/or myocardial scar. Figure 6.1 shows different ECG patterns of fQRS in patients with SCD. Since these electrical changes are present in other pathologies, such as HCM and ARVD/C, fQRS may also be detectable in other conditions; therefore, like many other risk factors fQRS is not very disease-specific. Demonstration of fQRS also depends on the ECG recording techniques such as low-pass filter setting that is generally used at 100 or 150 Hz. It may be missed or over-diagnosed under different settings. It should be interpreted in the presence of relevant clinical diagnosis.[22]

In summary, the potential uses of fQRS include prediction of SCD, presence of postmyocardial infarction, identification of high-risk patients with Brugada syndrome, risk stratification of patients for ICD, and identification of potential ablation targets.

The Reykjavik study of risk factors for out-of-hospital cardiac arrest in a large patient cohort of 8006 men and 9435 women found the following

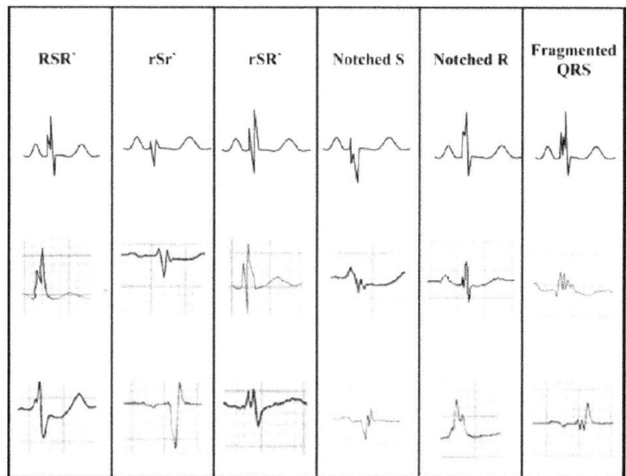

Figure 6.1. fQRS (RSR = pattern and its variants). The different morphologies of fQRS, which include various RSR = patterns, are shown. Note that if RSR = patterns are present in right precordial leads (leads V_1 and V_2) with QRS 100 ms (incomplete RBBB), or QRS 120 ms (complete RBBB) and in left precordial lead (RSR = in lead I, V_5, and V_6) with QRS 120 ms (left BBB), they are defined as complete or incomplete BBB and excluded from the definition of fQRS, whereas if the RSR = pattern is present in the midprecordial lead or in inferior leads, they are defined as fQRS. Modified with permission.[22]

ECG abnormalities: presence of Q-wave, QRS axis deviation, increased voltage, ST-segment depression, T-wave abnormalities, AV block, bundle branch block (BBB), atrial fibrillation (AF), and flutter.[23]

Table 6.1 shows the monogenic disorders associated with SCD.

Risk Factors for SCD

Risk factors for SCD have been discussed in detail in several chapters. It is beyond the scope of this chapter. The purpose here to discuss the value of ECG as a part of the risk stratification for SCD.[26–32]

It is important to link the risk factors to the specific syndrome and pathology and demonstrate cause and relation. Some risk factors have a weak link and others have a strong correlation. The multivariate analysis can help identify the degree of significance of a given risk factor to a specific condition.[27,29]

ECG Markers of SCD in Patients with Hypertension and LVH

Lewis noticed the importance of LVH and its relation to other conditions at the beginning of the twentieth century.[33]

Definition of LVH

The normal left ventricle (LV) mass is 135 g and the mass index is 71 g/m^2 for men. In women, the respective values are 99 g and 62 g/m^2. LVH is usually defined as being 2 standard deviations above normal. The prevalence of LVH by ECG, as reported by Framingham Heart Study, was 2.9% in men and 1.5% in women; whereas the echocardiographic (Echo) detection of LVH was 14.2% for men and 17.6% for women. The prevalence of ECG- and Echo-detected LVH is higher in African Americans than in Caucasians.[34]

LVH has multiple and diverse etiologies and reflects the manifestation of many cardiac and noncardiac diseases as summarized in Table 6.2.

Table 6.1. Monogenic disorders associated with SD.

Inherited Channelopathies	Inherited Cardiomyopathies
1. Long QT syndrome	1. HCM
2. Brugada syndrome	2. ARVD/C
3. Short QT syndrome	3. DCM
4. Timothy syndrome	4. Restrictive cardiomyopathy
5. Andersen-Tawil syndrome	5. (nonhypertrophic, nondilated)
6. Catecholaminergic polymorphic VT	6. Noncompaction cardiomyopathy
	7. Glycogen storage disease A. Fabry disease B. PRKAG2 C. Danon disease
	8. Mitochondrial myopathies
	9. Noonan syndrome
	10. Myofibrillar myopathies
	11. Naxos syndrome
	12. Carvajal syndrome

VT, ventricular tachycardia; PRKAG2, protein kinase, AMP-activated, gamma-2 noncatalytic subunit. Adapted with permission.[24,25]

ECG Criteria

LVH is characterized by the sum of (S wave in lead V_1 + R wave in lead V_5 or V_6) ≥ 3.5 mV in V_1 + RV_5 or R wave in V_5 or V_6 >2.6mV (Sokolow–Lyon voltage criteria).

Cornell voltage criteria: For men, S wave in lead V_3 + R wave in aVL > 28 mm (2.8 mV). For women, S wave in lead V_3 + R wave in lead aVL > 20 mm (2.0 mV).[46]

ECG Manifestation of Hypertension

Long-term hypertension produces a LVH pattern consistent with LVH criteria as discussed above, and a downsloping, convex ST segment with inverted asymmetrical T-wave at the opposite direction of QRS axis in leads V_5 or V_6. Furthermore, P-wave abnormalities are also identified. These changes increase the risk of HF, SCD, and AF. Thus, new-onset AF in hypertensive patients with LVH puts these patients at a higher risk of SCD.[47] Aggressive hypertension management may result in resolution of some of these ECG changes. Specifically, regression of LVH can often be observed. Furthermore, in patients with hypertension and LVH, regression of LV mass during antihypertensive therapy is associated with lower rates of clinical endpoints.[48–51] Similarly, regression of ECG LVH in patients with hypertension is associated with decreased incidence of new-onset AF.[52]

ECG manifestations of LVH:[9]

1. Increased QRS voltage.
2. Increased QRS prolongation: the results of the LIFE study show that QRS duration predicts SCD in hypertensive patients.
3. Left-axis deviation.
4. Repolarization abnormalities (ST-T wave abnormalities).
5. Left atrial abnormality.

This may be a normal variant in athletes and the young. Electrical axis is generally horizontal and occasionally left-axis deviation (LAD). The LVH is usually measured as 2 standard deviations above normal. Normalization to height might be more accurate. The diagnostic value of LVH by ECG is 2.4%. Thus, this criterion is not very specific.[53–55]

Table 6.2. Etiologies and ECG characteristics of LVH.

Diseases	ECG	Comments
1. Hypertension[35]	LVH, nonspecific ST-T wave abnormalities	Increases the risk of AF, VA, and SCD; Echo: Concentric LVH
2. Hypertensive heart disease[35]	LVH, LAE, non-specific ST-T wave abnormalities	Echo: Concentric LVH, LAE, diastolic dysfunction
3. Aortic stenosis	LVH, non-specific ST-T wave abnormalities	Echo: Concentric LVH, LAE; MRI: Mid-wall fibrosis by LGE; Ischemia during treadmill testing
4. Obesity	LVH, non-specific ST-T wave abnormalities	Echo: Diastolic dysfunction, LAE
5. HCM[36]	LVH, Q wave[37], anterior T-wave inversion	Echo: Asymmetric LVH (Septal hypertrophy); MRI: Fibrosis by LGE MRI; Contrast-enhanced MRI
6. LV non-compaction[39]	LVH, LBBB, non-specific ST-T wave abnormalities, AF, VA (up to 60%)	Echo: LVH, increased trabeculation, noncompaction pattern; MRI: LGE
Physiological LVH		
7. Athlete's heart[40]	LVH, LAE, ST-T wave abnormalities	Echo: LVH, enlarged LV cavity, normalized detraining
Infiltrative Cardiomyopathies		
8. Amyloidosis[41]	Low voltage QRS, LAE, LAD, AV block	Echo: LVH; ECG Echo mismatch; MRI CMR
9. Sarcoidosis[43]	AV block, LAD, RBBB, LBBB	Cardiac PET; MRI
10. Hemochromotasis[44]	LVH, non-specific ST-T wave abnormalities, AF, RVH, LAE	Echo; MRI
Metabolic disorders		
11. Fabry disease[45]	LVH; nonspecific ST-T wave abnormalities, RVH; heart block	Echo; MRI
12. Pompe disease[25]	LVH; RVH; heart block	Echo; MRI
13. Danon disease[24,25]	LVH; RVH; heart block	Echo; MRI

AV, atrioventricular; AF, atrial fibrillation; Echo, echocardiogram; LAE, left atrial enlargement; LGE, late enhancement; LVH, left ventricular hypertrophy; MRI, magnetic resonance imaging; PET, positron emission tomography; RVH, right ventricular hypertrophy; SCD, sudden cardiac death; VA, ventricular arrhythmias.

Echocardiographic Criteria

The current Echo criteria for LVH is ≥134 g/m^2 in men and ≥110 g/m^2 in women. Normalization to height and body surface might be more accurate. LVH occurs in 15% to 20% of hypertensive patients.

Left ventricular mass (g) = 1.05 [(LVEDD + IVS + PW)^3 – LVEDD^3]. Left ventricular mass was divided by body surface area to obtain the left ventricular mass index (LVMI). LVH was defined as LVMI ≥ 150 g/m^2 according to the data from Framingham Heart Study. The diagnostic yield of LVH by Echo is 17.4%. (IVS = Intraventricular Septum)[55–57]

Hypertensive Heart Disease (HHD)

HHD is defined as the anatomical and physiological changes (adaptations) of heart muscles, coronary arteries, and great vessels to hypertension. These changes in heart structure and function results in LVH, hemodynamic changes (i.e., left atrial enlargement, diastolic dysfunction, functional mitral regurgitation), and neurohormonal changes, which promote fibrosis and atrial and ventricular arrhythmias (VAs).[35,58]

HHD occurs in association with elevated arterial blood pressure. Its manifestations include increased LV mass, diastolic dysfunction, left atrial enlargement, coronary flow abnormalities, and interstitial fibrosis.

Echocardiographically, HHD demonstrates LVH evidence of diastolic dysfunction and left atrial enlargement.[58]

ECG predictors of SCD in patients with LVH:

1. Prolonged PR interval.
2. Incomplete or complete right or left bundle branch block (RBBB or LBBB).
3. Bi-fascicular block.
4. QT interval prolongation and dispersion.
5. ST-T wave abnormalities.[59]
6. QRS duration.
7. Late potentials.
8. fQRS.
9. VAs on Holter monitoring.

10. HRV.
11. Programmed electrical stimulation.

Arrhythmias that are seen in patients with LVH include AF, ventricular extrasystoles, couplets, nonsustained ventricular tachycardia (VT), sustained VT, and SCDs. LVH increases the overall mortality by 59% over 12 years. LVH significantly increases the risk of CAD (by 3- to 4-fold), SCD (by 6- to 8-fold for men and 3-fold for women), CHF by 10-fold, cerebrovascular accidents, and VAs. ECG-LVH is an independent risk factor and prognostic significance for incident AF.[60] During 4 years follow-up in the Framingham Heart Study, each 50 g/m increase in LV mass was associated with a 1.49 increase in relative risk of cardiovascular disease for men and 1.57 for women. The effect on cardiovascular mortality was even more striking, with a 1.73 relative risk for each 50 g/m for men and 2.12 for women.[34,61]

Causes of LVH include:

Concentric LVH: Systemic pressure overload: (1) hypertension (the most common cause); (2) aortic stenosis; and (3) static exercise.

Eccentric LVH: Left ventricular volume overload: (1) aortic; (2) mitral regurgitation; and (3) DCM.

Other risk factors: LVH and AF in hypertensive patients include age, race (LVH in African Americans), gender, salt intake, weight (obesity), diabetes, hypercholesterolemia, renin-angiotensin-aldosterone system, level of diurnal and nocturnal systolic blood pressure during 24-hour monitoring, left atrial diameter, left ventricular mass, catecholamines, genetic and environmental factors, maximum duration, and dispersion of the P wave of the ECG.[61]

Why Is LVH Arrhythmogenic?

1. *Electrogenesis of VAs in patients with LVH:* Hemodynamic effects, pressure overload, volume overload, and contraction–excitation feedback.[62]
2. *Neuroendocrine effect:* Catecholamines, renin-angiotensin system activation, and electrolyte depletion.

LVH produces microvascular myocardial ischemia. Silent ischemia is present in 90% of cases and is correlated with the presence of LVH. Wall stress, increased levels of catecholamines, CHF, and diastolic dysfunction are also produced by LVH; all of which can potentially produce enlarged myocytes. Hypokalemia, genetic factors, environmental factors, and myocardial fibrosis are among other risk factors. The above contributing risks alone or in combination may potentially trigger early after-depolarization and delayed after-depolarization, T wave or repolarization alternans, increased automaticity, and reentry leads to SCD. Figure 6.2 summarizes the electromechanical

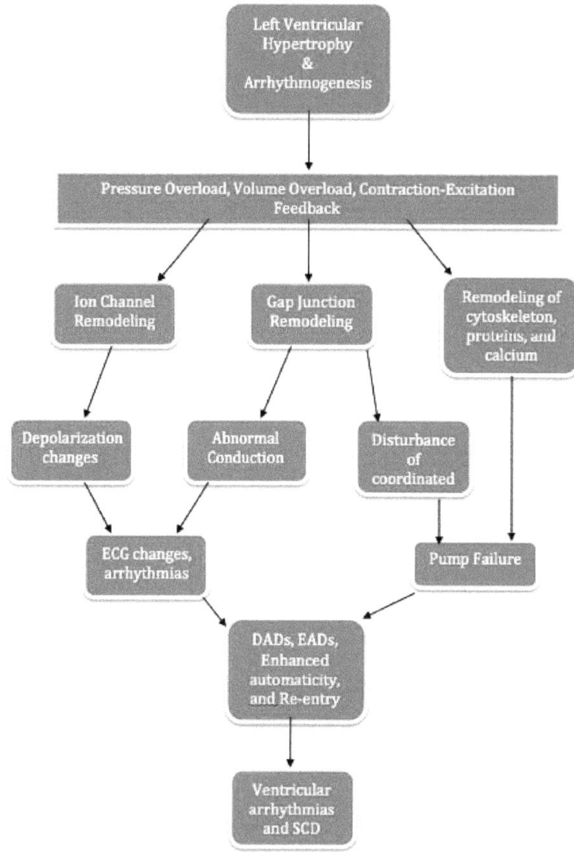

Figure 6.2. The potential mechanisms of relationship between LVH and arrhythmogenesis. DAD, delayed after-depolarizations; EAD, early after-depolarizations; SCD, sudden cardiac death. Modified with permission.[62]

pathways of LVH arrhythmogenesis. Summarized in one sentence, LVH is recognized as a silent killer; however, it is preventable and treatable.[49,63]

The natural history of severe LVH usually ends with HF where the presence of above arrhythmias has a poor prognosis. Benjamin and Levy once said: "LVH is a lethal attribute and is associated with a doubling in mortality."[34]

Differential Diagnosis of LVH[64]

1. Physiological hypertrophy, which is often seen in athletes with LVH.
2. HCM.
3. LVH due to infiltrative cardiomyopathies such as cardiac amyloidosis, sarcoidosis, and mitochondrial myopathy.

Figure 6.3 illustrates an algorithm and appropriate use of imaging tests for the differential diagnosis of LVH.[64]

Similarly, Namdar et al reported on the specific ECG patterns in differentiation of HHD, HCM, aortic stenosis, amyloidosis, and Fabry disease.[65]

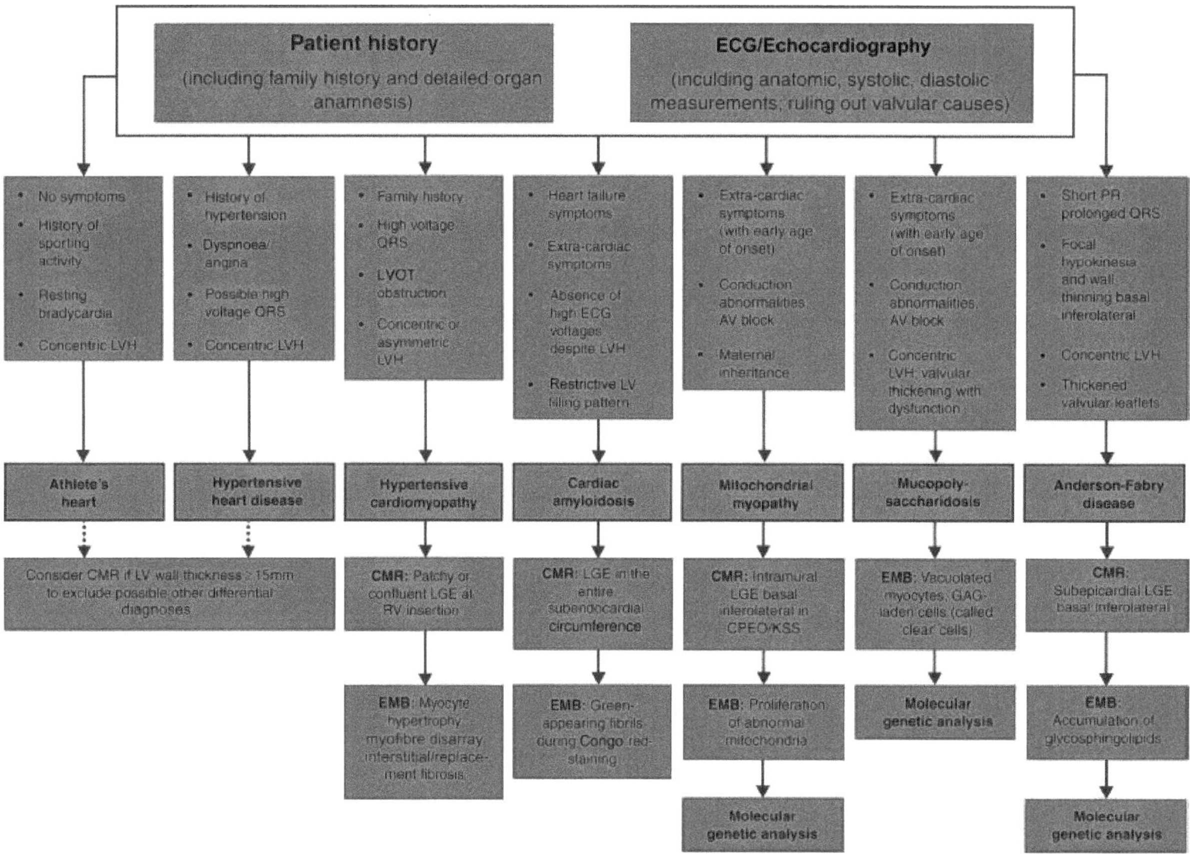

Figure 6.3. Diagnostic approach to the underlying diagnosis of (nonvalvular) LVH. AV, atrioventricular; CMR, cardiac magnetic resonance; CPEO, chronic progressive external ophthalmoplegia; EMB, endomyocardial biopsy; GAG, glycosaminoglycans; KSS, Kearns-Sayre syndrome; LGE, late gadolinium enhancement; LV, left ventricular; LVH, left ventricular hypertrophy; LVOT, left ventricular outflow tract; RV, right ventricular. Modified with permission.[64]

ECG Markers of SCD in Patients with CAD

It has been long recognized that resting ECG abnormalities are common in patients with CAD and allied syndromes; i.e., acute and sub-acute myocardial infractions and ischemia. It is a useful test for risk stratification and prediction of cardiovascular events. The resting ECG has already been implemented into the risk-factor models for CAD. The ECG is also very useful to evaluate the response to medical and interventional therapies in these patients. The ECG changes in CAD are summarized below.

ECG abnormalities:

1. Q or QS-wave abnormalities.
2. LVH.
3. Prolonged QRS duration.
4. QT prolongation and QT dispersion.[66]
5. fQRS.[12,14]
6. Complete or incomplete BBB.
7. Left anterior hemiblock is an independent predictor of total and cardiac mortality in patients with suspected CAD who have no history of MI.[67]
8. AF and/or atrial flutter.
9. Significant ST-T wave abnormalities.

Auer et al reported on the association of major and minor ECG abnormalities in patients with CAD and subsequent cardiovascular events. The study revealed that both minor and major ECG abnormalities were associated with increased risk of cardiovascular events in those patients.[68]

Soliman et al reported on how a detailed clinical and ECG analysis can differentiate ECG predictors separating atherosclerotic SCD from incident CAD. Although both syndromes share common risk factors such as hypertension, race, ethnicity, obesity, heart rate, QTc, and ST-T wave abnormalities, the magnitude of T-wave inversion in any ECG lead group and the level of ST elevation in V_2 have the potential to separate between the risk of SCD and CAD.[69]

ECG Markers of SCD in Patients with HF

HF is now one of the epidemics of the twenty-first century in medicine[70] and is a common cause of SCD.

Both HF with decreased systolic function and those with preserved systolic function (diastolic dysfunction) have diverse and often multiple etiologies; thus, single markers are neither usually sensitive nor specific. Multiple previous studies have demonstrated evidence of a relationship between HF and SCD. There are no reliable ECG findings specific for HF or those predictive of SCD. Interestingly, QRS duration is a good predictor of response and outcome to CRT.[71] However, the following abnormalities are often noticed, and they depend on the underlying etiologies and substrate of HF.

1. LVH is an independent risk of developing new-onset CHF in patients with hypertension.[48]
2. Evidence of prior myocardial infarction (presence of Q-wave).
3. QRS prolongation (≥120 ms): progressive increase in the QRS duration worsens the prognosis of HF. 14% to 47% of patients with HF show QRS prolongation on their ECGs.[71]
4. Intraventricular conduction delay.
5. BBB (more LBBB than RBBB).
6. Nonspecific ST-T wave abnormalities.
7. Wide QRS/T angle and low TV_5 amplitude.[72–74] Similarly, this measurement is useful to predict incident HF in patients with or without BBB.[75]
8. Wide $\theta(T_p|T_{ref})$, wide θ(R|STT), and increased QRS nondipolar voltage in women and wide $\theta(T_p|T_{ref})$, increased epicardial repolarization time, prolonged T_pT_e interval and T-wave complexity in men were independent predictors of incident HF.[76]
9. QT and QTc prolongation.
10. Presence of atrial and VAs.
11. J wave and fQRS in the inferior leads are associated with increased risk of SCD in patients with chronic HF in both dilated nonischemic as well as ischemic cardiomyopathy.[15]

Although VAs are not a specific marker for SCD, they increase all-cause mortality.[77]

A study by Shamim et al reported that intraventricular conduction delay and QTc prolongation were strong predictors of increased mortality.[78]

HRT is reported to be a powerful risk predictor for HF and arrhythmic death in patients with class II and III CHF.[79]

ECG Markers of SCD in Patients with HCM

HCM is characterized by a thickened LV, but not dilated LV in the absence of cardiac or noncardiac conditions, such as hypertension, aortic valve stenosis, and athlete's heart.

HCM is the most common genetic disease of the heart (autosomal dominant) and is a disease of sarcomere protein genes. It has a prevalence of 1 in 500 among the general population. SCD in HCM occurs in 1% to 2% per year in adult patients and 2% to 6% per year in children and adolescents.[44,80,81] The diagnosis of HCM is based on the detection of increased LV-wall thickness by any imaging modality.

ECG Characteristics of HCM[82]

The ECG is abnormal in 90% of symptomatic patients and is characterized in the following list.

1. LVH by voltage criteria.
2. Marked ST-T wave abnormalities and T-wave inversion in lateral precordial leads (coved ST-segment elevation in lateral chest leads).
3. Deep, narrow Q waves in aVL, and V_6 (≥40 ms).
4. Diminished R wave in lateral precordial leads.
5. LAE.

Abnormal Q waves (Q wave >3 mm in depth and/or >40 ms in athletes in 2 leads except aVR) are one of the most common ECG abnormalities in young patients with HCM. Interestingly, the Q waves may disappear with increasing age, especially when concentric LVH develops.[37,83] In about 6% of patients with clinical presentation and Echo evidence of HCM, the ECG may be normal upon presentation. This subset of patients appears to have a less severe phenotype with better cardiovascular outcome.[84]

The pathophysiological mechanisms of the Q wave in HCM are not fully understood; however, it is assumed that it may be related to the ratio of the upper anterior septal thickness and other regions of the LVs and right ventricles (RVs). Wider Q waves in this subset of patients are reported to be associated with late gadolinium enhancement (LGE).[85] In 5% of the patients, the ECG may be normal especially in the early phases of the disease.

Figure 6.4 illustrates typical ECG (panel A), long-axis Echo (panel B), and magnetic resonance imaging (MRI) of a patient with HCM (panel C).

The most important differential diagnosis is athlete's heart and LVH due to hypertension (see Chapter 4). In this case, other noninvasive imaging techniques, such as Echo and cardiac MRI, are valuable.[86] HCM patients show an unusual pattern of LV hypertrophy with a small LV cavity (<35 mm), LAE, abnormal LV filling, positive family history, abnormal genetic profile, whereas patients with athletic heart demonstrate LV cavity of >55 mmHg, have normal LV filling, no family history, and negative HCM genetic profile. Bizarre ECG patterns and LAE are often seen in athletic individuals.[87] Interestingly, with detraining, most of these changes will normalize in athletes.

Risk factors associated with an increased risk of sudden death (SD) in HCM[88,89]:

1. Family history of HCM with SCD.
2. History of syncope or presyncope.

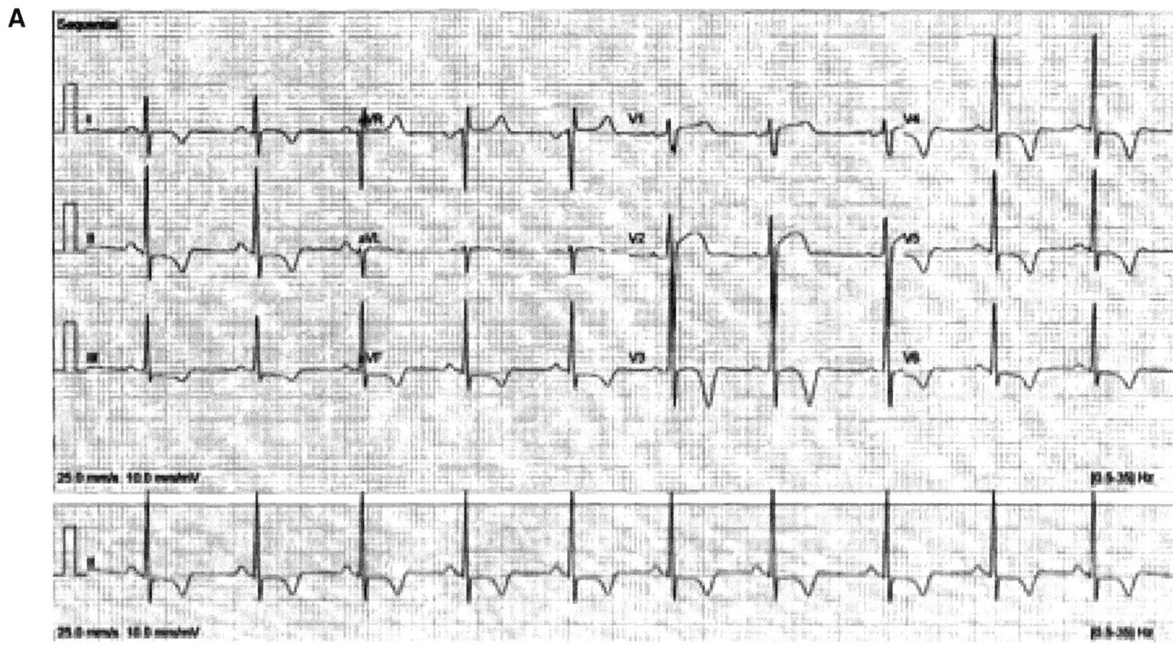

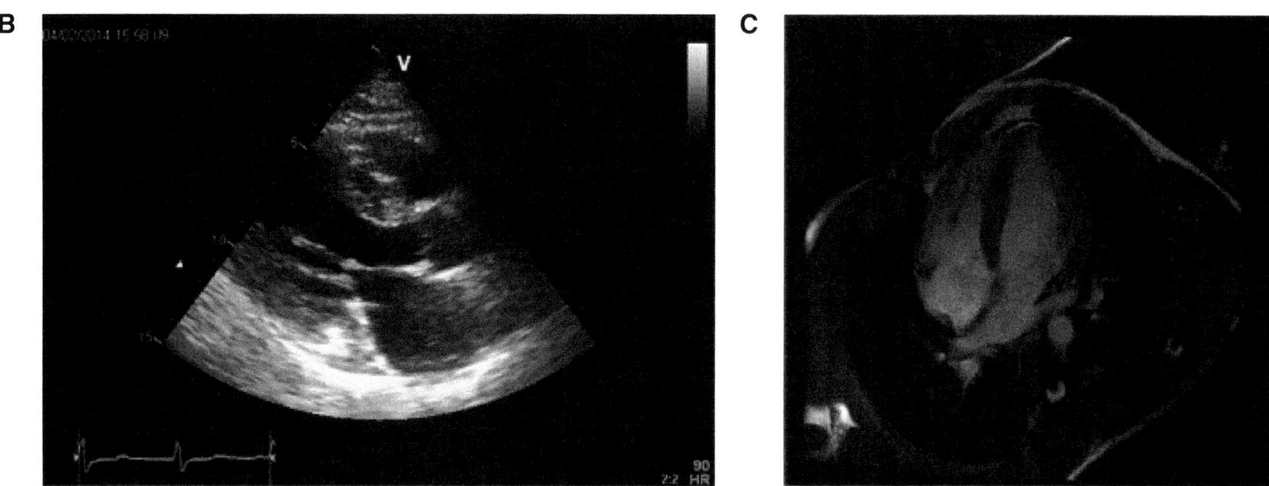

Figure 6.4. ECG, Echo, and MRI in a patient with HCM. **A**: 12-Lead ECG of a patient with HCM shows marked LVH with marked negative T wave in V_3 to V_6 and I, II, III, and aVF leads. **B**. Echocardiogram of the same patient as in panel A. Parasternal long-axis view showing significant septal hypertrophy of 19 mm and of a posterior wall of 4 mm. **C**. Cardiac MRI long-axis view showing septal hypertrophy.

3. Massive LV hypertrophy (septal wall thickness > 30 mm).
4. Survived SCD.
5. Nonsustained VT.
6. Abnormal blood pressure response to exercise.

ECG markers of HCM and SCD:

1. Massive LVH: Specific patterns of LVH is not predictive of cardiac events and SCD; however, mild, localized wall thickness is generally associated with lower risk independent of its location.[90]
2. Frequent PVCs and nonsustained VT.
3. AF (incidence is about 20%).
4. fQRS[91,92]
5. ECG amplitudes: HCM patients with cardiac arrest and/or SCD have substantially higher ECG amplitudes compared to HCM patients without such history.[93]
6. LAE.

Risk stratification of SCD in HCM (Figure 6.5)[36]

Patients with the highest risk profile

1. History of cardiac arrest, sustained VT, or sustained ventricular fibrillation (VF).
2. Family history of HCM and SCD.
3. History of unexplained syncope or near-syncope.
4. Repetitive nonsustained VT.
5. Massive LVH more than 30 mm.

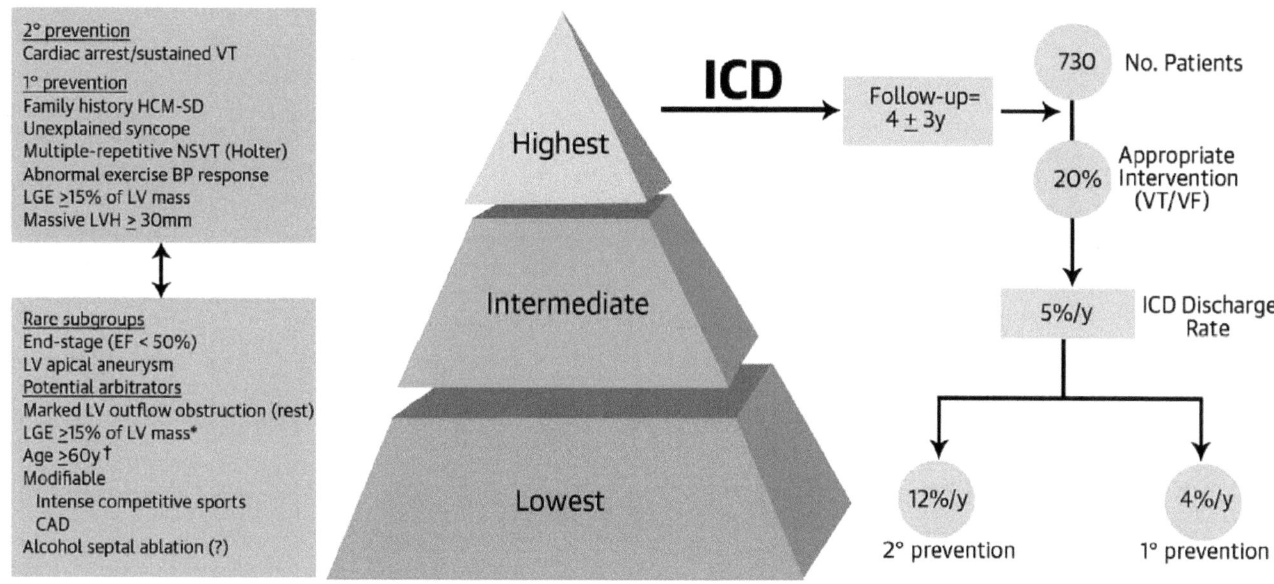

Figure 6.5. Risk stratification model in patients with HCM. Pyramid profile of risk stratification model currently used to identify patients at the highest SD risk who may be candidates for ICDS and SD prevention. Major and minor risk markers appear in boxes at the left. At the right are the results of ICD therapy in 730 children, adolescents, and adults assembled from 2 registry studies. Extensive LGE is a novel primary risk marker that can also be used as an arbitrator when conventional risk assessment is ambiguous. SD events are uncommon after 60 years of age, even with conventional risk factors. BP, blood pressure; CAD, coronary artery disease; EF, ejection fraction; ICD, implantable cardioverter-defibrillator; LV, left ventricular; LGE, late gadolinium enhancement; LVH, left ventricular hypertrophy; NSVT, nonsustained VT; SD, sudden death; VT/VF, ventricular tachycardia/ventricular fibrillation; y, years. Modified with permission. *Extensive LGE is a novel primary risk marker that can also be used as an arbitrator when conventional risk assessment is ambiguous. †SD events are uncommon after 60 years of age, even with conventional risk factors [36]

6. Abnormal exercise blood pressure response.
7. LGE.
8. Progression to HF.
9. HCM-specific mutations.
10. AF.

Patients with medium- to low-risk profile

1. Mild to moderate LVH.
2. Myocardial bridging.[94]
3. Left ventricular apical aneurysm.
4. Left ventricular outflow obstruction.
5. Intense physical exertion.

For full details, the readers are referred to the recent 2014 ESC guidelines on diagnosis and management of HCM.[80]

Recent data suggest that noninvasive contrast-enhanced cardiovascular magnetic resonance imaging surrogate for myocardial fibrosis can be used as a risk predictor for cardiovascular event and SCD.[38,95] However, in asymptomatic individuals, myocardial bridging does not appear to increase the risk of cardiac events.[96]

Other imaging techniques, biomarkers, and genetic tests are being used to confirm the diagnostic, prognostic, and differential diagnosis value of ECG findings. Needless to say, none of the tests are 100% accurate. At present, the overall yield of genetic testing in the largest cohort of HCM patients is about 34%.[38,97]

ECG Markers of SCD in Patients with DCM

Definition

DCM is characterized by impaired systolic left ventricular function and HF with diverse etiologies, such as valvular heart disease, viral infections, excess alcohol, hypertension, and postpartum. In many cases, the etiology remains unknown and is referred to as idiopathic DCM.[98] Idiopathic DCM is characterized by unexplained LV dilatation, impaired systolic left ventricular function, and HF. Both HF and arrhythmias in idiopathic DCM have a genetic basis and is beyond the discussion of this review.

For the purpose of this review, idiopathic DCM is referred to as DCM.

The ECG of Patients with DCM

The resting ECG shows PR interval prolongation, low voltage, nonspecific intraventricular conduction delay or LBBB morphology, and ST-T wave abnormalities. Lateral leads show fQRS, lack of inferior Q-waves, and lead V_6 S/R ratio.

S-to-R ratios of equal or more than 0.25 are highly suggestive of DCM patterns. Atrial and VAs may be detected on the ECG or during long-term monitoring.[99] Intracardiac electrogram recordings demonstrate prolonged HV interval.

Arrhythmias in DCM include sinus node dysfunction, AF, conduction abnormalities, VT, VF, and SCD.

ECG of Patients During VT

Most VTs are due to bundle branch reentry VT (BBre-VT) demonstrate a typical LBBB pattern or less often a RBBB pattern. Some patients may have both morphologies of tachycardia. BBre-VT may be similar in morphology to the QRS morphology during sinus rhythm. Figure 6.6 shows an example of BBre-VT. The diagnostic criteria for BBre-VT has been discussed elsewhere.[100–102]

VTs and SCDs are common in this group of patients. LBBB reentry VT is a common mechanism in these patients; however, nonBBre-VTs are often inducible.

SCD due to VT are reported in up to 60% of patients with DCM. The remaining patients often present with progressive HF. First- and second-degree AV block is also seen in the patients with DCM and increases the risk of SCD. Multiform premature ventricular complexes, ventricular couplets, and nonsustained VT are very common in patients with DCM. AF indicates a poor prognosis in these patients. Other abnormal ECG variables are abnormal signal average ECG, QT dispersion, and micro T-wave alternans.

Many nonBBre-VTs arise from the epicardium and the ECG markers are well described elsewhere and are not the purpose of this communication.[99]

Risk Stratification

Presence of the following indicates high risk of SCD with DCM.

1. History of SCD.
2. Conduction disturbances and BBB.
3. LVEF ≤ 35%.
4. Presence of VAs.
5. AF.
6. History of syncope.
7. Family history of SCD prior to the age of 35.
8. Lack of β-blocker use.[103]

Whereas, signal-averaged ECG, baro-reflex sensitivity, HRV, and T-wave alternans were not among significant risk predictors for arrhythmic events.[104]

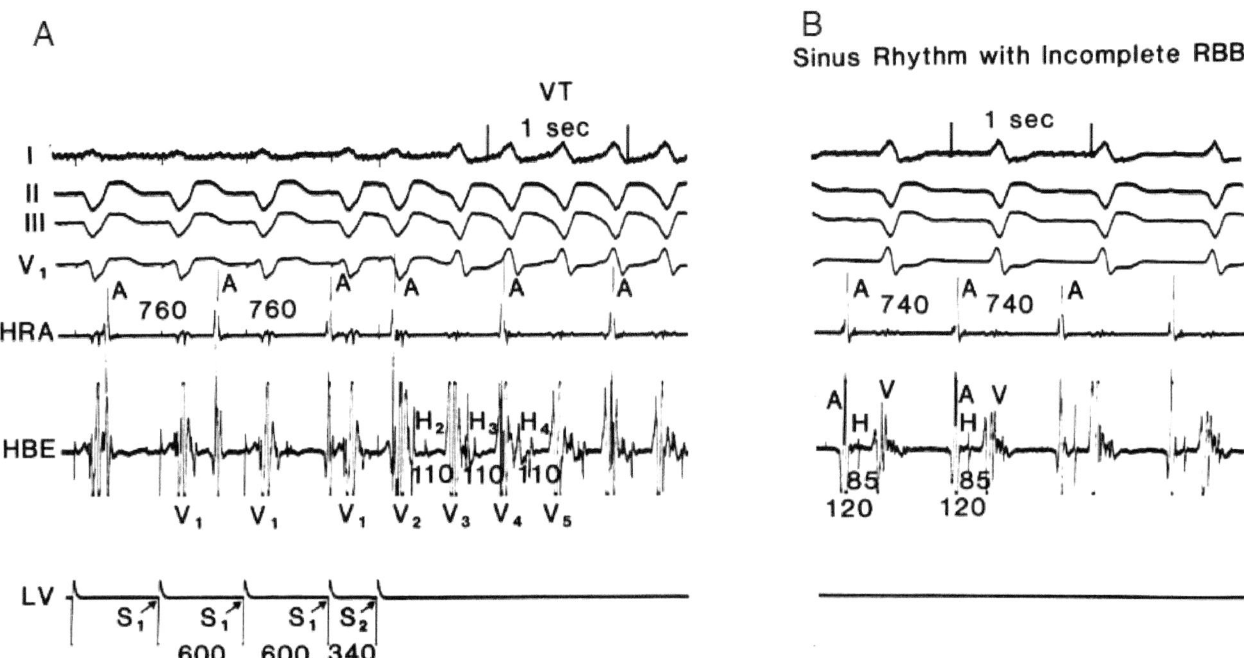

Figure 6.6. Inducible VT in a patient with DCM. A: Induction of BBre-VT during program stimulation. Note that there is a HIS bundle deflection preceding each ventricular electrogram. The HV-interval measures 110 ms. B: Sinus rhythm shows incomplete RBBB morphology and the HV-interval measures 85 ms. Note that the VT morphology is with RBBB and left-axis deviation similar to the one in sinus rhythm. Tracings are arranged as lead I, II, III, V_1, high right atrium (HRA), HIS bundle electrogram (HBE), and left ventricular stimulus artifact (LV). Note ventriculoatrial dissociation during VT.

ECG Markers of SCD in Patients with ARVD/C

Definition

ARVD/C is a genetic form of infiltrative cardiomyopathy and is characterized by fibrofatty infiltration/replacement of the RV and/or LV. ARVD/C is now classified under the umbrella of arrhythmogenic cardiomyopathies. It may present with: (1) concealed phase, which includes subtle RV changes with or without VT and SD may occur; (2) overt electrical and structural disorders, which include symptomatic VT, where VF and SCD may occur; (3) RV failure; and (4) final stage with LV failure, this stage may mimic DCM. Its presentation ARVD/C accounts for about 20% of cases of SCD in young athletes and its prevalence is higher in Mediterranean and Middle Eastern regions than other areas. Several reviews have described the diagnostic criteria for ARVD/C which includes a combination of major and minor criteria that are beyond the discussion of this communication. ARVD/C is characterized by: (1) global or regional dysfunctional and structural alterations in RV, LV, or both; (2) specific tissue characterization; (3) depolarization and repolarization abnormalities; (4) CHF; (5) arrhythmias (ventricular specific to ARVD/C and atrial related to its progression); and (6) family history.[105–107] Its clinical presentation is with VA, CHF, syncope, and SCD. In patients with documented ARVD/C, the cause of death are SCD in 29%, progressive HF in 59%, extra-cardiac causes in 8%, and unknown in 4%.[108,109] The diagnostic criteria (major and minor) of ARVD/C is discussed in detail elsewhere.[110,111]

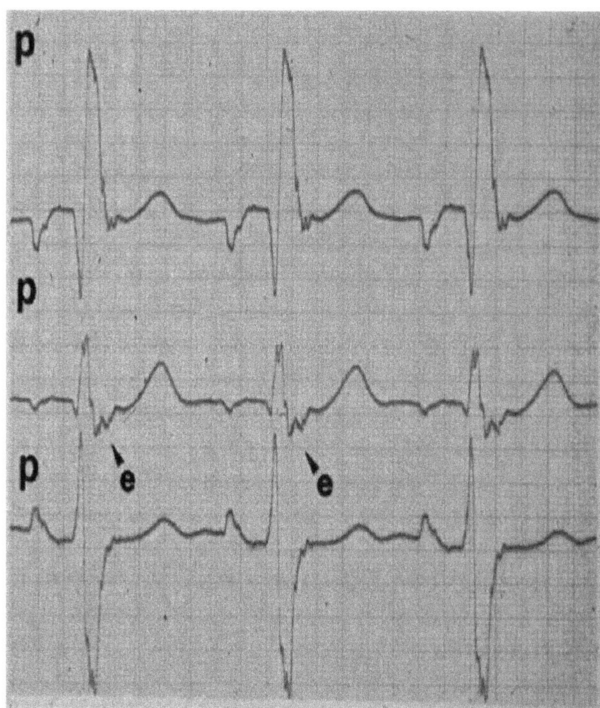

Figure 6.7. Example of an epsilon wave ("e" arrows) at the tail end of the QRS in a patient with ARVD/C. Three ECG leads are presented (*p* = P waves). Courtesy: Guy Fontaine.

ECG Characteristics of ARVD/C

Approximately 40% to 50% of patients with ARVD/C have a normal ECG in the early phase of the disease. However, after 6 years of the initial presentation, almost all patients will demonstrate one or more of the several ECG findings that are discussed below.

- RV enlargement.
- Right precordial ECG abnormalities.
    - T-wave inversion in V_1 to V_3 (46%–85% of the cases), broad S-wave upstroke.
    - QRS prolongation ≥110 ms (in 64% of cases).
    - Epsilon wave (in 25%–33% of cases)[112,110,108,113] (Figure 6.7).
    - QRS and QT dispersion.
    - Prolonged S-wave upstroke in V_1 to V_3 (Delayed S-wave upstroke) is the most frequent ECG finding in ARVD/C and is considered as a diagnostic ECG marker.[110]
    - fQRS more than ≥120 ms.
    - The differential diagnosis of ECG patterns of ARVD/C includes Brugada syndrome, acute myocardial infarction, myocarditis, and hypotheramia.

The ECG criteria has been discussed in detail elsewhere.[109,114-116]

ECG Characteristics of VT in Patients with ARVD/C

VT in patients with ARVD/C generally shows LBBB and superior axis morphology (Figure 6.8A). Multiple VT morphologies are often detected in spontaneous or induced VTs.

An important differential diagnosis is VT from RV outflow tracked origin VT (RVOT-VT). VT with LBBB/superior axis rules out RVOT-VT.[117]

The QRS duration of VTs in ARVD/C is generally longer than those from those with RVOT-VT. This differential diagnosis has significant therapeutic implications, as RVOT-VTs are amenable to radiofrequency ablation with high success rate, whereas VTs in ARVD/C are more difficult to ablate and have high recurrence rate. Hoffmayer et al proposed an ECG scoring system to differentiate RVOT-VT from VTs due to ARVD/C.[117] Such a transition at V_6 was exclusively seen in ARVD/C patients.[118]

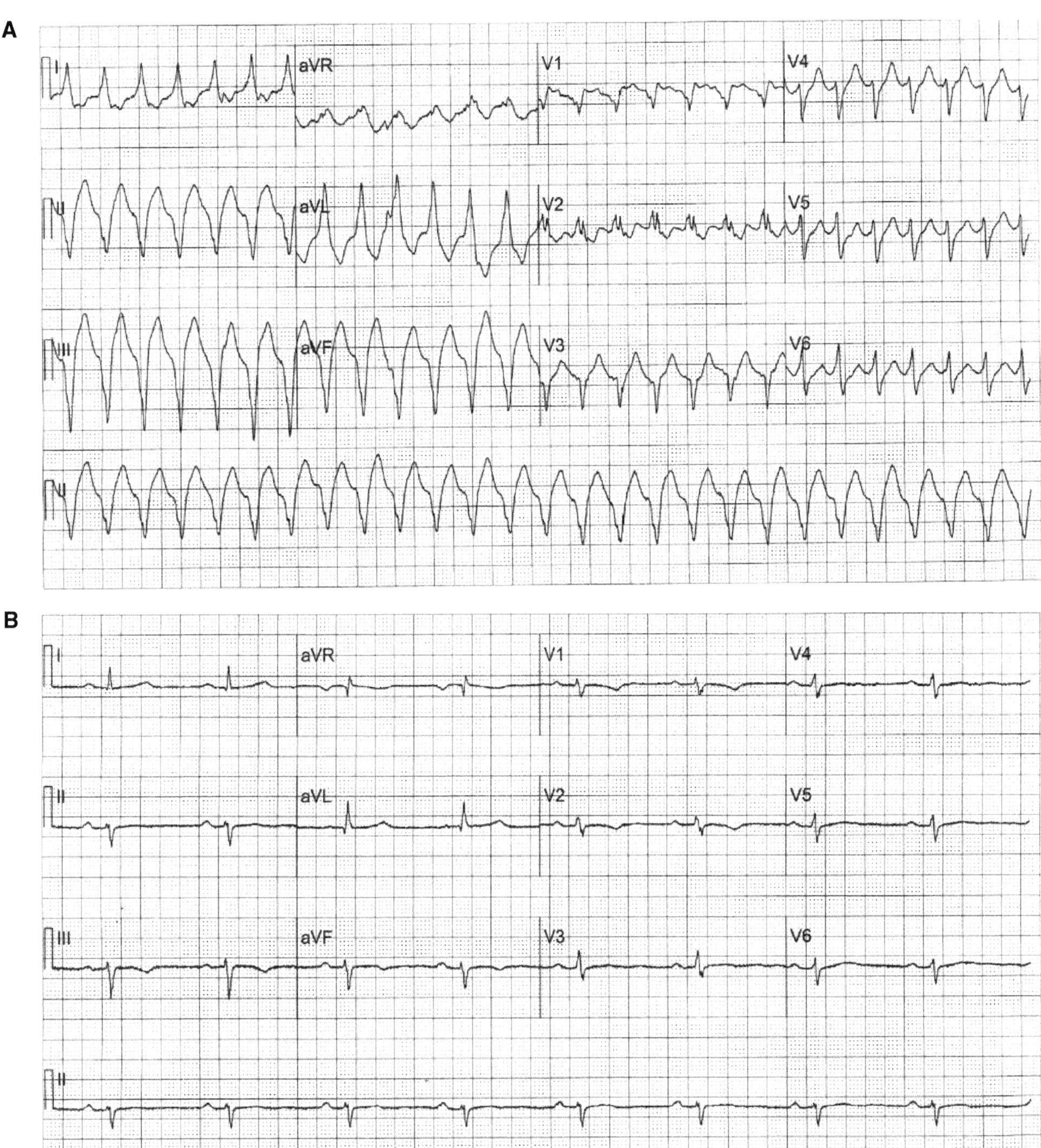

Figure 6.8. Twelve-lead ECG of VT in a patient with ARVD/C. **A.** A 12-lead ECG of a 61-year-old male with VT, LBBB morphology, and left-axis deviation. **B.** A 12-lead ECG of the same patient during sinus rhythm. Courtesy: Frank Marcus, University of Arizona Health Sciences Hospital, Tucson, AZ.

Risk stratification, predictors of VAs, and SCD in patients with ARVD/C[107,119–121] (Figure 6.9):

- History of cardiac arrest or syncope.
- Family history of ARVD/C or unexplained SCD.
- Extensive RV dysfunction and right HF.
- LV involvement.
- Intolerable or pleomorphic VT.
- Syncope.
- Endurance exercise.
- Unsuccessful antiarrhythmic drug treatment.
- Epsilon wave or late potential (signal-averaged ECG).
- QRS dispersion (>40 ms).

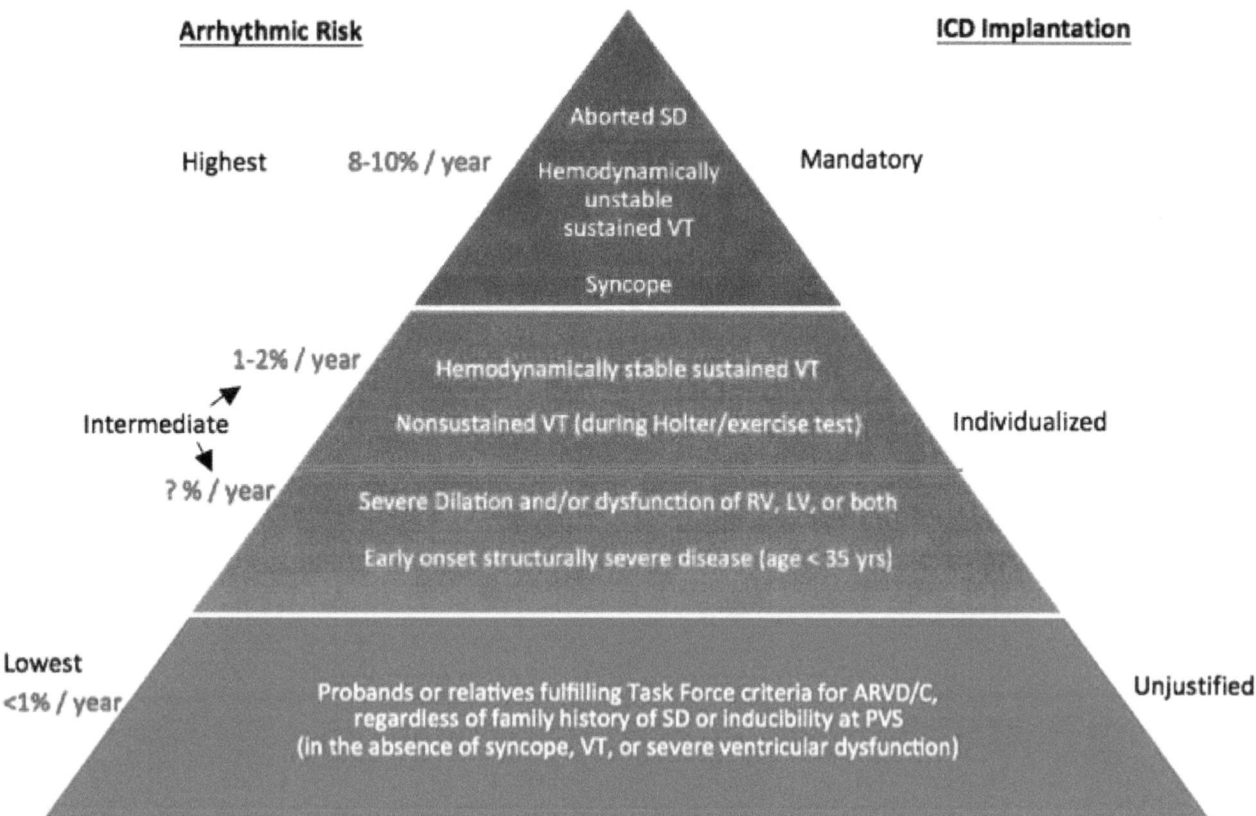

Figure 6.9. Risk-stratification model of patients with ARVD/C. Arrhythmic risk-stratification pyramid and current indications for implantation of an ICD based on observational studies on ICD therapy in ARVC/D. The best candidates for ICD therapy are patients with prior cardiac arrest and those with VT with hemodynamically unstable VT (i.e., associated with syncope or shock); syncope which remains unexplained after exclusion of noncardiac causes and vasovagal mechanisms is also considered a valuable predictor of SD and represents *per se* an indication for ICD implantation. ICD implantation for primary prevention in the general ARVC/D population seems to be unjustified. Patients with ARVC/D with no sustained VT or VF, asymptomatic probands, and relatives do not benefit from ICD therapy, regardless of familial SD or inducibility at programmed ventricular stimulation (PVS). Patients with well tolerated sustained or nonsustained VT on Holter or exercise testing have an intermediate arrhythmic risk. In this patient subgroup, the decision for implanting an ICD needs to be individualized; antiarrhythmic drug therapy (including β-blockers) and/or catheter ablation seems to be a reasonable first-line therapy. Whether, in the absence of syncope or significant VAs, severe dilation and/or dysfunction of the RV, LV or both, as well as early-onset structurally severe disease (age <35 years) require prophylactic ICD remains to be determined. Modified with permission.[122]

- fQRS.
- T-wave inversion beyond V_3 ≥120 ms.
- History of CHF.
- Young age at diagnosis.
- Any induced VT or VF.

Cardiac magnetic resonance is of great value in diagnosis of ARVD/C, and is currently included in the diagnostic criteria and guidelines.[123-124]

ECG markers of SCD in Patients with Cardiac Sarcoidosis

Sarcoidosis is a granulomatous disease of unknown etiology. It generally affects the lymph nodes, lungs, and the heart. Patients with cardiac sarcoidosis may present with heart block, VAs, SCD, and HF.[125–127]

ECG findings in patients with cardiac sarcoidosis include[43,128]:

1. Sinus node dysfunction.
2. Complete heart block (most common in up to 30% of patients), which may be the first presentation of cardiac sarcoidosis.
3. Second-degree heart block.
4. RBBB or LBBB (RBBB is more common and is observed in 12%–61% of patients).
5. Left-axis deviation.
6. VAs: PVCs, nonsustained VTs, sustained VTs (with multiple morphologies of spontaneous or induced VT).
7. VT/VF storm.
8. SCD.
9. Supraventricular arrhythmias: AF, atrial flutter, paroxysmal atrial tachycardia.

10. Pseudoinfarction: localized infiltration of granulomatous inflammation into the heart may mimic a transmural ECG pattern of myocardial infarction (depending on its location).

VAs account for the cause of SCD in 25% to 65% of patients with cardiac sarcoidosis.

Cardiac positron emission tomography (^{18}F-FDG PET) is a very useful, noninvasive imaging modality to detect cardiac involvement in sarcoidosis and the response to therapy. It is also very useful in identifying patients at high risk of VT and SCD.[129] Similarly, cardiac MRIs can also detect cardiac involvement in sarcoidosis and may be useful for risk stratification. Measurement of LGE is useful to assess the amount of fibrosis and scar tissue size.

The Heart Rhythm Society has recently published the expert consensus statement on the diagnosis and management of arrhythmias associated with cardiac sarcoidosis, including diagnostic ECG and diagnostic imaging workup.[130]

ECG Markers of SCD in Patients with Cardiac Amyloidosis

Definition

Cardiac amyloidosis is a common complication of systemic amyloidosis, secondary to immunoglobulin light-chain disease of plasma cells. Cardiac amyloidosis is the cause of death in 50% to 75% of systemic amyloidosis cases and poses a poor prognosis. The diagnosis is confirmed by cardiac biopsy; however, cardiac MRI provides significant diagnostic information. Cardiac amyloidosis typically presents with increased left ventricular wall thickness of more than 12 mm by Echo, whereas ECG shows low-voltage amplitude. Macroscopically, atrial dilatation with normal or near-normal left ventricular size is present. In some cases, mild to moderate LVH may exist and in this case the differential diagnosis is with HCM. Cardiac amyloidosis may cause both arrhythmias and HF; the latter is also seen in patients with preserved as well as reduced LV systolic function.[131]

Another form of amyloidosis is senile type, where small amounts of amyloid deposits are detected in the ventricles of 50% to 80% of patients aged >80 years. The Echo and ECG findings of senile amyloidosis are similar to other types of amyloidosis. The main differential diagnosis is HHD and HCM. Three-dimensional Echo is a useful technique to differentiate HCM from other causes of LVH.[41,132,133]

Recent investigations suggest that coronary microvascular dysfunction may be related to abnormalities in myocardial structure and function in cardioid amyloidosis. As such, workup for myocardial ischemia may help differentiate between LVH from cardiac amyloidosis.[134]

ECG Manifestations of Cardiac Amyloidosis

Normal- to low-voltage ECG pattern is observed in cardiac amyloidosis, with left anterior fascicular block, nonspecific ST-T wave abnormalities, and presence of LVH by ECG and thickened LV by Echo (low voltage-to-mass ratio).[41] Low-voltage QRS is a marker for high risk of SCD.[135] In some cases, the ECG may be normal or without low voltage.[136]

Cardiac MRI is quite useful in confirming the diagnosis as well as risk stratification of patients with cardiac amyloidosis.[137,138]

Anderson-Fabry Disease (Commonly Known as Fabry Disease)

Fabry disease is among metabolic disorders that cause cardiomyopathy. It is a genetic X-chromosome-linked (male-dominant) disease. Fabry disease is due to lysosomal storage secondary to α-galactosidase A deficiency. It is a multiorgan disease with cardiac involvement and produces cardiomyopathy with LVH and RVH. In its earlier stages, the ECG shows a short PR interval (in 40% of patients). Other ECG changes include nonspecific ST-T wave abnormalities. Arrhythmias are common in advanced stages, such as heart block; AF (17%); VA (8%); SCD; and rarely VT storm in patients with severe concentric LVH.[45,139,140] Figure 6.10A and B illustrate ECG examples of 2 patients with Fabry disease.

Syncope

Syncope is a very heterogeneous syndrome. The ECG findings in syncope depend on the etiology and on the underlying structural heart disease. Broadly speaking, most patients without heart disease have normal ECG with the exception of inherited channelopathies and manifest accessory pathways, whereas in patients with structural heart disease such as HCM, DCM, ARVD/C, etc., ECG may be of diagnostic value.[141,142] In approximately 5% of patients with the first episode of syncope, ECG is useful to establish the diagnosis. On the other hand, in patients with abnormal ECG such as presence of Q waves, scar, significant LVH, and Wolff-Parkinson-White ECG pattern, the ECG will be abnormal. Careful examination of ECG is useful to plan the workup of patients with recurrent syncope and avoid unnecessary, costly tests.[142] In general, the ECG has a low diagnostic yield in young individuals with syncope, especially those without structural heart disease.[141]

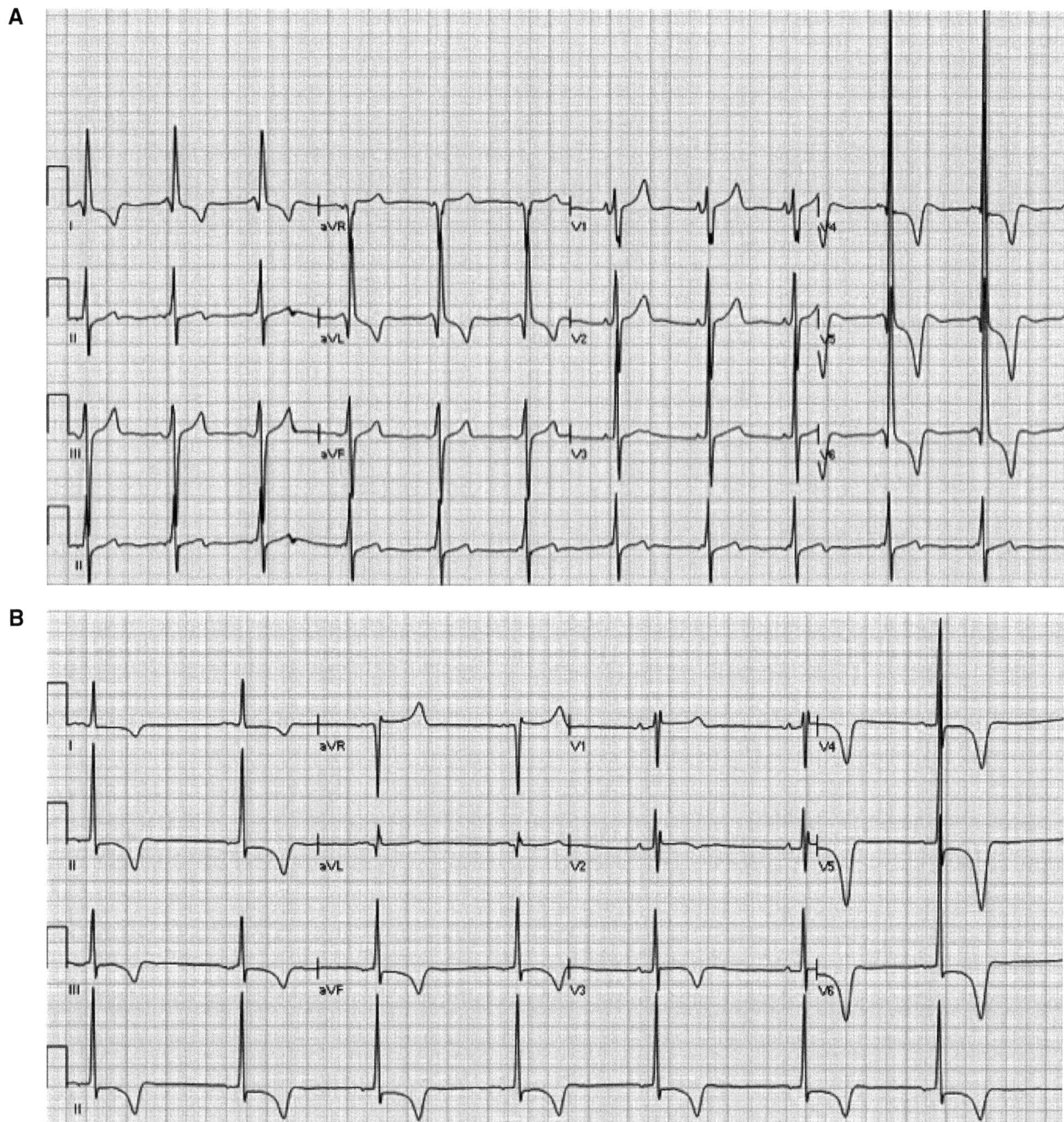

Figure 6.10. Two ECG examples of Fabry disease. **A.** A 55-year-old male with Fabry disease [Heart rate 67 beats per minute, PR 84 ms, QRS 130 ms, QT/QTc 430/455 ms]. **B.** A 59-year-old female with Fabry disease [heart rate 43 beats per minute, PR 178 ms, QRS 94 ms, QT/QTc 552/466 ms]. Note presence of LVH and T-wave abnormalities in both cases. Courtesy: Dr Reginald Nadaeu, University of Montreal, QC.

ECG Manifestations of Cancer-induced Cardiomyopathies

Cardiac complications during cancer therapy have been increasingly recognized to the point that the cardio-oncology department has emerged. Most cancer therapies cause cardiomyopathy with deleterious effect on LV systolic dysfunction and at times produce arrhythmias. The most common ECG findings are ST-T wave abnormalities, signs of myocardial ischemia, and cardiac arrhythmias. The most common chemotherapy medication that produces cardiac toxicity is anthracyclines, such as doxorubicin, which are well known to produce cardiomyopathy.[143]

This topic is further discussed in Chapter 18.

ECG Manifestations of Other Conditions

1. *LV Noncompaction:* LVH, AF, VA.[39]
2. *Myocarditis:* Nonspecific ST-T wave abnormalities may mimic acute MI or pericarditis with ST segment elevation, ST segment depression, PR

depression, pathologic Q waves. VAs have been reported as high as 55%.[144]

3. *Alcoholic and cocaine-associated cardiomyopathies:* Sinus tachycardia, early repolarization abnormalities (up to 32%), LVH (up to 16%), and normal ECG (in only 32%). AF and VT are not uncommon.[145]
4. *Chagas cardiomyopathy:* The ECG is the most single important test in Chagas cardiomyopathy. Sinus bradycardia, sick sinus syndrome, nonspecific ST-T wave abnormalities, low QRS voltage, abnormal Q waves, intraventricular conduction defect (IVCD), LBBB, RBBB, second- and third-degree AV block, LAD, AF, VA (PVCs, nonsustained and sustained VT). SCD in patients with normal ECG is rare.[146] Due to the significant arrhythmias caused by Chagas disease, it is considered as an arrhythmogenic cardiomyopathy. Patients with normal ECG have an excellent medium-term survival.[147]
5. *Peripartum and postpartum cardiomyopathy:* Sinus tachycardia, LVH (in 66%), nonspecific ST-T wave abnormalities (96%), AF, VA (PVCs, nonsustained VTs) (up to 20%–60% of patients), BBB. In those patients that develop HF, their ECG is rarely normal.[148,149]
6. *Diabetes mellitus:* The ECG in patients with diabetes mellitus demonstrates several ECG abnormalities depending on the extent and duration of diabetes. The common findings are sinus tachycardia, decreased T-wave amplitude, nonspecific ST-T wave abnormalities, prolonged QT and QTc intervals, and increased QT dispersion. Some of these abnormalities may reflect autonomic neuropathy and imbalance that are seen in patients with advanced diabetes mellitus, such as abnormal baroreflex dysfunction and abnormal HRV. LVH is seen in patients with diabetic cardiomyopathy and some of the ST-T wave abnormalities may be related to silent ischemia.[150]
7. *Hemochromatosis:* A systemic iron storage disease with cardiac involvement. The ECG is usually nondiagnostic in early stages and shows LVH; whereas in advanced cases, it shows low QRS complex voltage and nonspecific ST-T wave abnormalities, atrial tachyarrhythmias with AF being the most common. VAs are usually seen when left ventricular systolic dysfunction progresses. AV conduction abnormalities are also seen in advanced stages including first-, second-, and third-degree AV block. Echo and cardiac MRI are excellent screening tools in patients with suspected and established diagnosis of hemochromatosis.[44,151]

SUMMARY

Since most of the pathologies discussed above share basic structural and electrical abnormalities, many of the ECG features are common among them. Multivariate risk models should be implemented to increase the sensitivity, specificity, positive, and negative predictive values of each variable. Further imaging technologies and genetic testing may help to identify patients at higher risk. This algorithm should also help to select patients for primary and secondary preventative measures such as ICD and CRT implantation.

Like chest x-ray is the window to the body, ECG has the luxury of being the window to the heart and remains the cardiologists' best friend.[152] ECG can look at the specific conditions like the ones discussed in this review, but also major abnormalities such as global T-wave changes that are specific for left main coronary disease, acute cerebrovascular events, acute pulmonary embolism, and pulmonary edema.[153] Whereas minor changes may be perceived as such, a study of a large cohort of older adults revealed that minor nonspecific ST-T wave abnormalities were associated with a significant and important increase of cardiovascular events and primary arrhythmic death.[154]

FUTURE DIRECTIONS AND CHALLENGES

ECG Is at the Crossroad

SCD and its related etiologies are complex and diverse. ECG remains the first diagnostic and prognostic tool that is widely available, noninvasive, reproducible, inexpensive, and the results are available immediately faster than any laboratory test or even a simple chest x-ray.[155] If ECG is interpreted carefully, it is possible to differentiate between normal and abnormal conditions. In order to improve its diagnostic yield, the time has come to study the genotype–phenotype association of different symptoms with corresponding ECGs. It is hoped that in the near future, the association of ECG with other biomarkers, genetic testing, and imaging modalities, we can detect the preclinical and high-risk mutation carriers. We need to put into place the proper framework to link risk factors to SCD and include environmental and genetic profiles together. It's important to continue to improve the diagnostic and prognostic performance of the ECG in special subgroups such as HF, gender, and ethnic specific, etc. Gender and racial differences are now implemented into the ECG analysis risk model. For example, ECG predictors of CAD events and mortality in postmenopausal women have important implications compared to other groups.[72,156]

The ECG as discussed in this review is useful in many monogenic disorders associated with SCD such as inherited channelopathies: long and short QT syndrome, Brugada syndrome, Andersen-Tawil syndrome, catecholaminergic polymorphic VT, idiopathic VF, early repolarization syndrome. These are well discussed in previous chapters.

Inherited channelopathies:

- Long QT syndrome.
- Short QT syndrome.
- Brugada syndrome.
- Andersen-Tawil syndrome.
- Catecholaminergic polymorphic VT.
- Idiopathic VF.
- Early repolarization syndrome.

Cardiomyopathies:

- HCM.
- DCM.
- ARVD/C.
- Noncompaction cardiomyopathy.
- Restrictive cardiomyopathy.
- Amyloidosis.
- Fabry disease.
- Other diseases.[24,26,157]

Some of the risk factors discussed above are modifiable, and many of them are nonmodifiable. It may be that in the near future with advanced genetic modification and mutations, some of the nonmodifiable risk factors may become amendable.

The application of new imaging technologies, especially cardiac MRI and its correlation to the ECG finding will confirm the ECG findings with specific pathologies. They will be helpful to differentiate even the subsets of cardiomyopathies and the like.

Finally, as most of the pathologies discussed in this section share common risk factors, etiologies, and ECG changes such as SCD and CAD, the future challenge is to develop risk models that can differentiate between the different diseases.[69] This is where other noninvasive technologies may be useful. Table 6.3 summarizes the specific ECG abnormalities in different cardiac and systemic diseases with the potential application of imaging modalities to confirm the ECG findings. Future studies that correlate the noninvasive technologies with ECG in the specific diseases will certainly increase sensitivity, specificity, and predictive value of the ECG. Cardiac MRI appears to be a useful imaging modality that can help differentiate etiologies of LVH, HF, and the like, where the ECG provides nonspecific markers.[158,159] Combining ECG variables with patient-specific profiles may improve the diagnostic yield of the test. For example, correction of QRS voltage by body mass index in patients with LVH and hypertension improves the performance of ECG for the diagnosis of LVH in this group of patients.[160] O'Mahony et al recently reported a novel clinical risk prediction model for SCD in patients with HCM. This model is based on patient's age, family history of SCD, magnitude of the LV wall thickness, LV fractional shortening, left atrial dimensions, maximal LV outflow gradient, presence of nonsustained VT, and unexplained syncope. Applying this risk prediction model to patients with HCM may provide accurate individualized estimates for the probability of SCD in this patient cohort.[161]

The evolution of the ECG changes by age needs to be considered when making recommendations. T-wave inversions of ≥2 mm are considered to be normal "juvenile pattern" by age 12 (prepuberty); however, athletic activities and screening become an

Table 6.3. Specific ECG abnormalities in different cardiac and systemic diseases.

Cardiac Diseases	Electrocardiographic parameters	Major findings: Imaging modalities for differential diagnosis and noninvasive imaging modalities
SCD	fQRS; T-wave alternans; LVH; QRS prolongation	fQRS increases risk of SCD, VT, and ICD discharges
HF	fQRS; QRS prolongation; wide QRS/T angle; IVCD; BBB.	Echo; MRI
DCM	fQRS; PR prolongation; IVCD; LBBB	Echo; MRI
ARVD/C	fQRS; Epsilon wave; T-wave inversion; V_1 to V_3; QRS duration >110 ms in V_1 to V_3; Incomplete RBBB; QRS and QT dispersion; prolonged S-wave upstroke in V_1 to V_3 (delayed S-wave upstroke)	Echo; MRI
Sarcoidosis	Sinus node dysfunction; AV block; LAD; right BBB; VA; AF; VT; VF storm	SPECT; cardiac PET; MRI

Abbreviations: AF, atrial fibrillation; ARVD/C, arrhythmogenic right ventricular dysplasia/cardiomyopathy; AV, atrioventricular; BBB, bundle branch block; Echo, echocardiogram; fQRS, fragmented QRS; ICD, implantable cardioverter defibrillator; IVCD, intraventricular conduction defect; LAD, left atrial enlargement; LGE, late gadolinium enhancement; LVH, left ventricular hypertrophy; MRI, magnetic resonance imaging; PET, positron emission tomography; RBBB, right bundle branch block; SCD, sudden cardiac death; SPECT, single-photon emission computerized tomography; VT, ventricular tachycardia; VF, ventricular fibrillation.

important issue for the participants. In this case, Echo may be useful to discriminate normal variant T-wave inversions in early detection of cardiomyopathies.[162]

Early detection and in particular preclinical state of the disease is very important and the current noninvasive imaging as well as biomarkers will provide such capabilities that may be useful in early treatment that can potentially change the prognosis and outcome. In an excellent review by Wellens et al, they point out the value of the ECG-derived risk stratification model for SCD. The most important challenge for the future is to improve the positive and negative predictive values of ECG in SCD.[163] For example, measurement of propeptide of type I procollagen (PICP) as a marker for sarcomere-mutation carriers of HCM without overt disease may be useful in identification of preclinical HCM and HF.[164,165] Similarly, early fetal detection of cardiomyopathies by Echo appears to be useful in predicting adverse perinatal outcomes.[166]

Furthermore, advanced imaging technologies would help to improve the definition and diagnostic yield of ECG in the future. For example, cardiac MRI and its advanced sequences have been used to define the different patterns of LVH.[167–169]

As we learn more about ECGs, new markers will be discovered for the diagnosis and risk stratification of high-risk patients such as the new finding of narrow and tall QRS complex as a potential marker of SCD.[170]

LIMITATIONS OF THE ECG

Resting ECGs have several inherent limitations that lower the sensitivity and specificity and predictive value of the test, which includes the following:

1. Presence of borderline and normal variants.
2. Abnormalities that may be within normal range for a subgroup of patients such as those related to age, gender, and race or as those seen in athletes and African-Americans. Chandra et al recently reported on the prevalence of ECG abnormalities in young individuals and found that one in five young people who are in training program demonstrate sinus bradycardia, first-degree AV block, incomplete RBBB, early repolarization patterns, or isolated QRS voltage criteria for LVH.
3. Certain ECG abnormalities that are present in many diverse pathologies and thus lowers the specificity of the test such as presence of fQRS in CAD, HCM, DCM, and HF, which reflects a specific electrophysiological properties such as conduction delays that is a requirement for reentry arrhythmias and causes SCD/VT/VF in many cases.
4. Many of the ECG abnormalities are nonspecific, therefore additional testing and/or biomarkers may help to improve the sensitivity and specificity of the ECG markers and avoid unnecessary invasive procedures. This approach will certainly improve the cost effectiveness of invasive therapies.[171,172] Therefore, in normal ECG a patient suspected of certain pathologies should not be excluded from a disease. Normal ECG in patients with syncope as discussed above or rarely in patients with ARVD/C, HCM, and others should not rule out the presence of disease.[173,174]

REFERENCES

1. Chou R, Arora B, Dana T, et al. Screening asymptomatic adults with resting or exercise electrocardiography: a review of the evidence for the U.S. preventative services task force. *Ann Intern Med.* 2011;155:375–385.
2. Strauss DG, Mewton N, Verrier RL, et al. Screening entire health system ECG databases to identify patients at increased risk of death. *Circ Arrhythm Electrophysiol.* 2013;6:1156–1162.
3. Hohnloser S. T-wave alternans: Electrocardiographic characteristics and clinical value. In: Shenasa M, Josephson ME, Estes NAM III, eds. *The ECG Handbook: Contemporary Challenges.* Minneapolis, MN: Cardiotext Publishing; 2015.
4. Teodorescu C, Reinier K, Uy-Evanado, et al. Prolonged QRS duration on the resting ECG is associated with sudden death in coronary disease, independent of prolonged ventricular repolarization. *Heart Rhythm.* 2011;8:1562–1567.
5. Kurl S, Makikallio TH, Rautaharju, P, Kiviniemi V, Laukkanen JA. Duration of QRS complex in resting electrocardiogram is a predictor of sudden cardiac death in men. *Circulation.* 2012;125:2588–2594.
6. Iuliano S, Fisher SG, Karasik PE, Fletcher RD, Singh SN. QRS duration and mortality in patients with congestive heart failure. *Am Heart J.* 2002;143:1085–1091.
7. Bode-Schnurbus L, Bocker D, Block M, et al. QRS duration: A simple marker for predicting cardiac mortality in ICD patients with heart failure. *Heart.* 2003;89:1157–1162.
8. Zimetbaum PJ, Buxton AE, Batsford W, et al. Electrocardiographic predictors of arrhythmic death and total mortality in the multicenter unsustained tachycardia trial. *Circulation.* 2004;110:766–769.
9. Morin DP, Oikarinen L, Viitasalo M, et al. QRS duration predicts sudden cardiac death in hypertensive patients undergoing intensive medical therapy: The LIFE study. *Eur Heart J.* 2009;30:2908–2914.
10. Badheka AO, Singh V, Patel NJ, et al. QRS duration on electrocardiography and cardiovascular mortality (from the National Health and Nutrition Examination Survey-III). *Am J Cardiol.* 2013;112:671–677.
11. Strauss DG, Poole JE, Wagner GS, et al. An ECG index of myocardial scar enhances prediction of defibrillator shocks: An analysis of the sudden cardiac death in heart failure trial. *Heart Rhythm.* 2011;8:38–45.

12. Chatterjee S, Changawala N. Fragmented QRS complex: A novel marker of cardiovascular disease. *Clin Cardiol.* 2010;33:68–71.
13. Das MK, Suradi H, Maskoun W, et al. Fragmented wide QRS on a 12-lead ECG: A sign of myocardial scar and poor prognosis. *Arrhythmia Electrophysiol.* 2008;1:258–268.
14. Das MK, Saha C, Masry HE, et al. Fragmented QRS on a 12-lead ECG: a predictor of mortality and cardiac events in patients with coronary artery disease. *Heart Rhythm.* 2007;4:1385–1392.
15. Pei J, Li N, Gao Y, et al. The J wave and fragmented QRS complexes in inferior leads associated with sudden cardiac death in patients with chronic heart failure. *Europace.* 2012;14,1180–1187.
16. Femenia F, Arce M, Van Grieken J, et al. Fragmented QRS as a predictor of arrhythmic events in patients with hypertrophic obstructive cardiomyopathy. *J Interv Card Electrophysiol.* 2013;38:159–165.
17. Santangeli P, Russo AD, Pieroni M, et al. Fragmented and delayed electrograms within fibrofatty scar predict arrhythmic events in arrhythmogenic right ventricular cardiomyopathy: results from a prospective risk stratification study. *Heart Rhythm.* 2012;9:1200–1206.
18. Das KM, Maskoun W, Shen C, et al. Fragmented QRS on twelve-lead electrocardiogram predicts arrhythmic events in patients with ischemic and nonischemic cardiomyopathy. *Heart Rhythm.* 2010;7:74–80.
19. Ahn MS, Kim JB, Joung B, Lee MH, Kim SS. Prognostic implications of fragmented QRS and its relationship with delayed contrast-enhanced cardiovascular magnetic resonance imaging in patients with non-ischemic dilated cardiomyopathy. *Int J Cardiol.* 2013;167:1417–1422.
20. Assenza GE, Valente AM, Geva T, et al. QRS duration and QRS fractionation on surface electrocardiogram are markers of right ventricular dysfunction and atrialization in patients with Ebstein anomaly. *Eur Heart J.* 2013;34:191–200.
21. Morita H, Kusano KF, Miura D, et al. Fragmented QRS as a marker of conduction abnormality and a predictor of prognosis of Brugada syndrome. *Circulation.* 2008;118:1697–1704.
22. Das MK, Zipes DP. Fragmented QRS: A predictor of mortality and sudden cardiac death. *Heart Rhythm.* 2009;6:S8–S14.
23. Thorgeirsson G, Thorgeirsson G, Sigvaldason H, Witteman J. Risk factors for out-of-hospital cardiac arrest: The Reykjavik study. *Eur Heart J.* 2005;26:1499–1505.
24. Tan BY, Judge DP. A clinical approach to a family history of sudden death. *Circ Cardiovasc Genet.* 2012;5:697–705.
25. Kelly M, Semsarian C. Multiple mutations in genetic heart disease. *Circ Cardiovasc Genet.* 2009;2:182–190.
26. Deo R, Albert CM. Epidemiology and genetics of sudden cardiac death. *Circulation.* 2012;125:620–637.
27. Goldberger JJ. Evidence-based analysis of risk factors for sudden cardiac death. *Heart Rhythm.* 2009;6:S2–S7.
28. Watanabe E, Tanabe T, Osaka M, et al. Sudden cardiac arrest recorded during Holter monitoring: Prevalence, antecedent electrical events, and outcomes. *Heart Rhythm.* 2014;11:1418–1425.
29. Zipes DP, Wellens HJJ. Sudden cardiac death. *Circulation.* 1998;98:2334–2351.
30. Chugh SS, Reinier K, Teodorescu C, et al. Epidemiology of sudden cardiac death: Clinical and research implications. *Prog Cardiovasc Dis.* 2008;51:213–228.
31. Rubart M, Zipes DP. Mechanisms of sudden cardiac death. *J Clin Invest.* 2005;115:2305–2315.
32. George AL, Jr. Molecular and genetic basis of sudden cardiac death. *J Clin Invest.* 2013;123:75–83.
33. Lewis T. Observations upon ventricular hypertrophy with special reference to preponderance of one or the other chamber. *Heart.* 1914;5:367–402.
34. Benjamin E, Levy D. Why is left ventricular hypertrophy so predictive of morbidity and mortality? *Am J Med Sci.* 1999;317:168–175.
35. Raman SV. The hypertensive heart: an integrated understanding informed by imaging. *J Am Coll Cardiol.* 2010;55:91–96.
36. Maron BJ, Ommen SR, Semsarian C, et al. Hypertrophic cardiomyopathy: present and future, with translation into contemporary cardiovascular medicine. *J Am Coll Cardiol.* 2014;64:83–99.
37. Rao U, Agarwal A. Importance of Q waves in early diagnosis of hypertrophic cardiomyopathy. *Heart.* 2011;97:1993–1994.
38. Chan RH, Maron BJ, Olivotto I, et al. Prognostic value of quantitative contrast-enhanced cardiovascular magnetic resonance for the evaluation of sudden death risk in patients with hypertrophic cardiomyopathy. *Circulation.* 2014;130:484–495.
39. Sarma RJ, Chana A, Elkayam U. Left ventricular noncompaction. *Prog Cardiovasc Dis.* 2010;52:264–273.
40. Pelliccia A, Maron MS, Maron BJ. Assessment of left ventricular hypertrophy in a trained athlete: Differential diagnosis of physiologic athlete's heart from pathologic hypertrophy. *Prog Cardiovasc Dis.* 2012;54:387–396.
41. Dubrey SW, Hawkins PN, Falk RH. Amyloid diseases of the heart: Assessment, diagnosis, and referral. *Heart.* 2011;97:75–84.
42. Maceira AM, Joshi J, Prasad SK, et al. Cardiovascular magnetic resonance in cardiac amyloidosis. *Circulation.* 2005;111:186–193.
43. Nery PB, Leung E, Birnie DH. Arrhythmias in cardiac sarcoidosis: Diagnosis and treatment. *Curr Opin Cardiol.* 2012;27:181–189.
44. Arbustini E, Narula N, Dec W, et al. The MOGE(S) classification for a phenotype–genotype nomenclature of cardiomyopathy. *J Am Coll Cardiol.* 2013;62:2046–2072.
45. Yousef Z, Elliott PM, Cecchi F, et al. Left ventricular hypertrophy in Fabry disease: A practical approach to diagnosis. *Eur Heart J.* 2013;34:802–808.
46. Macfarlane PW. Is electrocardiography still useful in the diagnosis of cardiac chamber hypertrophy and dilatation? *Cardiol Clin.* 2006;24:401–411.
47. Okin PM, Bang CN, Wachtell K, et al. Relationship of sudden cardiac death to new-onset atrial fibrillation in hypertensive patients with left ventricular hypertrophy. *Circ Arrhythm Electrophysiol.* 2013;6:243–251.
48. Okin PM, Devereux RB, Nieminen MS, et al. Electrocardiographic strain pattern and prediction of new-onset congestive heart failure in hypertensive

patients: the Losartan Intervention for Endpoint reduction in hypertension (LIFE) study. *Circulation.* 2006;113:67–73.

49. Okin PM, Devereux RB, Jern S, et al. Regression of electrocardiographic left ventricular hypertrophy during antihypertensive treatment and the prediction of major cardiovascular events. *JAMA.* 2004;292:2343–2349.
50. Devereux RB, Wachtell K, Gerdts E, et al. Prognostic significance of left ventricular mass change during treatment of hypertension. *JAMA.* 2004;292:2350–2356.
51. Okin PM, Devereux RB, Liu JE, et al. Regression of electrocardiographic left ventricular hypertrophy predicts regression of echocardiographic left ventricular mass: The LIFE study. *J Hum Hypertens.* 2004;18:403–409.
52. Okin PM, Wachtell K, Devereux RB, et al. Regression of electrocardiographic left ventricular hypertrophy and decreased incidence of new-onset atrial fibrillation in patients with hypertension. *JAMA.* 2006;296:1242–1248.
53. Romhilt DW, Bove KE, Norris RJ, et al. A critical appraisal of the electrocardiographic criteria for the diagnosis of left ventricular hypertrophy. *Circulation.* 1969;40:185–195.
54. Pewsner D, Juni P, Egger M, et al. Accuracy of electrocardiography in diagnosis of left ventricular hypertrophy in arterial hypertension: Systematic review. *Br Med J.* 2007;335:711–720.
55. Sundstrom J, Lind L, Arnlov J, et al. Echocardiographic and electrocardiographic diagnoses of left ventricular hypertrophy predict mortality independently of each other in a population of elderly men. *Circulation.* 2001;103:2346–2351.
56. Levy D, Savage DD, Garrison RJ, et al. Echocardiographic criteria for left ventricular hypertrophy: the Framingham Heart Study. *Am J Cardiol.* 1987;59:956–960.
57. Yuda S, Khoury V, Marwick TH. Influence of wall stress and left ventricular geometry on the accuracy of dobutamine stress echocardiography. *J Am Coll Cardiol.* 2002;40:1311–1319.
58. Rosenberg MA, Manning WJ. Diastolic dysfunction and risk of atrial fibrillation: a mechanistic appraisal. *Circulation.* 2012;126:2353–2362.
59. Larsen CT, Dahlin J, Blackburn H, et al. Prevalence and prognosis of electrocardiographic left ventricular hypertrophy, ST segment depression and negative T-wave: The Copenhagen City Heart Study. *Eur Heart J.* 2002;23:315–324.
60. Chrispin J, Jain A, Soliman EZ, et al. Association of electrocardiographic and imaging surrogates of left ventricular hypertrophy with incident atrial fibrillation: MESA (Multi-Ethnic Study of Atherosclerosis). *J Am Coll Cardiol.* 2014;63:2007–2013.
61. Artham SM, Lavie CJ, Milani RV, et al. Clinical impact of left ventricular hypertrophy and implications for regression. *Prog Cardiovasc Dis.* 2009;52:153–167.
62. Kahan T, Bergfeldt L. Left ventricular hypertrophy in hypertension: Its arrhythmogenic potential. *Heart.* 2005;91:250–256.
63. Gardin JM, Lauer MS. Left ventricular hypertrophy: the next treatable, silent killer? *JAMA.* 2004;292:2396–2398.
64. Yilmaz A, Sechtem U. Diagnostic approach and differential diagnosis in patients with hypertrophied left ventricles. *Heart.* 2014;100:662–671.
65. Namdar M, Steffel J, Jetzer S, et al. Value of electrocardiogram in the differentiation of hypertensive heart disease, hypertrophic cardiomyopathy, aortic stenosis, amyloidosis, and Fabry disease. *Am J Cardiol.* 2012;109:587–593.
66. Liew R. Electrocardiogram-based predictors of sudden cardiac death in patients with coronary artery disease. *Clin Cardiol.* 2011;34:466–473.
67. Biagini E, Elhendy A, Schinkel AFL, et al. Prognostic significance of left anterior hemiblock in patients with suspected coronary artery disease. *J Am Coll Cardiol.* 2005;46:858–863.
68. Auer B, Bauer DC, Marques-Vidal P, et al. Association of major and minor ECG abnormalities with coronary heart disease events. *JAMA.* 2012;307:1497–1505.
69. Soliman EZ, Prineas RJ, Case LD, et al. Electrocardiographic and clinical predictors separating atherosclerotic sudden cardiac death from incident coronary heart disease. *Heart.* 2011;97:1597–1601.
70. Braunwald E. Shattuck lecture – cardiovascular medicine at the turn of the millennium: Triumphs, concerns, and opportunities. *N Engl J Med.* 1997;337:1360–1369.
71. Kashani A, Barold SS. Significant of QRS complex duration in patients with heart failure. *J Am Coll Cardiol.* 2005;46:2183–2192.
72. Rautaharju P, Kooperberg C, Larson JC, LaCroix A. Electrocardiographic abnormalities that predict coronary heart disease events and mortality in postmenopausal women: The Women's Health Initiative. *Circulation.* 2006;113:473–480.
73. Rautaharju P, Kooperberg C, Larson J, et al. Electrocardiographic predictors of incident congestive heart failure and all-cause mortality in postmenopausal women: The Women's Health Initiative. *Circulation.* 2006;113:481–489.
74. Okin PM. Electrocardiography in women: taking the initiative. *Circulation.* 2006;113:464–466.
75. Zhang ZM, Rautaharju PM, Prineas RJ, et al. Usefulness of electrocardiographic QRS/T angles with versus without bundle branch blocks to predict heart failure (from the Atherosclerosis Risk in Communities Study). *Am J Cardiol.* 2014;114:412–418.
76. Rautaharju PM, Zhang ZM, Haisty WK, et al. Electrocardiographic predictors of incident heart failure in men and women free from manifest cardiovascular disease (from the Atherosclerosis Risk in Communities [ARIC] Study). *Am J Cardiol.* 2013;112:843–849.
77. Teerlink JR, Jalaluddin M, Anderson S, et al. Ambulatory ventricular arrhythmias in patients with heart failure do not specifically predict an increased risk of sudden death. *Circulation.* 2000;101:40–46.
78. Shamim W, Francis DP, Yousufuddin M, et al. Intraventricular conduction delay: a prognostic marker in chronic heart failure. *Int J Cardiol.* 1999;70:171–178.
79. Cygankiewicz I, Zareba W, Vazquez R, et al. Heart rate turbulence predicts all-cause mortality and sudden death in congestive heart failure patients. *Heart Rhythm.* 2008;5:1095–1102.

80. Elliott PM, Anastasakis A, Borger MA, et al. 2014 ESC Guidelines on diagnosis and management of hypertrophic cardiomyopathy: The task force for the diagnosis and management of hypertrophic cardiomyopathy of the European Society of Cardiology (ESC). *Eur Heart J.* 2014;35:2733–2779.
81. Olivotto I, Cecchi F, Poggesi C, Yacoub MH. Patterns of disease progression in hypertrophic cardiomyopathy: An individualized approach to clinical staging. *Circ Heart Fail.* 2012;5:535–546.
82. Montgomery JV, Harris KM, Casey SA, et al. Relation of electrocardiographic patterns to phenotypic expression and clinical outcome in hypertrophic cardiomyopathy. *Am J Cardiol.* 2005;96:270–275.
83. Konno T, Shimizu M, Hidekazu I, et al. Diagnostic value of abnormal Q waves for identification of preclinical carriers of hypertrophic cardiomyopathy based on a molecular genetic diagnosis. *Eur Heart J.* 2004;25:246–251.
84. McLeod CJ, Ackerman MJ, Nishimura RA, et al. Outcome of patients with hypertrophic cardiomyopathy and a normal electrocardiogram. *J Am Coll Cardiol.* 2009;54:229–233.
85. Dumont CA, Monserrat L, Soler R, et al. Interpretation of electrocardiographic abnormalities in hypertrophic cardiomyopathy with cardiac magnetic resonaonce. *Eur Heart J.* 2006;27:1725–1731.
86. Puntmann VO, Jahnke C, Gebker R, et al. Usefulness of magnetic resonance imaging to distinguish hypertensive and hypertrophic cardiomyopathy. *Am J Cardiol.* 2010;106:1016–1022.
87. Maron BJ, Pelliccia A. The heart of trained athletes: Cardiac remodeling and the risks of sports including sudden death. *Circulation.* 2006;114:1633–1644.
88. Monserrat L, Elliott PM, Gimeno JR, et al. Non-sustained ventricular tachycardia in hypertrophic cardiomyopathy: An independent marker of sudden death risk in young patients. *J Am Coll Cardiol.* 2003;42:873–879.
89. Hess OM. Risk stratification in hypertrophic cardiomyopathy fact or fiction? *J Am Coll Cardiol.* 2003;42:880–881.
90. Spirito P, Bellone P, Harris KM, et al. Magnitude of left ventricular hypertrophy and risk of sudden death in hypertrophic cardiomyopathy. *N Engl J Med.* 2000;342:1778–1785.
91. Femenía F, Arce M, Arrieta M, Baranchuk A. Surface fragmented QRS in a patient with hypertrophic cardiomyopathy and malignant arrhythmias: Is there an association? *J Cardiovasc Dis Res.* 2012;3:32–35.
92. Kang KW, Janardhan AH, Jung KT, et al. Fragmented QRS as a candidate marker for high-risk assessment in hypertrophic cardiomyopathy. *Heart Rhythm.* 2014;11:1433–1440.
93. Ostman-Smith I, Wisten A, Nylander E, et al. Electrocardiographic amplitudes: A new risk factor for sudden death in hypertrophic cardiomyopathy. *Eur Heart J.* 2010;31:439–449.
94. Basso C, Thiene G, Mackey-Bojack S, et al. Myocardial bridging: A frequent component of the hypertrophic cardiomyopathy phenotype lacks systematic association with sudden cardiac death. *Eur Heart J.* 2009;30:1627–1634.
95. McKenna WJ, Nagueh SF. Cardiac magnetic resonance imaging and sudden death risk in patients with hypertrophic cardiomyopathy. *Circulation.* 2014;130:455–457.
96. Olivotto I, Cecchi F, Yacoub MH. Myocardial bridging and sudden death in hypertrophic cardiomyopathy: Salome drops another veil. *Eur Heart J.* 2009;30:1549–1550.
97. Bos JM, Will ML, Gersh BJ, et al. Characterization of a phenotype-based genetic test prediction score for unrelated patients with hypertrophic cardiomyopathy. *Mayo Clin Proc.* 2014;89:727–737.
98. Jefferies JL, Towbin JA. Dilated cardiomyopathy. *Lancet.* 2010;375:752–762.
99. Chia KKM, Hsia HH. Ventricular tachycardia in non-ischemic dilated cardiomyopathy: electrocardiographic and intracardiac electrogram correlation. *Card Electrophysiol Clin.* 2014;6:535-552.
100. Asirvatham SJ, Stevenson WG. Bundle branch reentry. *Circ Arrhythm Electrophysiol.* 2013;6:e92–e94.
101. Kusa S, Taniguchi H, Hachiya H, et al. Bundle branch reentrant ventricular tachycardia with wide and narrow QRS morphology. *Circ Arrhythm Electrophysiol.* 2013;6:e87–e91.
102. Nogami A, Olshansky B. Bundle branch reentry tachycardia. In: Zipes DP, Jalife J, eds. *Cardiac Electrophysiology: From Cell to Bedside.* Philadelphia, PA: Elsevier; 2014:835-847.
103. Lakdawala NK, Winterfield JR, Junke BH. Dilated cardiomyopathy. *Circ Arrhythm & Electrophysiol.* 2013;6:228–237.
104. Grimm W, Christ M, Bach J, Muller HH, Maisch B. Noninvasive arrhythmia risk stratification in idiopathic dilated cardiomyopathy: Results of the Marburg cardiomyopathy study. *Circulation.* 2003;108:2883–2891.
105. Hauer RNW, Cox MGPJ, Groeneweg JA. Impact of new electrocardiographic criteria in arrhythmogenic cardiomyopathy. *Front Physiol.* 2012;3:352.
106. Saguner AM, Duru F, Brunckhorst CB. Arrhythmogenic right ventricular cardiomyopathy: a challenging disease of the intercalated disc. *Circulation.* 2013;128:1381–1386.
107. Basso C, Corrado D, Marcus FI, Nava A, Thiene G. Arrhythmogenic right ventricular cardiomyopathy. *Lancet.* 2009;373:1289–1300.
108. Hulot JS, Jouven X, Empana JP, Frank R, Fontaine G. Natural history and risk stratification of arrhythmogenic right ventricular dysplasia/cardiomyopathy. *Circulation.* 2004;110:1879–1884.
109. Mcrae, III, AT, Chung MK, Asher CR. Arrhythmogenic right ventricular cardiomyopathy: A cause of sudden death in young people. *Cleve Clin J Med.* 2001;68:459–467.
110. Nasir K, Bomma C, Tandri H, et al. Electrocardiographic features of arrhythmogenic right ventricular dysplasia/cardiomyopathy according to severity: a need to broaden diagnostic criteria. *Circulation.* 2004;110:1527–1534.
111. Kies P, Bootsma M, Bax J, Schalij MJ, van der Wall EE. Arrhythmogenic right ventricular dysplasia/

cardiomyopathy: Screening, diagnosis, and treatment. *Heart Rhythm.* 2006;3:225–234.
112. Quarta G, Ward D, Esteban MTT, et al. Dynamic electrocardiographic changes in patients with arrhythmogenic right ventricular cardiomyopathy. *Heart.* 2010;96:516–522.
113. Fontaine G, Fontaliran F, Hebert JL, et al. Arrhythmogenic right ventricular dysplasia. *Annu Rev Med.* 1999;50:17–35.
114. Marcus FI, McKenna WJ, Sherrill D, et al. Diagnosis of arrhythmogenic right ventricular cardiomyopathy/dysplasia: Proposed modification of the task force criteria. *Circulation.* 2010;121:1533–1541.
115. te Riele AS, James CA, Rastegar N, et al. Yield of serial evaluation in at-risk family members of patients with ARVD/C. *J Am Coll Cardiol.* 2014;64:293–301.
116. Marcus F, Mestroni L. Family members of patients with ARVC: who is at risk? At what age? When and how often should we evaluate to determine risk? *J Am Coll Cardiol.* 2014;64:302–303.
117. Hoffmayer KS, Bhave PD, Marcus GM, et al. An electrocardiographic scoring system for distinguishing right ventricular outflow tract arrhythmias in patients with arrhythmogenic right ventricular cardiomyopathy from idiopathic ventricular tachycardia. *Heart Rhythm.* 2013;10:477–482.
118. Hoffmayer KS, Machado ON, Marcus GM, et al. Electrocardiographic comparison of ventricular arrhythmias in patients with arrhythmogenic right ventricular cardiomyopathy and right ventricular outflow tract tachycardia. *J Am Coll Cardiol.* 2011;58:831–838.
119. Buja G, Estes, III, M, Wichter T, et al. Arrhythmogenic right ventricular cardiomyopathy/dysplasia: risk stratification and therapy. *Prog Cardiovasc Dis.* 2008;50:282–293.
120. Basso C, Corrado D, Bauce B, Thiene G. Arrhythmogenic right ventricular cardiomyopathy. *Circ Arrhythm Electrophysiol.* 2012;5:1233–1246.
121. Link MS, Laidlaw D, Polonsky B, et al. Ventricular arrhythmias in the North American multidisciplinary study of ARVC. *J Am Coll Cardiol.* 2014;64:119–125.
122. Corrado D, Basso C, Pilichou K, Thiene G. Molecular biology and clinical management of arrhythmogenic right ventricular cardiomyopathy/dysplasia. *Heart.* 2011;97:530–539.
123. te Riele AS, Bhonsale A, James CA, et al. Incremental value of cardiac magnetic resonance imaging in arrhythmic risk stratification of arrhythmogenic right ventricular dysplasia/cardiomyopathy-associated desmosomal mutation carriers. *J Am Coll Cardiol.* 2013;62:1761–1769.
124. Lindsay BD. Challenges of diagnosis and risk stratification in patients with arrhythmogenic right ventricular cardiomyopathy/dysplasia. *J Am Coll Cardiol.* 2013;62:1770–1771.
125. Evanchan JP, Crouser ED, Kalbfleisch SJ. Cardiac sarcoidosis: Recent advances in diagnosis and treatment and an argument for the need for a systematic multidisciplinary approach to management. *J Innov Cardiac Rhythm Manage.* 2013;4:1160–1174.
126. Dubrey SW, Falk RH. Diagnosis and management of cardiac sarcoidosis. *Prog Cardiovasc Med.* 2010;52:336–346.
127. Doughan AR, Williams BR. Cardiac sarcoidosis. *Heart.* 2006;92:282–288.
128. Fasano R, Rimmerman CM, Jaber WA. Cardiac sarcoidosis: a cause of infiltrative cardiomyopathy. *Cleve Clin J Med.* 2004;71:483–488.
129. Blankstein R, Osborne M, Naya M, et al. Cardiac positron emission tomography enhances prognostic assessments of patients with suspected cardiac sarcoidosis. *J Am Coll Cardiol.* 2014;63:329–336.
130. Birnie DH, Sauer WH, Bogun F, et al. HRS expert consensus statement on the diagnosis and management of arrhythmias associated with cardiac sarcoidosis. *Heart Rhythm.* 2014;11:1304–1323.
131. Mohammed SF, Mirzoyev SA, Edwards WD. Left ventricular amyloid deposition in patients with heart failure and preserved ejection fraction. *J Am Coll Cardiol Heart Failure.* 2014;2:113–122.
132. Falk RH. Cardiac amyloidosis: A treatable disease, often overlooked. *Circulation.* 2011;124:1079–1085.
133. Caselli S, Pelliccia A, Maron M, et al. Differentiation of hypertrophic cardiomyopathy from other forms of left ventricular hypertrophy by means of three-dimensional echocardiography. *Am J Cardiol.* 2008;102:616–620.
134. Dorbala S, Vangala D, Bruyere J, et al. Coronary microvascular dysfunction is related to abnormalities in myocardial structure and function in cardiac amyloidosis. *J Am Coll Cardiol Heart Failure.* 2014;2:358–367.
135. Kristen AV, Perz JB, Schonland SO, et al. Non-invasive predictors of survival in cardiac amyloidosis. *Eur J Heart Fail.* 2007;9:617–624.
136. Lee GY, Kim K, Choi JO, et al. Cardiac amyloidosis without increased left ventricular wall thickness. *Mayo Clin Proc.* 2014;89:781–789.
137. Syed IS, Glockner JF, Feng D, et al. Role of cardiac magnetic resonance imaging in the detection of cardiac amyloidosis. *JACC Cardiovasc Imag.* 2010;3:155–164.
138. Austin BA, Tang WH, Rodriguez ER, et al. Delayed hyper-enhancement magnetic resonance imaging provides incremental diagnostic and prognostic utility in suspected cardiac amyloidosis. *JACC Cardiovasc Imag.* 2009;2:1369–1377.
139. O'Mahony C, Elliott P. Anderson-Fabry disease and the heart. *Prog Cardiovasc Dis.* 2010;52:326–335.
140. Linhart A, Kampmann C, Zamorano JL, et al. Cardiac manifestations of Anderson-Fabry disease: results from the international Fabry outcome survey. *Eur Heart J.* 2007;28:1228–1235.
141. Sun BC, Hoffman JR, Mower WR, et al. Low diagnostic yield of electrocardiogram testing in younger patients with syncope. *Ann Emerg Med.* 2008;51:240–246.
142. Perez-Rodod J, et al. Progonstic value of the electrocardiogram in patients with syncope: Data from the Group for Syncope Study in the Emergency Room (GESINUR). *Heart Rhythm.* 2014;11:2035-2044.143. Curigliano G, Mayer EL, Burstein HJ, Winer EP, Goldhirsch A. Cardiac toxicity from systemic cancer

therapy: a comprehensive review. *Prog Cardiovasc Dis.* 2010;53:94–104.

143. Takemura G, Fujiwara H. Doxorubicin-induced cardiomyopathy from the cardiotoxic mechanisms to management. *Prog Cardiovasc Dis.* 2007;49:330–352.
144. Blauwet LA, Cooper LT. Myocarditis. *Prog Cardiovasc Dis.* 2010;52:274–288.
145. Awtry EH, Philippides GJ. Alcoholic and cocaine-associated cardiomyopathies. *Prog Cardiovasc Dis.* 2010;52:289–299.
146. Biolo A, Ribeiro AL, Clausell N. Chagas Cardiopathy – where do we stand after a hundred years? *Prog Cardiovasc Dis.* 2010;52:300–316.
147. Nunes MCP, Dones W, Morillo CA, Encina JJ, Ribeiro AL. Chagas disease: An overview of clinical and epidemiological aspects. *J Am Coll Cardiol.* 2013;62:767–776.
148. Sliwa K, Hilfiker-Kleiner D, Petrie MC, et al. Current state of knowledge on aetiology, diagnosis, management, and therapy of peripartum cardiomyopathy *Euro J Heart Fail.* 2010;12:767–777.
149. Tibazarwa K, Sliwa K. Peripartum cardiomyopathy in Africa: Challenges in diagnosis, prognosis, and therapy. *Prog Cardiovasc Dis.* 2010;52:317–325.
150. Stern S, Sclarowsky S. The ECG in diabetes mellitus. *Circulation.* 2009;120:1633–1636.
151. Gulati V, Harikrishnan P, Palaniswama C, et al. Cardiac involvement in hemochromatosis. *Cardiol. Rev.* 2014;22:56–68.
152. Stern S. Electrocardiogram: still the cardiologist's best friend. *Circulation.* 2006;113:e753–e756.
153. Afolabi-Brown O, Morris DL, Figueredo VM. Global T-wave inversion on electrocardiogram: what is the differential? *Rev Cardiovasc Med.* 2014;15:131–141.
154. Kumar A, Prineas RJ, Arnold AM, et al. Prevalence, prognosis, and implications of isolated minor nonspecific ST-segment and T-wave abnormalities in older adults: Cardiovascular health study. *Circulation.* 2008;118:2790–2796.
155. Wellens HJJ, Gorgels AP. The electrocardiogram 102 years after Einthoven. *Circulation.* 2004;109:562–564.
156. Okin PM, Kjeldsen SE, Julius S, Dahlof B, Devereux RB. Racial differences in sudden cardiac death among hypertensive patients during antihypertensive therapy: The LIFE study. *Heart Rhythm.* 2012;9:531–537.
157. Hughes SE, McKenna WJ. New insights into the pathology of inherited cardiomyopathy. *Heart.* 2005;91:257–264.
158. Karamitsos TD, Francis JM, Myerson S, Selvanayagam JB, Neubauer S. The role of cardiovascular magnetic resonance imaging in heart failure. *J Am Coll Cardiol.* 2009;54:1407–1424.
159. Armstrong AC, Gidding S, Gjesdal O, et al. LV mass assessed by echocardiography and CMR, cardiovascular outcomes, and medical practice. *J Am Cardiol Img.* 2012;5:837–848.
160. Angeli F, Verdecchia P, Iacobellis G, Reboldi G. Usefulness of QRS voltage correction by body mass index to improve electrocardiographic detection of left ventricular hypertrophy in patients with systemic hypertension. *Am J Cardiol.* 2014;114:427–432.
161. O'Mahony C, Jichi F, Pavlou M, et al. A novel clinical risk prediction model for sudden cardiac death in hypertrophic cardiomyopathy (HCM Risk-SCD). *Eur Heart J.* 2014;35:2010–2020.
162. Migliore F, Zorzi A, Michieli P, et al. Prevalence of cardiomyopathy in Italian asymptomatic children with electrocardiographic T-wave inversion at preparticipation screening. *Circulation.* 2012;125:529–538.
163. Wellens HJJ, Schwartz PJ, Lindemans FW, et al. Risk stratification for sudden cardiac death: current status and challenges for the future. *Eur Heart J.* 2014;35:1642–1651.
164. Ho CY, Lopez B, Coelho-Filho OR, et al. Myocardial fibrosis as an early manifestation of hypertrophic cardiomyopathy. *N Engl J Med.* 2010;363:552–563.
165. Coller JM, Campbell DJ, Krum H, Prior DL. Early identification of asymptomatic subjects at increased risk of heart failure and cardiovascular events: Progress and future directions. *Heart Lung Circ.* 2013;22:171–178.
166. Weber R, Kantor P, Chitiyat D, et al. Spectrum and outcome of primary cardiomyopathies diagnosed during fetal life. *J Am Coll Cardiol Heart Failure.* 2014;2:403–411.
167. Khouri MG, Peshock RM, Ayers CR, de Lemos JA, Drazner MH. A 4-tiered classification of left ventricular hypertrophy based on left ventricular geometry: The Dallas heart study. *Circ Cardiovasc Imaging.* 2010;3:164–171.
168. Chinali M, Aurigemma GP. Refining patterns of left ventricular hypertrophy using cardiac MRI. *Circ Cardiovasc Imaging.* 2010;3:129–131.
169. Giannakidis A, Rohmer D, Veress AI, Gullberg GT. Diffusion tensor magnetic resonance imaging-derived myocardial fiber disarray in hypertensive left ventricular hypertrophy: visualization, quantification and the effect on mechanical function. In: Shenasa M, Hindricks G, Borggrefe, Breithardt G, Josephson ME, eds. *Cardiac Mapping,* 4th ed. Palo Alto, CA: Wiley Blackwell; 2013:574–588.
170. Wolpert C, Veltmann C, Schimpf R, et al. Is a narrow and tall QRS complex an ECG marker for sudden death? *Heart Rhythm*;2008;5:1339–1345.
171. Chandra N, Bastiaenen R, Papdakis M, et al. Prevalence of electrocardiographic anomalies in young individuals. *J Am Coll Cardiol.* 2014;63:2028–2034.
172. Curtis AB, Bourji M. ECG screening is not warranted for the recreational athlete. *J Am Coll Cardiol.* 2014;63:2035–2036.
173. Tanawuttiwat T, Sager SJ, Hare JM, Myerburg RJ. Myocarditis and ARVC/D: variants or mimics? *Heart Rhythm* 2013;10:1544–1548.
174. te Riele AS, James CA, Bhonsale A, et al. Malignant arrhythmogenic right ventricular dysplasia/cardiomyopathy with a normal 12-lead electrocardiogram: a rare but underrecognized clinical entity. *Heart Rhythm.* 2013;10:1484–1491.

CHAPTER

7

Electrocardiographic Markers of Arrhythmic Events and Sudden Death in Channelopathies

Sergio Richter, MD, Josep Brugada, MD, PhD, Ramon Brugada, MD, and Pedro Brugada, MD, PhD

INTRODUCTION

Advanced progress in genetics and molecular biology has rendered it possible to define a series of inherited arrhythmogenic disorders linked to sudden cardiac death (SCD) in young individuals with structurally normal hearts: the long QT syndrome (LQTS), Brugada syndrome (BrS), short QT syndrome (SQTS), and catecholaminergic polymorphic ventricular tachycardia (CPVT). These diseases are linked to mutations in genes encoding cardiac ion-channel proteins or related regulatory peptides and affect the structure and function of cardiac ion channels (so-called *ion channelopathies*). Mutation-specific alterations in ionic currents and action potential (AP) shape may lead to abnormalities in cardiac impulse formation and conduction, paving the way for atrial and ventricular arrhythmias, with SCD as the most severe clinical manifestation. Since Keating's group made the seminal discovery of the first disease-causing genes for LQTS in the mid-1990s,[1–3] the characterization of ion channelopathies has provided important insights into the molecular pathogenesis of cardiac arrhythmias and defined an essential substrate for what has long been considered idiopathic ventricular fibrillation (VF) and sudden unexplained or infant death syndrome.

The ECG brings several cardiac electrophysiologic abnormalities to the surface and may even act as a genetic messenger when its simple waveforms reflect highly specific protein alterations in the heart. Apart from its outstanding role in the diagnosis of inherited arrhythmia syndromes, the surface ECG provides the most practical and powerful tool for risk stratification, particularly of asymptomatic individuals. However, there is a large variability in the phenotypic expression among individuals with any given channelopathy. This holds particularly true for the electrocardiographic picture and makes genotype–phenotype correlation and ECG-based risk stratification challenging tasks. The aim of this chapter is to summarize the electrocardiographic features and markers of arrhythmic risk in cardiac ion channelopathies.

The ECG Handbook of Contemporary Challenges © 2015 Mohammad Shenasa, Mark E. Josephson, N.A. Mark Estes III
Cardiotext Publishing, ISBN: 978-1-935395-88-1

BRUGADA SYNDROME

BrS is an arrhythmogenic disorder characterized by right precordial coved-type ST-segment elevation, conduction abnormalities, atrial arrhythmias, and life-threatening ventricular arrhythmias.[4] The worldwide prevalence of BrS is estimated to be 1:2000.[5] BrS is heterogeneous but in several instances is an inherited genetic disease caused by cardiac ion-channel mutations in up to 30% of phenotypically affected individuals. Twelve genes causally linked to BrS have been identified so far.[5] Loss-of-function mutations in *SCN5A*, the gene encoding the α-subunit of the cardiac sodium channel, account for the majority (>75%) of genotype-positive cases and constitute the genetic key player at present (BrS1).[6] The clinical manifestations of BrS are quite malignant, as they include unexpected syncope, nocturnal agonal respiration, and SCD in young and otherwise healthy individuals. These symptoms usually occur at rest, during sleep, fever, or vagotonic conditions. BrS predominantly manifests in male adults with arrhythmic events peaking in the fourth and fifth decade of life. Once symptomatic, patients are prone to experience future arrhythmic events. Therefore, ECG-based risk stratification is of particular importance to identify asymptomatic individuals at increased risk of SCD, which can be the first clinical manifestation without any warning signature.

ECG Features and Risk Stratification

The ECG hallmark and diagnostic cornerstone of BrS is coved-type ≥2 mm (0.2 mV) ST-segment elevation followed by an inverted T-wave in the right precordial leads V_1 to V_2 that present either spontaneously or after intravenous administration of a sodium-channel blocker (ajmaline, flecainide, procainamide, or pilsicainide) (Figure 7.1). This characteristic ECG pattern has been labeled type 1 Brugada ECG and is the only pattern diagnostic of the syndrome. In addition, nondiagnostic (types 2 and 3) patterns of right precordial ≥2 mm (0.2 mV) J-point and ST-segment elevation with saddleback-like configuration have long been described and linked to BrS. Since the type 3 pattern is unspecific and relatively prevalent in the general population (up to 2.3% in Asia), it has most recently been proposed to skip this pattern and consider only a single, saddleback-shaped type 2 pattern that combines ECG features of the previously defined type 2 and 3 patterns (Figure 7.2).[9]

Importantly, spontaneous right precordial J-point and ST-segment elevation is highly dynamic in extent and over time in virtually all patients with BrS.[10] This includes transient normalization and conversion from one to the other ECG pattern in the presence or absence of right bundle branch block (RBBB) (Figure 7.3). Moreover, a diagnostic coved-type pattern frequently

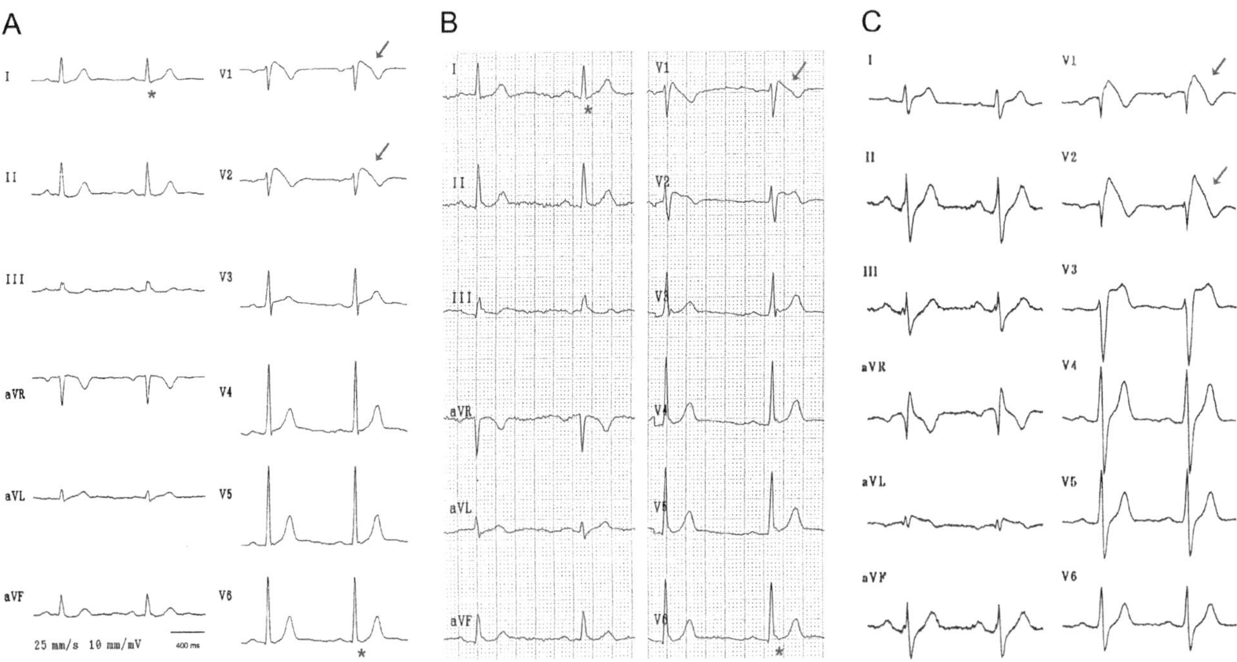

Figure 7.1. Examples of a spontaneous type 1 Brugada ECG characterized by coved-type ST-segment elevation in leads V_1 to V_2 (arrows). **A** and **B**. The lack of reciprocal S waves in leads V_6 and I indicates absence of incomplete RBBB (asterisks). **B**. Note the presence of inferolateral early repolarization and type 2 pattern in lead V_2 (*single-lead type 1 ECG*). **C**. Signs of a more severe ECG phenotype are present including concomitant ST-segment elevation in lead aVL, PR prolongation, true RBBB with marked left-axis deviation, and prominent R wave in lead aVR (*aVR sign*). Paper speed = 25 mm/s.

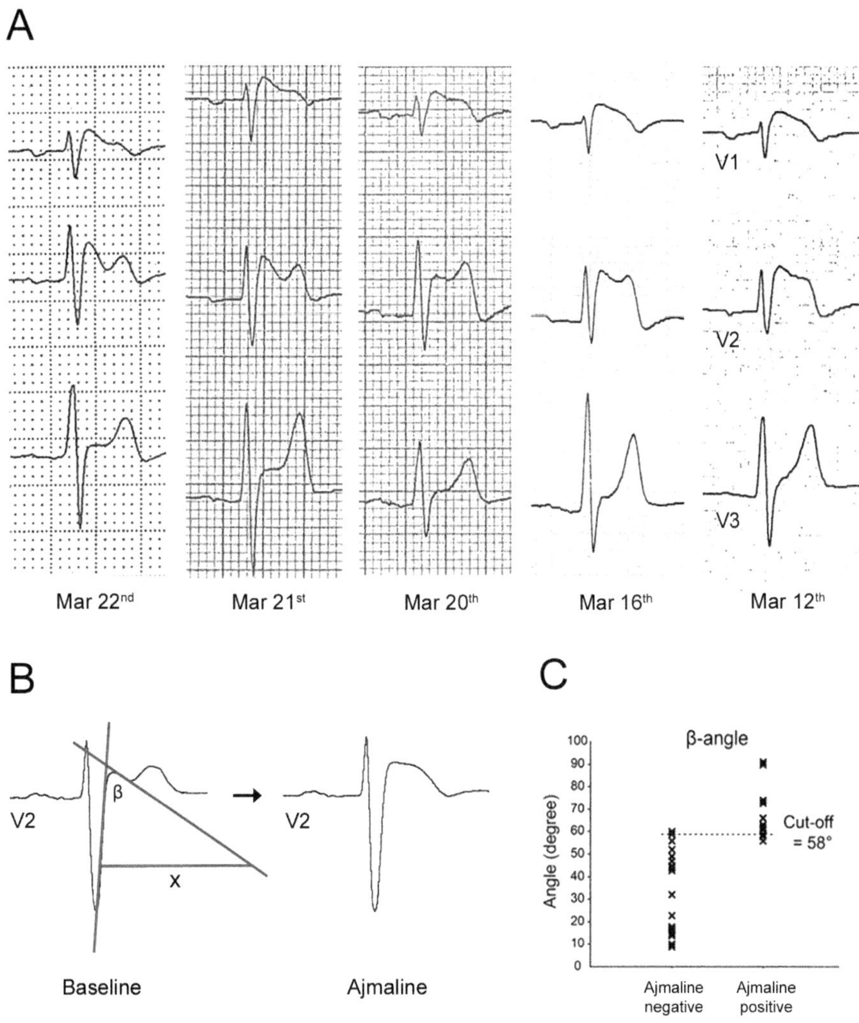

Figure 7.2. Characteristics of saddleback-type ST-segment elevation. **A.** Note the dynamic variations in J-point and ST-segment elevation and the spontaneous conversion from type 1 to type 2 pattern in lead V_2. **B** and **C.** Cut-off values for β >58° and *x* > 3.5 mm allow differentiation between incomplete RBBB and type 2 Brugada pattern and predict a positive response to ajmaline. β, angle between upslope of the S wave and downslope of the r′ (J) wave; *x*, duration of the base of the triangle at 5 mm from peak of the r′(J) wave. **C.** Modified with permission.[109]. Paper speed = 25 mm/s.

appears in only one standard right precordial lead (V_1 or V_2) with or without a concomitant saddleback-type pattern in one of the other right precordial leads (see Figure 7.1B).[11] We have recently shown that individuals with only so-called single-lead type 1 ECGs have a similar clinical profile and arrhythmic risk as Brugada patients with ECGs fulfilling the proposed 2002 consensus diagnostic ECG criteria.[11] Our findings were not surprising since detection of diagnostic coved-type ST-segment elevation strongly depends on the position of the recording lead in relation to the right ventricular outflow tract (RVOT), which harbors the critical arrhythmogenic substrate in BrS. Using magnetic resonance imaging (MRI), Veltmann et al[14] elegantly demonstrated that the RVOT projects to the third intercostal space in all cases and that leads placed in sternal and left parasternal positions at the third and fourth intercostal spaces revealed the highest yield to detect a spontaneous or drug-induced type 1 ECG. According to these and other new data, the diagnostic consensus ECG criteria have most recently been revised.[15] BrS is from now on diagnosed in the presence of spontaneous or drug-induced coved-type ST-segment elevation in ≥1 right precordial lead (V_1 to V_2) placed in a standard or modified sternal position at the fourth or third intercostal space after exclusion of other clinical conditions known to cause or contribute to right precordial coved-type ST-segment elevation mimicking the Brugada–ECG phenotype (so-called *Brugada phenocopies*[16]) (Table 7.1).

Proposed underlying mechanisms of the ECG phenotype and related arrhythmias are based on

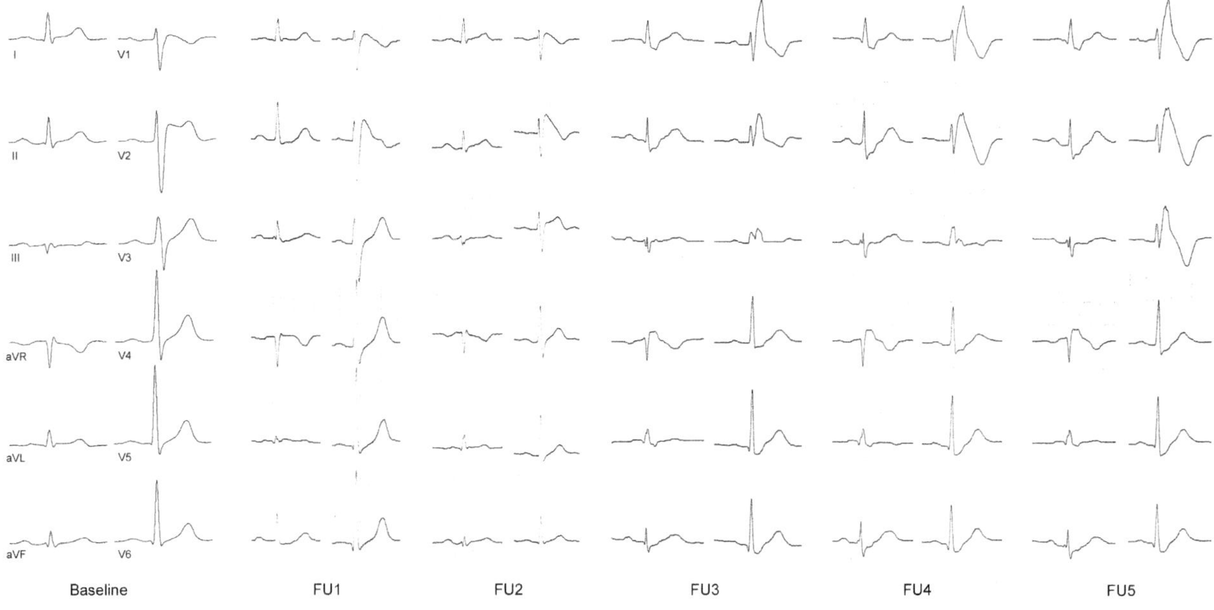

Figure 7.3. Selected 12-lead ECGs recorded during follow-up in a symptomatic male ICD recipient. Note the spontaneous variability of the Brugada ECG pattern in lead V_2 and time-dependent development of complete RBBB with and without spontaneous appearance of type 1 ST-segment elevation. Paper speed = 25 mm/s.

Table 7.1. **Causes of right precordial ST-segment elevation other than BrS.**

Acute myocardial ischemia (involving anterior septum or RV).
Prinzmetal's variant angina.
Acute (peri-) myocarditis.
Acute pulmonary embolism.
Dissecting aortic aneurysm.
Arrhythmogenic right ventricular cardiomyopathy.
Chagas disease.
Myotonic dystrophy type 1.
Friedreich's ataxia.
Duchenne muscular dystrophy.
Hemopericardium.
Pectus excavatum.
Mediastinal tumor.
External electrical cardioversion.
Early repolarization (particularly in athletes).
Electrolyte disturbances (i.e., hyperkalemia, hypercalcemia).
Cocaine intoxication.
Hypothermia.

an intrinsic and/or induced marked increase in dispersion of ventricular repolarization (*repolarization hypothesis*) and regional RVOT conduction slowing (*depolarization hypothesis*). According to the repolarization theory, an intrinsically prominent I_{to}-mediated AP notch and subsequent loss of AP dome in the RVOT epicardium but not endocardium give rise to a transmural voltage gradient resulting in ST-segment elevation and increased susceptibility to phase 2 reentry and VF.[13] In this regard, modulating factors (sympathovagal balance, body temperature, electrolyte imbalance, metabolic, and hormonal factors) and pharmacological drugs that create an outward shift in current active during phase 1 of the cardiac AP (basically $\downarrow I_{Na}$, $\uparrow I_{to}$, and $\downarrow I_{Ca\text{-}L}$) can provoke or aggravate transient J-point and ST-segment elevation, promote conduction slowing, and critically increase electrical vulnerability in affected individuals.[13] With the exception of sodium-channel blockers to unmask a type 1 Brugada ECG for diagnostic purpose (see Figure 7.2B), listed pharmacological drugs (www.brugadadrugs.org) should therefore be avoided in patients with BrS.[18] Indeed, the majority of individuals with the type 1 ECG signature do not develop ventricular arrhythmias throughout their lifetime when they refrain from these drugs and fever is aggressively managed. Nonetheless, a significant number of patients (20%–40%) experience arrhythmic events, which emphasizes the great challenge of risk assessment particularly in asymptomatic individuals and those with assumed neurally-mediated syncope.

The knowledge of the dynamics of the spontaneous ECG pattern has changed our way of thinking about the role of the baseline 12-lead ECG in decision making and risk stratification. The spontaneous presence of a type 1 ECG does not only facilitate recognition of an underlying arrhythmogenic disorder but also indicate an increased arrhythmic risk, particularly in individuals with unexplained syncope.[19–22] In fact, the vast majority of patients reported with arrhythmic events have a spontaneous type 1 ECG. Moreover, we have reported that even symptomatic patients may have a favorable outcome in cases where spontaneous type 1 ST-segment elevation has never been documented on any ECG recording.[10] Notably, spontaneous alterations in the type and amplitude (Δ ≥2 mm) of right precordial ST-segment elevation are associated with arrhythmic events.[23] Including recent follow-up data from the major Brugada registries, the annual event rate in asymptomatic patients with spontaneous type 1 ECG reaches up to 2.5%. On the other hand, there is a general agreement that arrhythmic risk is negligible in asymptomatic patients with only drug-induced type 1 ECG.[19–22] We now understand that detection of spontaneous and dynamic coved-type ST-segment elevation is crucial for ECG-based risk stratification. This calls for tools other than standard 12-lead ECG to improve prognostic yield such as repetitive modified right precordial lead recording, multichannel Holter-ECG recording, and exercise testing.

Specifically, the development or augmentation of coved-type ST-segment elevation during the recovery phase of exercise[24] (Figure 7.4) and the presence of QRS fragmentation in the right precordial leads (Figure 7.5) have been convincingly identified as strong indicators of arrhythmic risk. The existence of late potentials (LPs) and complex fractionated electrograms is a compelling marker of slow electrical impulse conduction within the ventricular myocardium.[27] In addition to a marked left QRS axis deviation (Rs pattern in lead I, rS pattern in inferior leads, $S_{II} > S_{III}$) and pronounced (≥0.3 mV) R wave in lead aVR (so-called *aVR sign*[28]) (see Figure 7.1C), critical degree of RVOT conduction delay may manifest on surface ECG as prolonged (>110 ms) and fragmented QRS complex (f-QRS) in the right precordial leads V_1 and V_2. Localized right precordial QRS prolongation is a well-recognized ECG feature in patients with spontaneous J-point and ST-segment elevation.[29–31] Sophisticated combined body-surface potential mapping and signal-averaged ECG (SAECG) recording localized terminal conduction delay to the RVOT and mapped remarkably delayed potentials to the area of maximum ST-segment elevation in the RVOT. LPs and dominant right precordial prolongation of filtered QRS duration are frequently observed in symptomatic patients with BrS. SAECG may therefore provide another useful ECG tool to identify patients at increased risk.

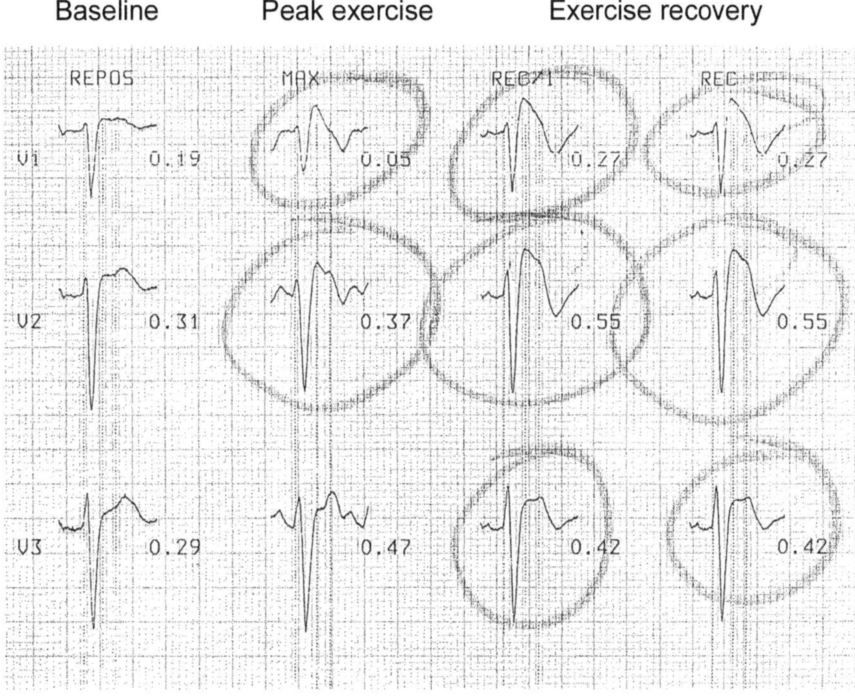

Figure 7.4. Effect of exercise on right precordial ST-segment elevation in a patient with syncope. Note the appearance of type 1 ST-segment elevation in leads V_1 and V_2 at peak exercise and further increase in amplitude during exercise recovery. Paper speed = 25 mm/s.

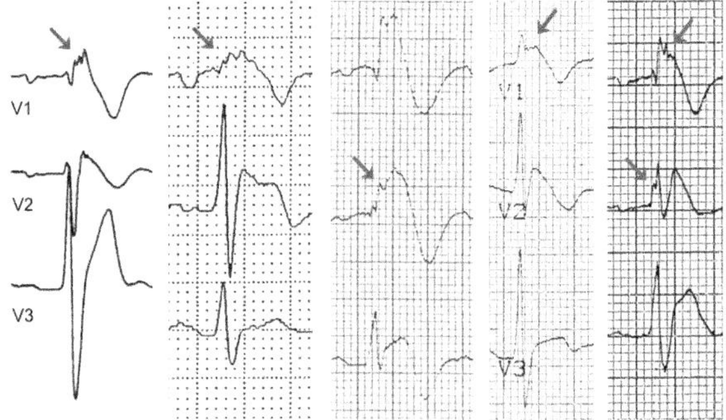

Figure 7.5. Different patterns of right precordial QRS fragmentation (arrows). Note the presence of spontaneous type 1 ST-segment elevation in all cases. Paper speed = 25 mm/s.

Localized QRS prolongation in the right precordial leads is basically the result of a prolonged S-wave upstroke and/or broad J wave (so-called *S terminal delay*) and has been proposed as an ECG marker to discriminate symptomatic from asymptomatic patients.[29] A cut-off value of ≥120 ms for the QRS duration in lead V_2 yielded the best prediction with an odds ratio of 2.5 for being symptomatic. Interestingly, Tatsumi et al[30] reported that symptoms were not only associated with QRS prolongation in lead V_2 and corresponding prolongation of the filtered QRS duration and low-amplitude signals on SAECG, but even more with daily fluctuations of these parameters. Prolonged QRS duration in lead V_2 may also be associated with an increased QT interval, QT dispersion, T_{peak}-T_{end} interval, and T_{peak}-T_{end} dispersion in the presence of spontaneous coved-type ST-segment elevation (Figure 7.6). These ECG features, in particular T_{peak}-T_{end} interval and T_{peak}-T_{end} dispersion are markers of an increased and inhomogeneous transmural dispersion of repolarization (TDR) and electrical instability. In this spirit, a corrected QT interval >460 ms in lead V_2 (but not in the inferolateral leads), T_{peak}-T_{end} interval ≥100 ms, and precordial T_{peak}-T_{end} dispersion >20 ms seem to be useful ECG risk markers in BrS.[36]

Perhaps the strongest indicator of an acutely increased TDR and electrical instability is the appearance of macroscopic T-wave alternans (TWA). Alternation in T-wave amplitude or polarity may occasionally occur during sodium channel-blocker administration and is usually associated with the development of coved-type ST-segment elevation in the right precordial or inferior leads. In a recent study by Tada et al,[38] drug-induced TWA proved to be an independent predictor of VF. Fortunately, macroscopic TWA virtually never occurs spontaneously in the absence of fever.[39] Experimental data from the wedge suggest that TWA may result from alternating loss of the epicardial AP dome or concealed phase 2 reentry within the epicardium on alternate beats.[40] The acute emergence of

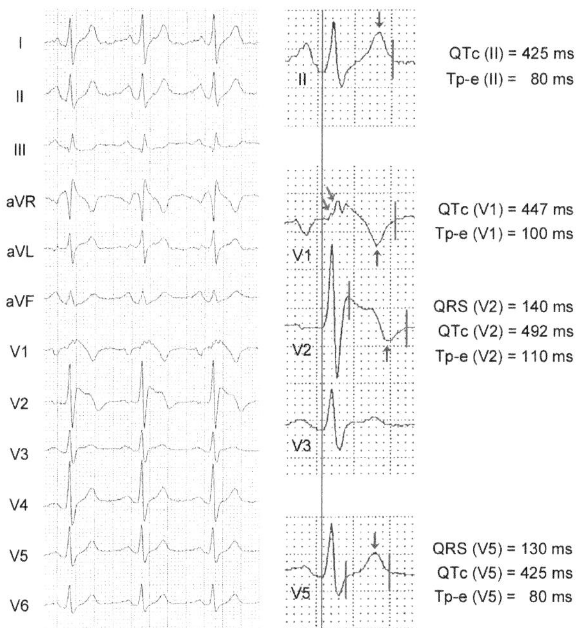

Figure 7.6. ECG signs of localized right ventricular depolarization and repolarization abnormalities. Note the prolonged and fractionated QRS complex in lead V_1 (red arrows) and markedly prolonged QTc and T_{peak}-T_{end} interval in lead V_2 in the presence of coved-type ST-segment elevation. T_{peak}-T_{end} dispersion is 30 ms. Selected intervals are given. Blue arrows indicate T_{peak}. Paper speed = 25 mm/s.

augmented J-waves in the inferior (and lateral) leads provides another potential ECG marker of an acutely increased electrical vulnerability and risk of imminent malignant ventricular arrhythmias in BrS (Figure 7.7).

Conduction abnormalities are frequently encountered in patients with BrS, particularly in those carrying a loss-of-function *SCN5A* mutation.[41] Common manifestations of associated conduction disease are signs of sinus node dysfunction, prolonged PR interval and HV conduction time, left QRS axis deviation, and QRS prolongation with or without RBBB and/or left fascicular block. Importantly, the presence of a prolonged PR interval (>200 ms) has been identified as an independent predictor of arrhythmic events.[42] Another important ECG manifestation in BrS is paroxysmal atrial fibrillation, which occurs in approximately 20% to 30% of affected individuals and may be the first presenting symptom. Its spontaneous appearance has been associated with an increased electrical vulnerability and occurrence of ventricular arrhythmias.

Many of the above-discussed ECG markers usually appear in conjunction with spontaneous coved-type ST-segment elevation and, as a consequence, are not very frequent in nature, considering that even in high-risk patients only 1 out of 4 (25%) 12-lead ECG recordings display spontaneous type 1 ST-segment elevation.[10] The low penetrance of *SCN5A* mutations

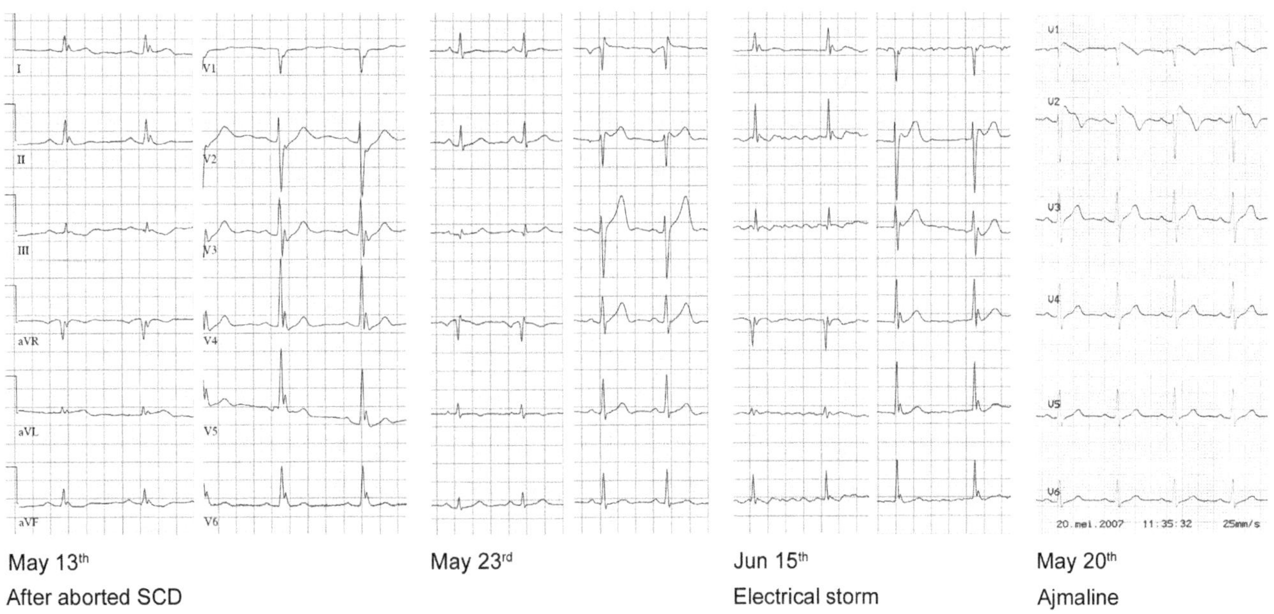

B

15/06/07 9:45:03

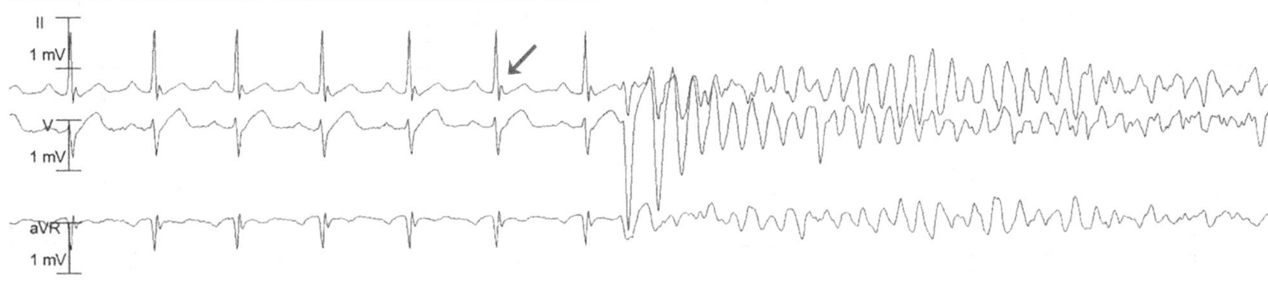

Figure 7.7. Example of malignant early repolarization associated with BrS. Selected ECGs from an Asian cardiac-arrest survivor who experienced recurrent VF. **A.** Note the dynamic nature of the ECG and emergence of augmented J waves in the inferolateral leads at time of arrhythmic events (May 13th and Jun 15th). Intravenous ajmaline unmasked type 1 ST-segment elevation in leads V_1 and V_2 (May 20th). Note the presence of AF during an electrical storm episode (Jun 15th). **B.** Spontaneous VF episode associated with inferior early repolarization (arrow). Paper speed = 25 mm/s.

and the high variability of the Brugada ECG phenotype throw a bit of a monkey wrench in risk stratifying affected individuals based on the ECG. A completely normal ECG recorded today may convert to a diagnostic and even prognostic one tomorrow. This raises anew the controversial issue of whether asymptomatic patients with a spontaneous type 1 ECG should undergo invasive risk stratification. Clearly, despite substantial discrepancies in outcome of inducible patients, all registries agree on the excellent negative predictive value of programmed ventricular stimulation (98%–99%).[45] In addition, the presence of a short ventricular effective refractory period (<200 ms) has most recently been identified as an independent predictor of arrhythmic events.[20] A prolonged HV interval (>60 ms) may further assist in decision making.[46] In view of the lack of sensitive data on other risk-stratification tools, we recommend making use of this information and offering an electrophysiologic study to (as yet) asymptomatic individuals with spontaneous type 1 ECG.[47] Table 7.2 summarizes the proposed ECG risk markers in BrS.

LONG QT SYNDROME

The congenital LQTS, the prototype of an arrhythmogenic ion-channel disease is characterized by prolongation of the QT interval and life-threatening ventricular arrhythmias. LQTS is estimated to be prevalent in

Table 7.2. **Proposed ECG risk markers in BrS.**

Spontaneous coved-type ST-segment elevation in leads V_1 to V_2(V_3).
Augmented ST-segment elevation during exercise recovery.
f-QRS in leads V_1 to V_2.
Prominent R wave (≥0.3 mV) in lead aVR ("aVR-sign").
Prolonged QRS duration in lead V_2 (≥120 ms).
Prolonged QTc interval in lead V_2 (>460 ms).
Increased T_{p-e} interval (≥100 ms) and precordial T_{p-e} dispersion (>20 ms).
Macroscopic TWA (after class I drug challenge).
Early repolarization pattern in inferior (lateral) leads.
Prolonged PR interval (>200 ms).

1:2000 apparently healthy living births and represents a frequent cause of SCD in the young.[48] As of today, molecular genetic studies have identified 13 LQTS variants caused by several mutations in genes encoding subunits of cardiac ion channels, related factors, and membrane adaptor proteins.[49] By far, *KCNQ1*, *KCNH2*, and *SCN5A* (LQT1-3) are the most common LQTS genes, accounting for >90% of genotype-positive cases.[49] Consequently, our knowledge on genotype–phenotype characteristics and risk stratification in LQTS mainly derives from large cohorts of individuals affected by these 3 LQTS variants.

ECG Features and Risk Stratification

The electrocardiographic hallmark of LQTS is a prolonged, rate-corrected QT (QTc) interval. In general, QTc intervals >440 ms are considered prolonged but may still be normal among females. The proposed cutoff values for a definitely abnormal QTc prolongation (using Bazett's formula) are >450 ms in adult men, >460 ms in infants and children, and >470 ms in adult women.[50] However, the QTc interval is not necessarily prolonged in genetically affected individuals: 10% (LQT3) to 37% (LQT1) have a normal QTc interval on resting 12-lead ECG (so-called *silent mutation carriers*) as a consequence of low penetrance. Accordingly, it has been proposed to diagnose LQTS in the presence of an unequivocally disease-causing mutation irrespective of the QTc interval.[15] Conversely, in the absence of secondary causes for QTc prolongation, LQTS is diagnosed in the presence of a QTc interval ≥500 ms.[15] In all other cases, the updated LQTS diagnostic (Schwartz) score, which includes gradual scoring for longer QTc intervals should be applied.[53] According to the recently proposed consensus criteria, the diagnosis of LQTS is highly probable with a LQTS score of ≥3.5.[15] Importantly, the Schwartz score is mainly comprised of ECG parameters, some of which strongly indicate an increased risk, in particular, of the spontaneous occurrence of torsades de pointes (TdP) polymorphic VT, the degree of QTc interval prolongation, and the appearance of morphologic T-wave alterations.

There is convincing evidence that the longer the QTc interval, the more severe is the ECG phenotype and the greater the risk for arrhythmic events. The risk is significantly high when the QTc interval exceeds 500 ms and becomes extremely high when the QTc interval outruns 550 to 600 ms. The recently proposed M-FACT risk score takes the strong prognostic value of such prolonged QTc intervals into consideration.[54] Importantly, an extreme prolongation of the QTc interval may occasionally cause 2:1 functional atrioventricular (AV) block, which usually manifests in the fetal or neonatal period (incidence up to 4.5%) and is associated with an extremely high risk of lethal arrhythmic events (Figure 7.8). A recent study on neonates with congenital LQTS and 2:1 AV block revealed an average QTc interval of 616 ms (range 531–830 ms).[62] Early recognition and treatment with β-blocker (± mexiletine) and cardiac pacing if necessary keyed to improve the outcome in this high-risk pediatric population. Basically, the presence of marked bradycardia caused by functional AV block or sudden sinus pauses (>1200 ms) has been regarded as a marker of risk for TdP events, particularly in affected children with LQT3.[63] Schwartz et al[64] observed that long sinus pauses are frequently followed by the appearance of a notch on the T wave and postulated that repetitive and TdP-triggering premature beats most likely arise from such notches. Indeed, ventricular repolarization is not only prolonged but also inhomogeneous in the majority of genetically affected LQTS patients, resulting in distinct and often gene-specific morphologic T-wave alterations, which are particularly evident in the precordial leads and contribute to diagnosis and ECG-based risk stratification in LQTS (Figure 7.9).

T-wave notching is rather typical for LQT2 and its appearance has been associated with a higher risk of arrhythmic events.[58] Notches on the T waves are believed to reflect the presence of subthreshold early afterdepolarizations (EADs). Prolongation of ventricular repolarization predisposes to the generation of secondary Ca^{2+}-triggered depolarizations during the plateau or early repolarization phase of the AP. However, an underlying substrate of increased dispersion of ventricular repolarization seems to be essential for EAD-mediated triggered activity to initiate TdP and maintain reentry.[69–71]

Clinically useful ECG markers of increased spatial and transmural dispersion of ventricular repolarization and electrical instability are an augmented QT

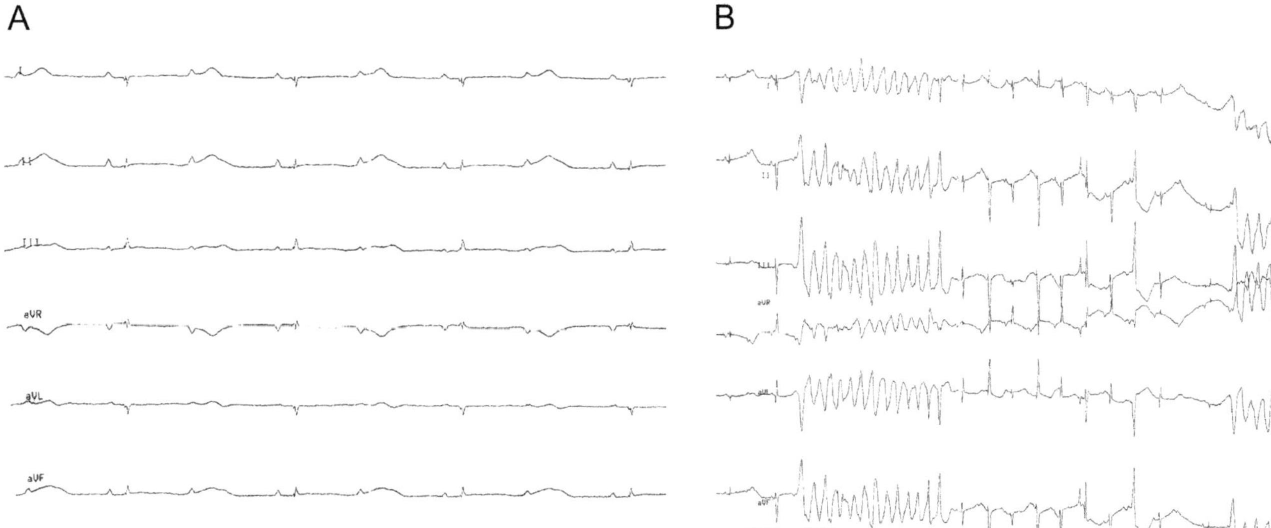

Figure 7.8. Functional 2:1 AV block caused by an extremely prolonged QTc interval (**A**) resulting in self-limiting episodes of TdP (**B**) in a newborn with congenital LQT3. Note that the absolute QT interval exceeds the sinus cycle length by far.

dispersion and prolonged T_{peak}-T_{end} interval. The proposed cut-off values to identify LQTS patients at increased risk are >100 ms for QT dispersion (QT_{max}-QT_{min}) and >6 for the QT dispersion index (standard deviation of QT/QT average × 100).[73] The consideration of the T_{peak}-T_{end} interval may extent the value of repolarization abnormalities beyond QT duration and dispersion, particularly in individuals with normal or borderline QTc interval. The T_{peak}-T_{end} interval is thought to provide a reasonable measure of TDR since it reflects both epicardial repolarization (T_{peak}) and repolarization of the M cells (T_{end}).[76] Recent studies identified an abnormally prolonged T_{peak}-T_{end} interval (>100 ms) as an independent predictor of SCD in patients with coronary artery disease or acquired bradyarrhythmias.[77,78] In cases of acquired LQTS,

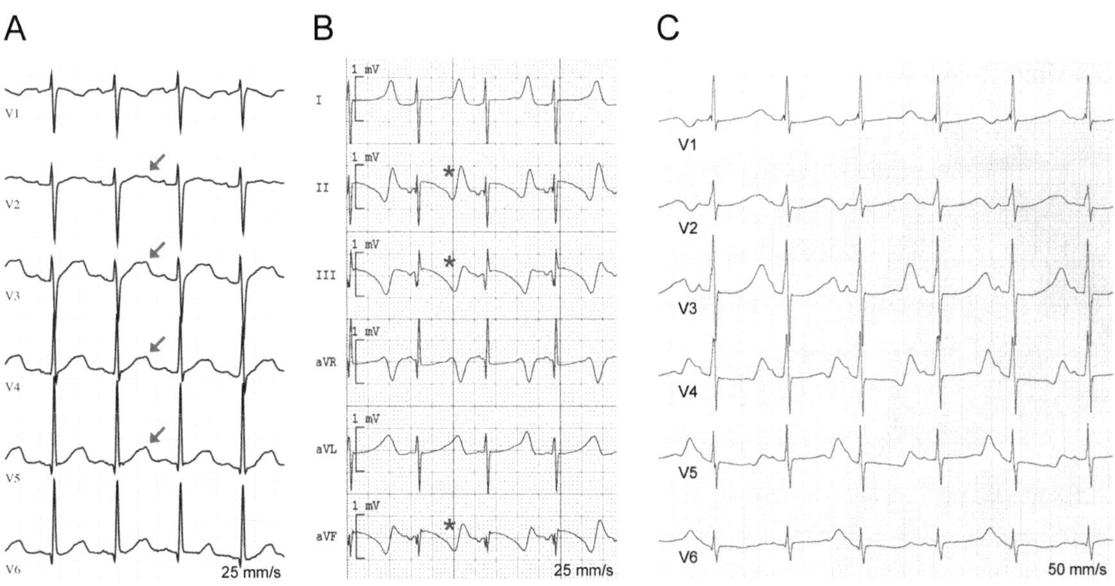

Figure 7.9. Different T-wave morphologies in genetically affected patients with LQTS. **A.** Note the notched T waves in the precordial leads (arrows) typically seen in LQT2. QTc = 521 ms. **B.** Biphasic T waves in the inferior leads (asterisks) in a patient with LQT3. Note the typical LQT3 T-wave pattern in lead I with late-onset T wave of normal duration and amplitude. QTc = 650 ms. **C.** Alternation in T-wave amplitude (V_3 to V_6) and polarity (V_1 to V_2) in concert with an extremely prolonged QTc interval (665 ms) in a patient with LQT3. Paper speed as indicated (5 mm/s).

the T_{peak}-T_{end} interval was found to be significantly longer in patients with TdP (>100 ms; mean 185 ± 46 ms) than without TdP.[74] In addition, a cut-off value >0.28 for the T_{peak}-T_{end}/QT ratio identified patients at risk for arrhythmic events in this study. Notably, Takenaka et al[75] showed that genetically affected LQT2 patients revealed significantly longer baseline T_{peak}-T_{end} intervals than LQT1 patients (191 ± 67 vs. 132 ± 52 ms) despite similarly prolonged QTc intervals, which may partially contribute to the generally higher risk (especially at rest) in LQT2 compared with LQT1. Conversely, in particular LQT1 patients exhibited significant prolongation of the QTc interval and corrected T_{peak}-T_{end} interval (215 ± 46 ms) in response to exercise,[75] strongly suggesting an exercise-related increase in TDR, which may in turn contribute to the high incidence of exercise-triggered arrhythmic events in LQT1 patients.[81]

Morphological T-wave abnormalities frequently seen in patients with congenital LQTS include biphasic and bifid (or notched) T-wave patterns (see Figure 7.9A and B). These T-wave alterations are believed to indicate electrical vulnerability and have been associated with arrhythmic events.[58] The most devastating ECG marker of acutely increased TDR and electrical instability is the appearance of macroscopic TWA (Figures 7.9C and 7.10A).[57] Alternation in T-wave amplitude or polarity is rarely present at rest but may occur during emotional stress or physical activity. Macroscopic alternans in T-wave polarity is invariably associated with marked QTc prolongation and often precedes TdP, which may degenerate into VF, and, accordingly, identifies patients at high risk for SCD (see Figure 7.10B). This holds particularly true when TWA becomes evident despite proper antiadrenergic therapy.[80] The mechanisms underlying TWA are not entirely elucidated. Data derived from the wedge strongly suggest that TWA is a result of beat-to-beat alternation of the M cell AP duration leading to exaggeration of TDR on alternate beats.[83]

Risk stratification in congenital LQTS is at times straightforward but still remains challenging in many affected individuals. As discussed in this section, the ECG may provide important clues to facilitate risk assessment. However, complexity is added by the fact that arrhythmic risk is age-dependent, gender- and genotype-related. Together with the presence of marked QTc prolongation >500 ms, the genetic background is one of the strongest independent predictors of cardiac events before and during antiadrenergic therapy. Noteworthy, the recessive Jervell and Lange-Nielsen syndrome (LQT1 + 5) variants and the extremely rare Timothy syndrome (LQT8) are highly malignant, manifest with arrhythmic events very early, and respond poorly to conventional therapy. Specifically, Timothy syndrome is associated with an inconceivably high mortality at very young age.[85] Of particular interest, affected children often present

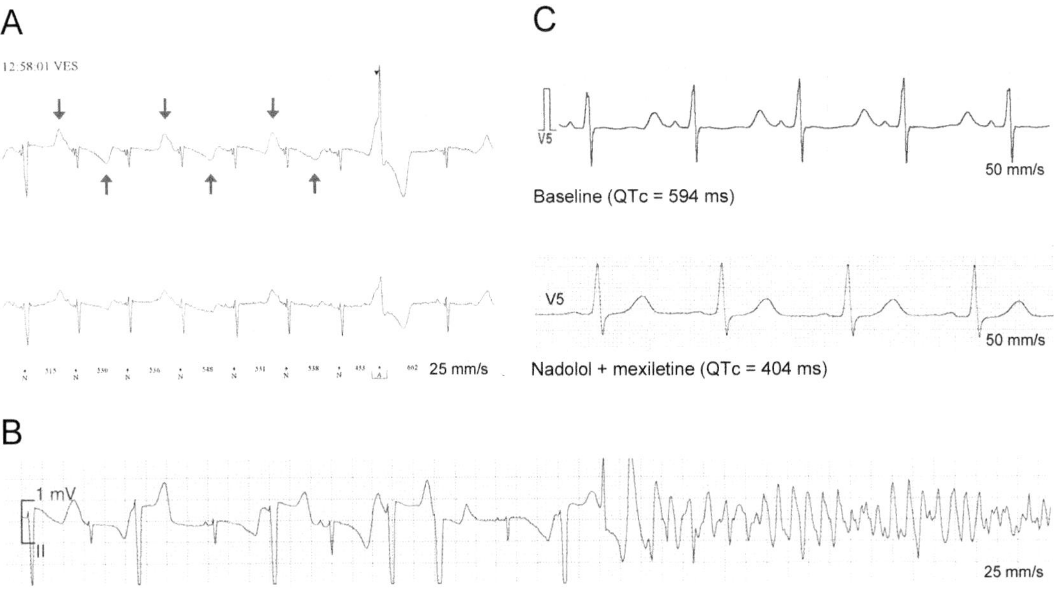

Figure 7.10. Example of macroscopic TWA (**A.** arrows) preceding ventricular ectopies and polymorphic VT degenerating into VF (**B**) in a newborn with congenital LQT3. **C.** Note the prolonged QTc interval (594 ms) and isoelectric ST segment at baseline. Combined β-blocker and sodium-channel blocker treatment resulted in suppression of ventricular arrhythmias and normalization of the QTc interval (404 ms). Paper speed as indicated.

Table 7.3. **Proposed ECG risk markers in LQTS.**

Marked QTc prolongation (>500 ms).
2:1 functional AV conduction block.
Spontaneous episodes of TdP.
Macroscopic TWA.
Biphasic or notched T waves in precordial (inferior) leads.
Prolonged T_{p-e} interval (>100 ms) and T_{p-e}/QT ratio (>0.28).
Increased QT dispersion (>100 ms) and QT dispersion index (>6).
Severe sinus bradycardia or pauses (>1200 ms).

with the strongest ECG risk markers, namely severe QTc prolongation, 2:1 functional AV block, and macroscopic TWA.[85] Table 7.3 summarizes the proposed ECG risk markers in congenital LQTS.

SHORT QT SYNDROME

The SQTS is characterized by an abnormally short cardiac repolarization and high vulnerability to atrial and life-threatening ventricular arrhythmias and SCD.[86–88] Mutations in 5 genes encoding cardiac potassium and calcium-channel proteins have been linked to SQTS.[87] This very rare, inherited arrhythmia syndrome affects predominantly young adult males with structurally normal hearts. The occurrence of arrhythmia-related symptoms is time-dependent, peaking in the third decade of life.[89] To date, only a limited number of affected individuals have been reported worldwide with the largest cohort including 73 SQTS patients identified in 47 families.[90] Hence, the natural history of this entity is poorly elucidated, which hampers in particular risk stratification of asymptomatic individuals and those without aborted cardiac arrest.

ECG Features and Risk Stratification

The eponymous ECG signature of SQTS is a (very) short QT interval (Figure 7.11). According to the recently proposed consensus criteria, SQTS is diagnosed in the presence of a QTc interval ≤330 ms and can be diagnosed in the presence of a QTc interval <360 ms in conjunction with a disease-causing mutation or at least one clinical factor in individuals without structural heart disease and excluded secondary causes of QTc shortening.[15] For diagnostic purpose, 12-lead ECG recording and QTc calculation (using Bazett's formula) should be performed at normal resting heart rates, since the QT interval does not appropriately adapt to changes in heart rate in SQTS patients.[91] This most likely prevents incorrect measurement of a pseudonormal QTc interval at

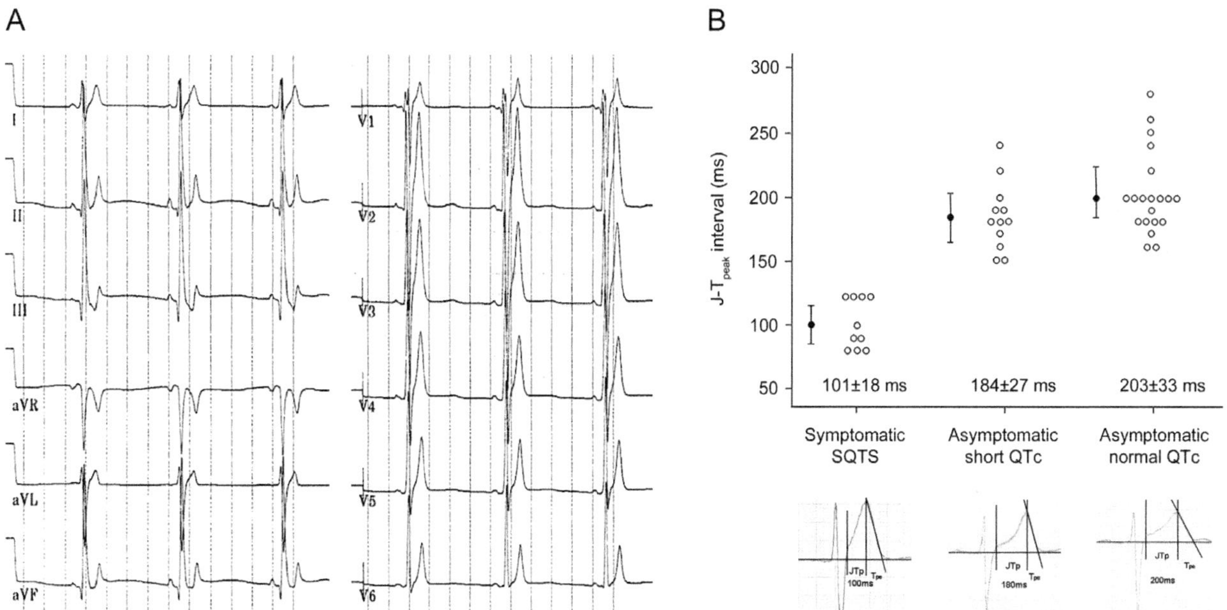

Figure 7.11. ECG features in SQTS. **A.** 12-lead ECG recorded during sinus rhythm at 65 bpm in a young patient with SQTS reveals a very short QTc interval (252 ms), tall, peaked, and symmetrical T waves in the precordial leads. Note the absence of an ST segment. Paper speed = 25 mm/s. Modified with permission.[110] **B.** An abbreviated J-T_{peak} interval is a very useful ECG marker to discriminate between SQTS patients at risk and asymptomatic individuals with short QT interval (cut-off 150 ms). Modified with permission.[92]

faster heart rates, which may lead to a false-negative diagnosis, particularly in pediatric patients.

In addition to a short QT interval, the resting 12-lead ECG typically reveals an abbreviated or even absent ST segment, and often tall, peaked, and symmetrical T waves in the precordial leads. U waves are usually small or not discernable (see Figure 7.11A). Paroxysmal AF is commonly observed and may be the first presenting symptom.[86]

The relative absence of an ST segment in patients with SQTS results in an extreme abbreviation of the interval from the J point to peak of the T wave (J-T_{peak} interval). Recent studies suggest that the presence of a markedly abbreviated J-T_{peak} interval helps to discriminate between SQTS patients at risk (J-T_{peak} <120 ms) and asymptomatic individuals with short QT interval (J-T_{peak} >150 ms) (see Figure 7.11B).[92–94] In support of these data, a previous community-based ECG study consistently revealed J-T_{peak} intervals >150 ms in healthy males (188 ± 11 ms) and females (214 ± 15 ms).[95]

Another important ECG feature in SQTS is an increased ratio of the (prolonged) T_{peak}-T_{end} interval to (shortened) QT interval (T_{peak}-T_{end}/QT ratio), one of the proposed ECG markers of augmented TDR and arrhythmogeneity. In this respect, Anttonen et al[92] found out that symptomatic SQTS patients had a significantly higher mean rate-corrected T_{peak}-T_{end}/QT ratio (0.30 ± 0.04; QTc 317 ± 27 ms) than asymptomatic individuals with equally short QT interval (0.24 ± 0.05; QTc 314 ± 14 ms) and healthy controls with normal QT interval (0.24 ± 0.04; QTc 405 ± 28 ms). It is of very great interest, and somehow surprising, that the QTc interval does not significantly differ between symptomatic and asymptomatic patients. Moreover, recent data from the largest SQTS registries actually suggest that even a very short QTc interval (<330 ms), assumed to represent a more severe ECG phenotype, is not a prognostic marker in SQTS, which is in striking contrast to the LQTS, where the extent of QTc prolongation definitely identifies patients at higher risk of life-threatening events, as described above. As a consequence, the proposed SQTS Gollob score that includes gradual scoring for shorter QTc intervals has not been widely accepted for diagnosis and risk stratification of affected individuals.

Importantly, SQTS may be associated with a type 1 Brugada ECG and early repolarization pattern. SQTS patients with loss-of-function mutations in genes encoding the cardiac L-type calcium channel (SQT4 + 5) exhibit spontaneous or drug-induced right precordial, coved-type ST-segment elevation in addition to a moderately shortened (330–360 ms) QTc interval.[100] It is tempting to speculate that this combined ECG phenotype (particularly with spontaneous type 1 pattern) bears a higher arrhythmogenic risk compared to the sole short QT phenotype seen in nonmutation carriers or carriers of single gain-of-function potassium channel mutations (SQT1-3). Early repolarization in the inferior and lateral leads is commonly observed in SQTS, and its appearance has been associated with arrhythmic events.[101]

These findings suggest that concomitant spontaneous abnormalities during the early phase of repolarization, such as prominent inferolateral J-point augmentation and right precordial coved-type ST-segment elevation, indicate an increased electrical instability and potential risk for arrhythmic events in SQTS. Table 7.4 depicts the proposed ECG risk markers in congenital SQTS.

CATECHOLAMINERGIC POLYMORPHIC VENTRICULAR TACHYCARDIA

CPVT is characterized by exercise- or emotional stress-induced polymorphic VT. CPVT manifests predominantly in children and adolescents without structural heart disease and frequently causes syncope and SCD at young age.[102–104] Molecular genetic studies have identified 2 CPVT variants caused by mutations in genes encoding the cardiac calcium-release channel (ryanodine receptor; *RyR2*) and a sarcoplasmic reticulum protein (calsequestrin; *CASQ2*), both of which critically involve calcium handling.[49] This inherited disorder is highly malignant and, when unrecognized or untreated, associated with a high mortality rate reaching 30% by the age of 30.[102] The overall prevalence of CPVT is estimated to be 1:10.000.[105]

ECG Features and Risk Stratification

The ECG hallmark of CPVT is a ventricular arrhythmia with typical bidirectional appearance,[106] which reproducibly appears during adrenergic stimulation such as physical activity, emotional stress, exercise testing, or isoproterenol infusion.[104] At first, ventricular ectopy progressively develops with exercise- or isoproterenol-induced sinus tachycardia (kick-off at 110–120 bpm). The frequency and complexity of the ventricular ectopy increase as heart rate further accelerates, finally leading to polymorphic and bidirectional

Table 7.4. **Proposed ECG risk markers in SQTS.**

Marked shortening of J-T_p interval (<120 ms).
Increased T_{p-e} interval (>100 ms) and corrected T_{p-e}/QT ratio.
Early repolarization pattern in inferior (lateral) leads .
Spontaneous type 1 Brugada pattern in leads V_1 to V_2 (SQT4 + 5).

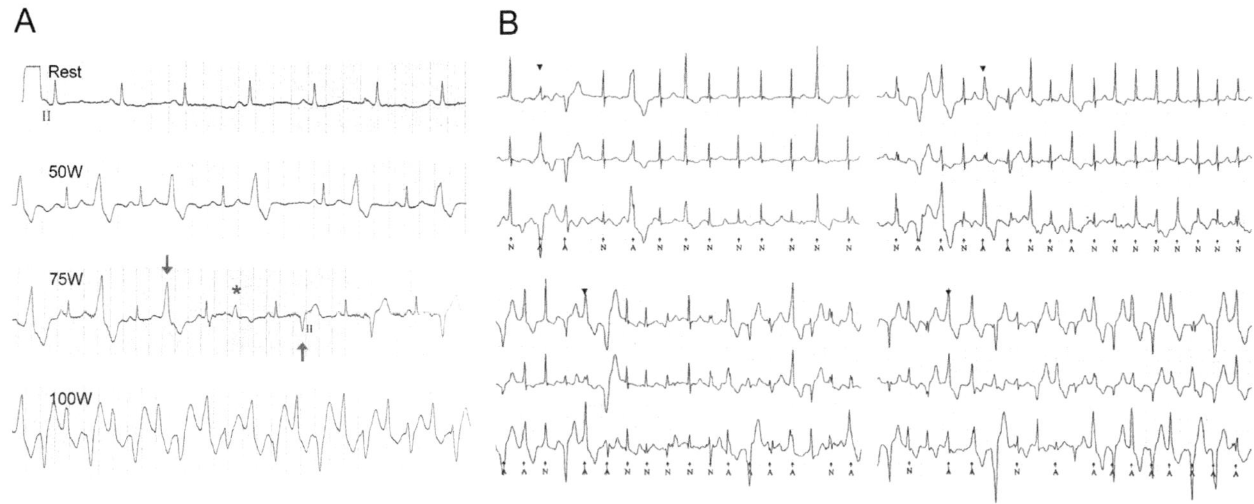

Figure 7.12. A. ECGs illustrating the successive emergence of ventricular ectopies and typical bidirectional VT in 2 distinct patients with CPVT during exercise testing (A) and acute emotional stress recorded by Holter monitoring (B). A. Note the fusion beat (asterisk) and change in QRS axis of the ventricular bigeminy (arrows) at 75 W preceding bidirectional VT with similar QRS morphologies. Paper speed = 25 mm/s.

VT (Figure 7.12), which may degenerate into VF.[107] Exercise-induced atrial tachyarrhythmias, including AF and ectopic atrial tachycardia, are frequently observed and may further trigger the occurrence of malignant ventricular arrhythmias (Figure 7.13).[108] The usually young and otherwise healthy CPVT patients present with a normal resting 12-lead ECG. In particular, the QTc interval is within normal limits or at most borderline in some cases. The baseline sinus heart rate may occasionally be lower than normal.

Thus far, no independent ECG predictor for arrhythmic events has been identified. However, the

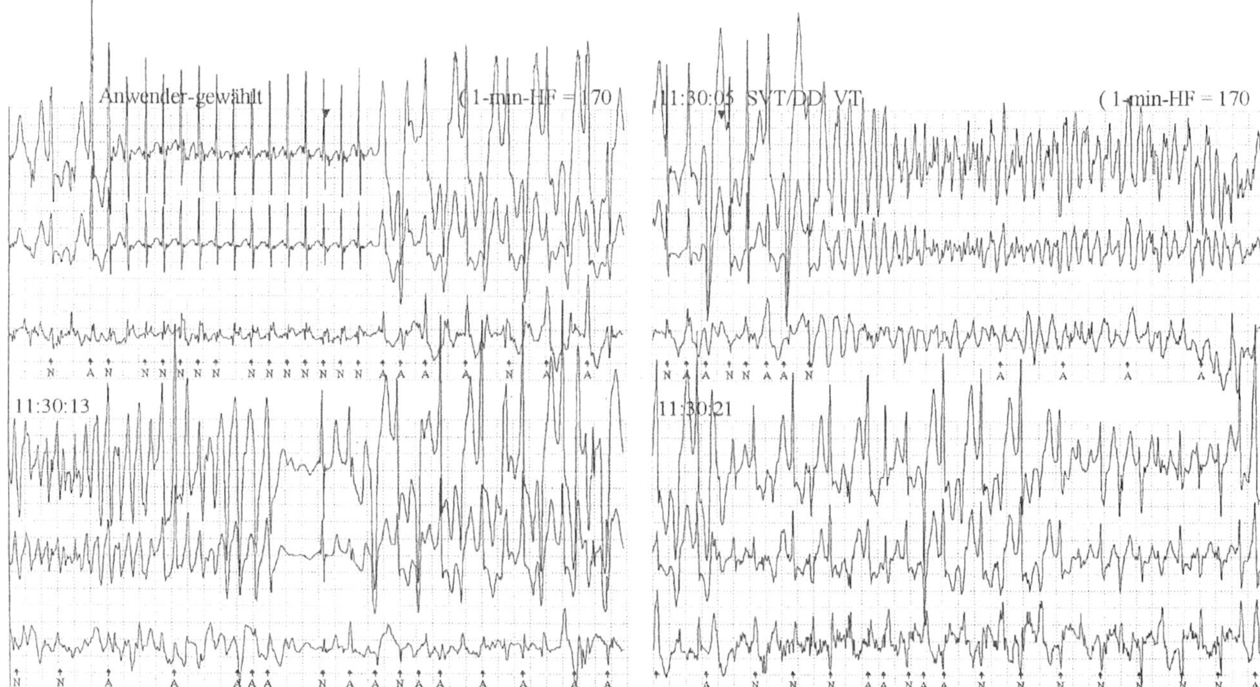

Figure 7.13. Holter monitor recording during an exercise-related syncopal episode in a young female with CPVT showing bidirectional VT degenerating into self-limiting VF. Note the temporary overdrive of the bidirectional VT by a very fast atrial tachycardia. Paper speed = 25 mm/s. Modified with permission.[111]

persistence of exercise-induced ventricular couplets or nonsustained runs of polymorphic VT despite proper β-blocker therapy has been associated with worse outcome.[103]

SUMMARY

- The surface ECG has an outstanding role in the diagnosis of inherited arrhythmia syndromes and provides the most practical and powerful tool for risk stratification.
- Spontaneous and exercise-induced dynamic type 1 ST-segment elevation and the presence of QRS fragmentation are useful ECG risk markers in BrS.
- The presence of a markedly prolonged QTc interval (>500 ms), 2:1 functional AV block, and macroscopic TWA provide strong risk indicators in LQTS.
- ECG markers of an increased and inhomogenous dispersion of ventricular repolarization (particularly indices with respect to T_{peak}-T_{end} interval, QT dispersion, and macroscopic TWA) indicate an increased electrical vulnerability and arrhythmic risk in BrS, LQTS, and SQTS.
- An abbreviated J-T_{peak} interval (<120 ms) provides a clinically useful ECG risk marker in SQTS.
- Thus far, no ECG risk markers have convincingly been identified in CPVT.

REFERENCES

1. Wang Q, Shen J, Splawski I, et al. SCN5A mutations associated with an inherited cardiac arrhythmia, long QT syndrome. *Cell.* 1995;80:805–811.
2. Curran ME, Splawski I, Timothy KW, et al. A molecular basis for cardiac arrhythmia: HERG mutations cause long QT syndrome. *Cell.* 1995;80:795–803.
3. Wang Q, Curran ME, Splawski I, et al. Positional cloning of a novel potassium channel gene: KVLQT1 mutations cause cardiac arrhythmias. *Nat Genet.* 1996;12:17–23.
4. Brugada P, Brugada J. Right bundle branch block, persistent ST segment elevation and sudden cardiac death: a distinct clinical and electrocardiographic syndrome. A multicenter report. *J Am Coll Cardiol.* 1992;20:1391–1396.
5. Mizusawa Y, Wilde AA. Brugada syndrome. *Circ Arrhythm Electrophysiol.* 2012;5:606–616.
6. Kapplinger JD, Tester DJ, Alders M, et al. An international compendium of mutations in the SCN5A-encoded cardiac sodium channel in patients referred for Brugada syndrome genetic testing. *Heart Rhythm.* 2010;7:33–46.
7. Wilde AA, Antzelevitch C, Borggrefe M, et al. Proposed diagnostic criteria for the Brugada syndrome: consensus report. *Circulation.* 2002;106:2514–2519.
8. Antzelevitch C, Brugada P, Borggrefe M, et al. Brugada syndrome: report of the second consensus conference: endorsed by the Heart Rhythm Society and the European Heart Rhythm Association. *Circulation.* 2005;111:659–670.
9. Bayes de Luna A, Brugada J, Baranchuk A, et al. Current electrocardiographic criteria for diagnosis of Brugada pattern: a consensus report. *J Electrocardiol.* 2012;45:433–442.
10. Richter S, Sarkozy A, Veltmann C, et al. Variability of the diagnostic ECG pattern in an ICD patient population with Brugada syndrome. *J Cardiovasc Electrophysiol.* 2009;20:69–75.
11. Richter S, Sarkozy A, Paparella G, et al. Number of electrocardiogram leads displaying the diagnostic coved-type pattern in Brugada syndrome: a diagnostic consensus criterion to be revised. *Eur Heart J.* 2010;31:1357–1364.
12. Meregalli PG, Wilde AA, Tan HL. Pathophysiological mechanisms of Brugada syndrome: depolarization disorder, repolarization disorder, or more? *Cardiovasc Res.* 2005;67:367–378.
13. Yan GX, Antzelevitch C. Cellular basis for the Brugada syndrome and other mechanisms of arrhythmogenesis associated with ST-segment elevation. *Circulation.* 1999;100:1660–1666.
14. Veltmann C, Papavassiliu T, Konrad T, et al. Insights into the location of type I ECG in patients with Brugada syndrome: correlation of ECG and cardiovascular magnetic resonance imaging. *Heart Rhythm.* 2012;9:414–421.
15. Priori SG, Wilde AA, Horie M, et al. HRS/EHRA/APHRS expert consensus statement on the diagnosis and management of patients with inherited primary arrhythmia syndromes: document endorsed by HRS, EHRA, and APHRS in May 2013 and by ACCF, AHA, PACES, and AEPC in June 2013. *Heart Rhythm.* 2013;10:1932–1963.
16. Baranchuk A, Nguyen T, Ryu MH, et al. Brugada phenocopy: New terminology and proposed classification. *Ann Noninvasive Electrocardiol.* 2012;17:299–314.
17. Wilde AA, Postema PG, Di Diego JM, et al. The pathophysiological mechanism underlying Brugada syndrome: depolarization versus repolarization. *J Mol Cell Cardiol.* 2010;49:543–553.
18. Postema PG, Wolpert C, Amin AS, et al. Drugs and Brugada syndrome patients: Review of the literature, recommendations, and an up-to-date website (www.brugadadrugs.org). *Heart Rhythm.* 2009;6:1335–1341.
19. Brugada J, Brugada R, Brugada P. Determinants of sudden cardiac death in individuals with the electrocardiographic pattern of Brugada syndrome and no previous cardiac arrest. *Circulation.* 2003;108:3092–3096.
20. Priori SG, Gasparini M, Napolitano C, et al. Risk stratification in Brugada syndrome: Results of the PRELUDE (PRogrammed ELectrical stimUlation preDictive valuE) registry. *J Am Coll Cardiol.* 2012;59:37–45.
21. Probst V, Veltmann C, Eckardt L, et al. Long-term prognosis of patients diagnosed with Brugada syndrome: Results from the FINGER Brugada Syndrome Registry. *Circulation.* 2010;121:635–643.

22. Delise P, Allocca G, Marras E, et al. Risk stratification in individuals with the Brugada type 1 ECG pattern without previous cardiac arrest: usefulness of a combined clinical and electrophysiologic approach. *Eur Heart J.* 2011;32:169–176.
23. Take Y, Morita H, Wu J, et al. Spontaneous electrocardiogram alterations predict ventricular fibrillation in Brugada syndrome. *Heart Rhythm.* 2011;8:1014–1021.
24. Makimoto H, Nakagawa E, Takaki H, et al. Augmented ST-segment elevation during recovery from exercise predicts cardiac events in patients with Brugada syndrome. *J Am Coll Cardiol.* 2010;56:1576–1584.
25. Morita H, Kusano KF, Miura D, et al. Fragmented QRS as a marker of conduction abnormality and a predictor of prognosis of Brugada syndrome. *Circulation.* 2008;118:1697–1704.
26. Take Y, Morita H, Toh N, et al. Identification of high-risk syncope related to ventricular fibrillation in patients with Brugada syndrome. *Heart Rhythm.* 2012;9:752–759.
27. Coronel R, Casini S, Koopmann TT, et al. Right ventricular fibrosis and conduction delay in a patient with clinical signs of Brugada syndrome: A combined electrophysiological, genetic, histopathologic, and computational study. *Circulation.* 2005;112:2769–2777.
28. Babai Bigi MA, Aslani A, Shahrzad S. aVR sign as a risk factor for life-threatening arrhythmic events in patients with Brugada syndrome. *Heart Rhythm.* 2007;4:1009–1012.
29. Junttila MJ, Brugada P, Hong K, et al. Differences in 12-lead electrocardiogram between symptomatic and asymptomatic Brugada syndrome patients. *J Cardiovasc Electrophysiol.* 2008;19:380–383.
30. Tatsumi H, Takagi M, Nakagawa E, et al. Risk stratification in patients with Brugada syndrome: analysis of daily fluctuations in 12-lead electrocardiogram (ECG) and signal-averaged electrocardiogram (SAECG). *J Cardiovasc Electrophysiol.* 2006;17:705–711.
31. Furushima H, Chinushi M, Hirono T, et al. Relationship between dominant prolongation of the filtered QRS duration in the right precordial leads and clinical characteristics in Brugada syndrome. *J Cardiovasc Electrophysiol.* 2005;16:1311–1317.
32. Hisamatsu K, Kusano KF, Morita H, et al. Relationships between depolarization abnormality and repolarization abnormality in patients with Brugada syndrome: Using body surface signal-averaged electrocardiography and body surface maps. *J Cardiovasc Electrophysiol.* 2004;15:870–876.
33. Postema PG, van Dessel PF, Kors JA, et al. Local depolarization abnormalities are the dominant pathophysiologic mechanism for type 1 electrocardiogram in Brugada syndrome a study of electrocardiograms, vectorcardiograms, and body surface potential maps during ajmaline provocation. *J Am Coll Cardiol.* 2010;55:789–797.
34. Ikeda T, Sakurada H, Sakabe K, et al. Assessment of noninvasive markers in identifying patients at risk in the Brugada syndrome: Insight into risk stratification. *J Am Coll Cardiol.* 2001;37:1628–1634.
35. Huang Z, Patel C, Li W, et al. Role of signal-averaged electrocardiograms in arrhythmic risk stratification of patients with Brugada syndrome: a prospective study. *Heart Rhythm.* 2009;6:1156–1162.
36. Castro Hevia J, Antzelevitch C, Tornes Barzaga F, et al. Tpeak-Tend and Tpeak-Tend dispersion as risk factors for ventricular tachycardia/ventricular fibrillation in patients with the Brugada syndrome. *J Am Coll Cardiol.* 2006;47:1828–1834.
37. Pitzalis MV, Anaclerio M, Iacoviello M, et al. QT-interval prolongation in right precordial leads: an additional electrocardiographic hallmark of Brugada syndrome. *J Am Coll Cardiol.* 2003;42:1632–1637.
38. Tada T, Kusano KF, Nagase S, et al. Clinical significance of macroscopic T-wave alternans after sodium channel blocker administration in patients with Brugada syndrome. *J Cardiovasc Electrophysiol.* 2008;19:56–61.
39. Morita H, Nagase S, Kusano K, et al. Spontaneous T wave alternans and premature ventricular contractions during febrile illness in a patient with Brugada syndrome. *J Cardiovasc Electrophysiol.* 2002;13:816–818.
40. Fish JM, Antzelevitch C. Cellular mechanism and arrhythmogenic potential of T-wave alternans in the Brugada syndrome. *J Cardiovasc Electrophysiol.* 2008;19:301–308.
41. Smits JP, Eckardt L, Probst V, et al. Genotype-phenotype relationship in Brugada syndrome: electrocardiographic features differentiate SCN5A-related patients from non-SCN5A-related patients. *J Am Coll Cardiol.* 2002;40:350–356.
42. Maury P, Rollin A, Sacher F, et al. Prevalence and prognostic role of various conduction disturbances in patients with the Brugada syndrome. *Am J Cardiol.* 2013;112:1384–1389.
43. Morita H, Kusano-Fukushima K, Nagase S, et al. Atrial fibrillation and atrial vulnerability in patients with Brugada syndrome. *J Am Coll Cardiol.* 2002;40:1437–1444.
44. Kusano KF, Taniyama M, Nakamura K, et al. Atrial fibrillation in patients with Brugada syndrome relationships of gene mutation, electrophysiology, and clinical backgrounds. *J Am Coll Cardiol.* 2008;51:1169–1175.
45. Viskin S, Rogowski O. Asymptomatic Brugada syndrome: a cardiac ticking time-bomb? *Europace.* 2007;9:707–710.
46. Kanda M, Shimizu W, Matsuo K, et al. Electrophysiologic characteristics and implications of induced ventricular fibrillation in symptomatic patients with Brugada syndrome. *J Am Coll Cardiol.* 2002;39:1799–1805.
47. Brugada J, Brugada R, Brugada P. Electrophysiologic testing predicts events in Brugada syndrome patients. *Heart Rhythm.* 2011;8:1595–1597.
48. Schwartz PJ, Stramba-Badiale M, Crotti L, et al. Prevalence of the congenital long QT syndrome. *Circulation.* 2009;120:1761–1767.
49. Ackerman MJ, Priori SG, Willems S, et al. HRS/EHRA expert consensus statement on the state of genetic testing for the channelopathies and cardiomyopathies this document was developed as a partnership between the Heart Rhythm Society (HRS) and the European Heart Rhythm Association (EHRA). *Heart Rhythm.* 2011;8:1308–1339.

50. Goldenberg I, Moss AJ, Zareba W. QT interval: How to measure it and what is "normal". *J Cardiovasc Electrophysiol.* 2006;17:333–336.
51. Priori SG, Napolitano C, Schwartz PJ. Low penetrance in the long QT syndrome: Clinical impact. *Circulation.* 1999;99:529–533.
52. Priori SG, Schwartz PJ, Napolitano C, et al. Risk stratification in the long QT syndrome. *N Engl J Med.* 2003;348:1866–1874.
53. Schwartz PJ, Crotti L. QTc behavior during exercise and genetic testing for the long QT syndrome. *Circulation.* 2011;124:2181–2184.
54. Schwartz PJ, Spazzolini C, Priori SG, et al. Who are the long QT syndrome patients who receive an implantable cardioverter-defibrillator and what happens to them? Data from the European Long QT Syndrome Implantable Cardioverter-Defibrillator (LQTS ICD) Registry. *Circulation.* 2010;122:1272–1282.
55. Sauer AJ, Moss AJ, McNitt S, et al. Long QT syndrome in adults. *J Am Coll Cardiol.* 2007;49:329–337.
56. Goldenberg I, Moss AJ, Peterson DR, et al. Risk factors for aborted cardiac arrest and sudden cardiac death in children with the congenital long QT syndrome. *Circulation.* 2008;117:2184–2191.
57. Schwartz PJ, Malliani A. Electrical alternation of the T-wave: Clinical and experimental evidence of its relationship with the sympathetic nervous system and with the long Q-T syndrome. *Am Heart J.* 1975;89:45–50.
58. Malfatto G, Beria G, Sala S, et al. Quantitative analysis of T wave abnormalities and their prognostic implications in the idiopathic long QT syndrome. *J Am Coll Cardiol.* 1994;23:296–301.
59. Zareba W, Moss AJ, Schwartz PJ, et al. Influence of genotype on the clinical course of the long QT syndrome. International Long QT Syndrome Registry Research Group. *N Engl J Med.* 1998;339:960–965.
60. Garson A, Jr., Dick M, 2nd, Fournier A, et al. The long QT syndrome in children. An international study of 287 patients. *Circulation.* 1993;87:1866–1872.
61. Trippel DL, Parsons MK, Gillette PC. Infants with long QT syndrome and 2:1 atrioventricular block. *Am Heart J.* 1995;130:1130–1134.
62. Aziz PF, Tanel RE, Zelster IJ, et al. Congenital long QT syndrome and 2:1 atrioventricular block: An optimistic outcome in the current era. *Heart Rhythm.* 2010;7:781–785.
63. Schwartz PJ, Spazzolini C, Crotti L. All LQT3 patients need an ICD: True or false? *Heart Rhythm.* 2009;6:113–120.
64. Schwartz P, Priori S, Napolitano C. The long QT syndrome. In: Zipes DP, Jalife J, eds. *Cardiac Electrophysiology: From Cell to Bedside.* 3rd ed. Philadelphia, PA: Saunders; 2000;597–615.
65. Moss AJ, Zareba W, Benhorin J, et al. ECG T-wave patterns in genetically distinct forms of the hereditary long QT syndrome. *Circulation.* 1995;92:2929–2934.
66. Zhang L, Timothy KW, Vincent GM, et al. Spectrum of ST-T-wave patterns and repolarization parameters in congenital long QT syndrome: ECG findings identify genotypes. *Circulation.* 2000;102:2849–2855.
67. Antzelevitch C, Sicouri S. Clinical relevance of cardiac arrhythmias generated by afterdepolarizations. Role of M cells in the generation of U waves, triggered activity and torsade de pointes. *J Am Coll Cardiol.* 1994;23:259–277.
68. Choi BR, Burton F, Salama G. Cytosolic Ca^{2+} triggers early afterdepolarizations and Torsade de Pointes in rabbit hearts with type 2 long QT syndrome. *J Physiol.* 2002;543:615–631.
69. Restivo M, Caref EB, Kozhevnikov DO, et al. Spatial dispersion of repolarization is a key factor in the arrhythmogenicity of long QT syndrome. *J Cardiovasc Electrophysiol.* 2004;15:323–331.
70. Akar FG, Yan GX, Antzelevitch C, et al. Unique topographical distribution of M cells underlies reentrant mechanism of torsade de pointes in the long QT syndrome. *Circulation.* 2002;105:1247–1253.
71. El-Sherif N, Caref EB, Yin H, et al. The electrophysiological mechanism of ventricular arrhythmias in the long QT syndrome. Tridimensional mapping of activation and recovery patterns. *Circ Res.* 1996;79:474–492.
72. Day CP, McComb JM, Campbell RW. QT dispersion: An indication of arrhythmia risk in patients with long QT intervals. *Br Heart J.* 1990;63:342–344.
73. Priori SG, Napolitano C, Diehl L, et al. Dispersion of the QT interval. A marker of therapeutic efficacy in the idiopathic long QT syndrome. *Circulation.* 1994;89:1681–1689.
74. Yamaguchi M, Shimizu M, Ino H, et al. T wave peak-to-end interval and QT dispersion in acquired long QT syndrome: A new index for arrhythmogenicity. *Clin Sci (Lond).* 2003;105:671–676.
75. Takenaka K, Ai T, Shimizu W, et al. Exercise stress test amplifies genotype-phenotype correlation in the LQT1 and LQT2 forms of the long QT syndrome. *Circulation.* 2003;107:838–844.
76. Yan GX, Antzelevitch C. Cellular basis for the normal T wave and the electrocardiographic manifestations of the long QT syndrome. *Circulation.* 1998;98:1928–1936.
77. Panikkath R, Reinier K, Uy-Evanado A, et al. Prolonged Tpeak-to-Tend interval on the resting ECG is associated with increased risk of sudden cardiac death. *Circ Arrhythm Electrophysiol.* 2011;4:441–447.
78. Topilski I, Rogowski O, Rosso R, et al. The morphology of the QT interval predicts torsade de pointes during acquired bradyarrhythmias. *J Am Coll Cardiol.* 2007;49:320–328.
79. Ruan Y, Liu N, Napolitano C, et al. Therapeutic strategies for long QT syndrome: Does the molecular substrate matter? *Circ Arrhythm Electrophysiol.* 2008;1:290–297.
80. Priori SG, Napolitano C, Schwartz PJ, et al. Association of long QT syndrome loci and cardiac events among patients treated with beta-blockers. *JAMA.* 2004;292:1341–1344.
81. Schwartz PJ, Priori SG, Spazzolini C, et al. Genotype-phenotype correlation in the long QT syndrome: Gene-specific triggers for life-threatening arrhythmias. *Circulation.* 2001;103:89–95.
82. Zareba W, Moss AJ, le Cessie S, et al. T wave alternans in idiopathic long QT syndrome. *J Am Coll Cardiol.* 1994;23:1541–1546.

83. Shimizu W, Antzelevitch C. Cellular and ionic basis for T-wave alternans under long QT conditions. *Circulation.* 1999;99:1499–1507.
84. Schwartz PJ, Spazzolini C, Crotti L, et al. The Jervell and Lange-Nielsen syndrome: natural history, molecular basis, and clinical outcome. *Circulation.* 2006;113:783–790.
85. Splawski I, Timothy KW, Sharpe LM, et al. Ca(V)1.2 calcium channel dysfunction causes a multisystem disorder including arrhythmia and autism. *Cell.* 2004;119:19–31.
86. Gussak I, Brugada P, Brugada J, et al. Idiopathic short QT interval: A new clinical syndrome? *Cardiology.* 2000;94:99–102.
87. Patel C, Yan GX, Antzelevitch C. Short QT syndrome: From bench to bedside. *Circ Arrhythm Electrophysiol.* 2010;3:401–408.
88. Brugada R, Hong K, Dumaine R, et al. Sudden death associated with short QT syndrome linked to mutations in HERG. *Circulation.* 2004;109:30–35.
89. Giustetto C, Schimpf R, Mazzanti A, et al. Long-term follow-up of patients with short QT syndrome. *J Am Coll Cardiol.* 2011;58(6):587–595.
90. Mazzanti A, Kanthan A, Monteforte N, et al. Novel insight into the natural history of short QT syndrome. *J Am Coll Cardiol.* 2014;63:1300–1308.
91. Wolpert C, Schimpf R, Giustetto C, et al. Further insights into the effect of quinidine in short QT syndrome caused by a mutation in HERG. *J Cardiovasc Electrophysiol.* 2005;16:54–58.
92. Anttonen O, Junttila MJ, Maury P, et al. Differences in twelve-lead electrocardiogram between symptomatic and asymptomatic subjects with short QT interval. *Heart Rhythm.* 2009;6:267–271.
93. Gollob MH, Redpath CJ, Roberts JD. The short QT syndrome: Proposed diagnostic criteria. *J Am Coll Cardiol.* 2011;57:802–812.
94. Villafane J, Atallah J, Gollob MH, et al. Long-term follow-up of a pediatric cohort with short QT syndrome. *J Am Coll Cardiol.* 2013;61:1183–1191.
95. Bidoggia H, Maciel JP, Capalozza N, et al. Sex-dependent electrocardiographic pattern of cardiac repolarization. *Am Heart J.* 2000;140:430–436.
96. Anttonen O, Vaananen H, Junttila J, et al. Electrocardiographic transmural dispersion of repolarization in patients with inherited short QT syndrome. *Ann Noninvasive Electrocardiol.* 2008;13:295–300.
97. Gupta P, Patel C, Patel H, et al. T(p-e)/QT ratio as an index of arrhythmogenesis. *J Electrocardiol.* 2008;41:567–574.
98. Veltmann C, Borggrefe M. Arrhythmias: a "Schwartz score" for short QT syndrome. *Nat Rev Cardiol.* 2011;8:251–252.
99. Bjerregaard P. Proposed diagnostic criteria for short QT syndrome are badly founded. *J Am Coll Cardiol.* 2011;58:549–550; author reply: 550–551.
100. Antzelevitch C, Pollevick GD, Cordeiro JM, et al. Loss-of-function mutations in the cardiac calcium channel underlie a new clinical entity characterized by ST-segment elevation, short QT intervals, and sudden cardiac death. *Circulation.* 2007;115:442–449.
101. Watanabe H, Makiyama T, Koyama T, et al. High prevalence of early repolarization in short QT syndrome. *Heart Rhythm.* 2010;7:647–652.
102. Leenhardt A, Lucet V, Denjoy I, et al. Catecholaminergic polymorphic ventricular tachycardia in children. A 7-year follow-up of 21 patients. *Circulation.* 1995;91:1512–1519.
103. Hayashi M, Denjoy I, Extramiana F, et al. Incidence and risk factors of arrhythmic events in catecholaminergic polymorphic ventricular tachycardia. *Circulation.* 2009;119:2426–2434.
104. Priori SG, Napolitano C, Memmi M, et al. Clinical and molecular characterization of patients with catecholaminergic polymorphic ventricular tachycardia. *Circulation.* 2002;106:69–74.
105. Leenhardt A, Denjoy I, Guicheney P. Catecholaminergic polymorphic ventricular tachycardia. *Circ Arrhythm Electrophysiol.* 2012;5:1044–1052.
106. Reid DS, Tynan M, Braidwood L, et al. Bidirectional tachycardia in a child. A study using His bundle electrography. *Br Heart J.* 1975;37:339–344.
107. Sumitomo N, Harada K, Nagashima M, et al. Catecholaminergic polymorphic ventricular tachycardia: Electrocardiographic characteristics and optimal therapeutic strategies to prevent sudden death. *Heart.* 2003;89:66–70.
108. Sumitomo N, Sakurada H, Taniguchi K, et al. Association of atrial arrhythmia and sinus node dysfunction in patients with catecholaminergic polymorphic ventricular tachycardia. *Circ J.* 2007;71:1606–1609.
109. Chevallier S, Forclaz A, Tenkorang J, et al. New electrocardiographic criteria for discriminating between Brugada types 2 and 3 patterns and incomplete right bundle branch block. *J Am Coll Cardiol.* 2011;58:2290–2298.
110. Schimpf R, Wolpert C, Gaita F, et al. Short QT syndrome. *Cardiovasc Res.* 2005;67:357–366.
111. Richter S, Gebauer R, Hindricks G, et al. A classic electrocardiographic manifestation of catecholaminergic polymorphic ventricular tachycardia. *J Cardiovasc Electrophysiol.* 2012;23:560.

CHAPTER

8

Early Repolarization Syndrome: Its Relationship to ECG Findings and Risk Stratification

Arnon Adler, MD, Ofer Havakuk, MD, Raphael Rosso, MD, and Sami Viskin, MD

HISTORICAL PERSPECTIVE

"...Occasionally, the S-T vector due to normal early repolarization (ER) forces is difficult to distinguish from the S-T vector due to acute pericarditis." With this casual phrase, Grant coined the term "early repolarization" in 1951.[1] Previous reports, by Shipley and Hallaran in 1936,[2] and by Myers et al in 1947,[3] described "J deflection of the terminal part of the QRS complex accompanied by ST segment elevation" in the ECG of young, otherwise healthy individuals. Accordingly, widespread recognition of the "benign nature of ER" remained undisputed.[4] This perception lasted for almost half a century. Then intriguing reports describing unexpected ventricular fibrillation (VF) in young, ostensibly healthy individuals with ER in their ECG began to appear, initially from the southeast Asia[5,6] and then from other countries as well. Originally, the data were scarce and somehow confusing; although clear-cut description of ER was sometimes depicted by the authors (as in "VF in a patient with prominent J waves and ST segment elevation in the inferior electrocardiographic leads"),[7] recognition that ER might be the one to blame for this malignant ventricular arrhythmias awaited.

In 1996, Yan and Antzelevitch described the cellular basis for the electrocardiographic J wave[8] followed by the cellular and ionic mechanisms for ER syndrome (ERS).[9] Their tissue model suggested a possible link between the highly arrhythmogenic Brugada syndrome (BrS) and the still considered benign ER pattern. Their studies highlighted the role of the transient outward (I_{to}) potassium current in creating potentially arrhythmogenic voltage gradient across the ventricular wall. However, clinical evidence incriminating this innocent electrocardiographic variant as arrhythmogenic would remain relatively scarce for one more decade.

In 2008, Haïssaguerre,[10] Nam,[11] and our group[12] reported, almost simultaneously, that in matched case-control series, ER is clearly associated with idiopathic VF. Haïssaguerre[10] and Nam[13] further provided data in favor of a cause-and-effect association with illustrations clearly demonstrating augmentation of the J-wave amplitude immediately prior to the onset

The ECG Handbook of Contemporary Challenges © 2015 Mohammad Shenasa, Mark E. Josephson, N.A. Mark Estes III
Cardiotext Publishing, ISBN: 978-1-935395-88-1

of VF. Soon thereafter, large population studies[14,15] reinforced these findings from a different angle by showing that asymptomatic individuals with ER apparently have a higher incidence of sudden death during long-term follow-up.

As explained in detail below, for patients with ER, the risk for spontaneous VF may be *slightly increased by a common disease* (in the case of ischemic VF during myocardial infarction) or may be *markedly increased by a rare disease* [Purkinje extrasystoles in idiopathic VF]. In both instances, however, the finite risk for the asymptomatic individual is small. The last point cannot be overemphasized: the overwhelming majority of asymptomatic individuals with ER will do well.

ELECTROCARDIOGRAPHIC DEFINITION

The electrocardiographic pattern known as "ER" consists of 2 ECG phenomena: J-point elevation and ST-segment elevation. At present, either of these phenomena are enough for the definition of ER. However, as outlined elsewhere,[16] until Haïssaguerre's seminal paper in 2008,[10] the ST-segment elevation was the main focus of ER discussions. Since then, attention has shifted to the J-point elevation as the more interesting component of ER (at least as far as arrhythmic risk is concerned). This change has caused considerable controversy regarding the definition of ER, with some experts calling for clear distinction between "J-point elevation" and "classic ER."[17] As these controversies are still unresolved, the definitions in the following section are based primarily on those used in recent studies and should be regarded in the context of the ongoing controversy.

J-Point Elevation

J-point elevation is usually defined as the elevation of the QRS–ST junction in at least 2 leads and of at least 0.1 mV.[10,14] Historically, to differentiate ER from BrS, only J-point elevation in inferior (leads II, III, and aVF) and anterolateral leads (leads I, aVL, and V_{4-6}) were considered. Recent data[18] suggests that this distinction is not always straightforward.[19]

The morphology of the J-point elevation can be either notching (a distinct, positive deflection at the end of the QRS sometimes referred to as "J wave") or slurring (gradual transition from QRS to ST segment) (Figure 8.1). Temporal fluctuations between these 2 morphologies may appear in some patients, while in others they may coexist in different leads (see Figure 8.1).

While these definitions (and figures) establish a robust foundation for the term "J-point elevation," they leave ample room for interpretation. The exact

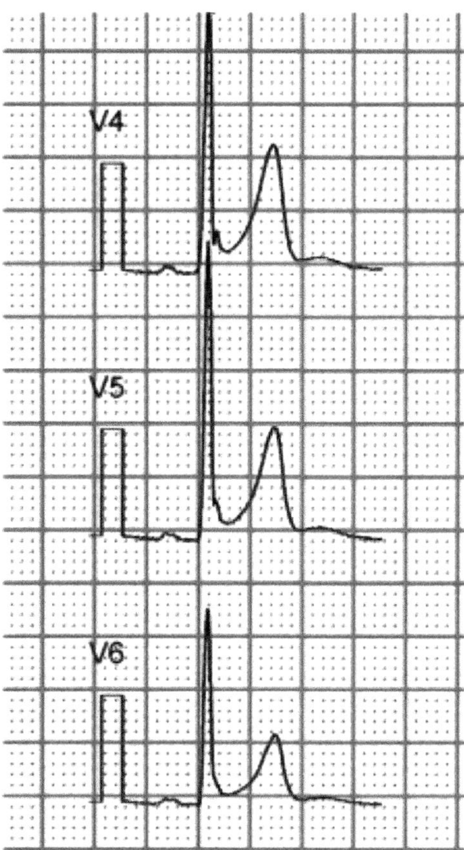

Figure 8.1. J-point elevation morphologies. Leads V_4 to V_6 in an ECG where an end QRS notch is present in V_4 is less marked in V_5 and has become a slur in V_6. Modified with permission.[20]

definition of slurring remains unresolved, as well as definition of QRS termination and a precise method for J-wave amplitude measurement (for further discussion on these controversies see Macfarlane et al[20]).

ST-Segment Elevation

Similarly to J-point elevation, at least 2 leads are required for the definition of ER. Here, too, 2 morphologies have been described: descending/horizontal ST segment and ascending ST segment (Figure 8.2). The definition used in recent studies for distinction between these morphologies was ST elevation > 0.1 mV, occurring 100 ms after the J-point for ascending and ≤ 0.1 mV for horizontal/descending.[21] As explained below, the "descending/horizontal" pattern has been associated with increased arrhythmic risk.[22]

Differential Diagnosis

The differential diagnosis of ER includes a wide range of medical conditions in which J-point elevation or ST-segment elevation may occur (Table 8.1). As can be appreciated from Figure 8.3, in most of these

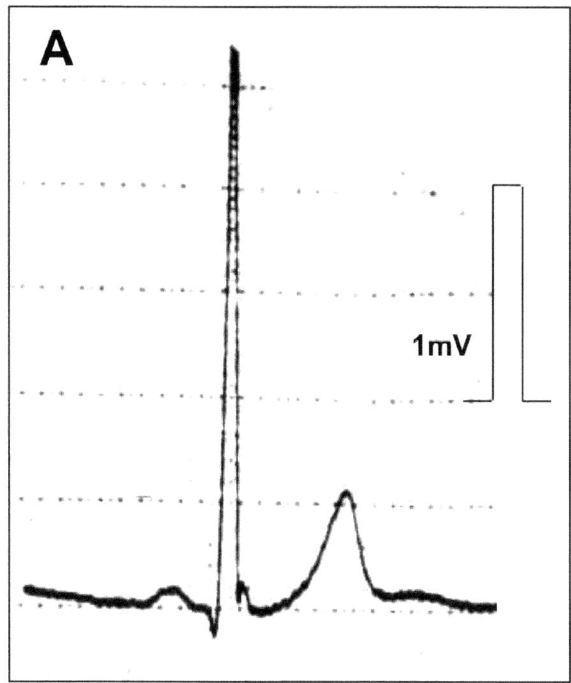

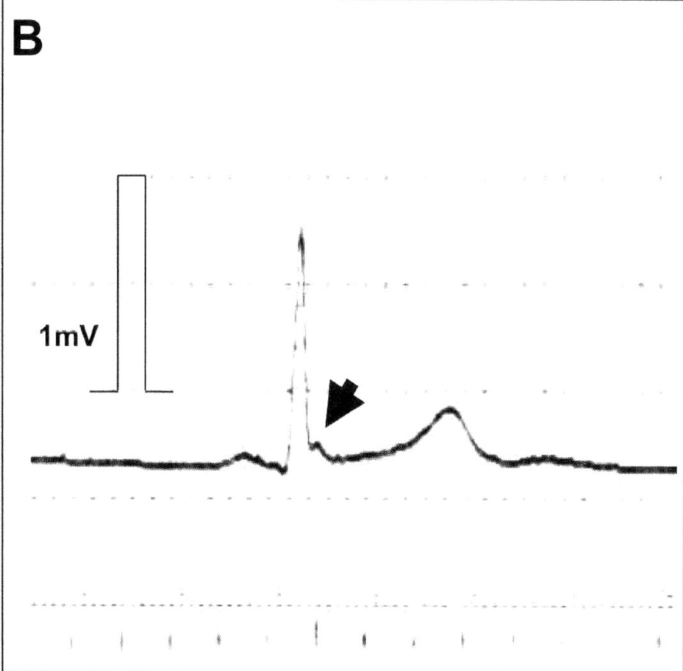

Figure 8.2. J-point elevation with different ST-segment morphologies. Rapidly ascending (A) and horizontal (B) ST-segment in leads displaying J-point elevation. Modified with permission from Rosso et al. Heart Rhythm 2012;9:225-9.

situations, the morphology of the J-point elevation is considerably different from that described in ER definitions above (i.e., slurring or notching). Furthermore, in many instances (e.g., typical acute ST-elevation myocardial infarction, hypothermia) the diagnosis is readily apparent. Nevertheless, exclusion of these imitators is the mandatory first step in the evaluation of any patient with ER.

BrS is of specific importance among the listed differential diagnoses because, as in the case of ERS (see below), it manifests as arrhythmic syncope or death in young individuals with no structural heart disease. Some have actually proposed regarding BrS and ERS as a single continuum of "J-wave syndromes."[23] Although the typical ECG in BrS (see Figure 8.3) differs from ERS in both morphology (J-point elevation with coved ST-segment elevation) and location

Table 8.1. **Differential diagnosis of ER.**

ST-segment myocardial infarction.
Old myocardial infarction.
Acute pericarditis.
Left ventricular hypertrophy.
Left bundle branch block (LBBB).
Hypokalemia.
Brugada Syndrome (BrS).
Arrhythmogenic right ventricular dysplasia.

(right precordial leads), in the minority of cases the Brugada pattern may also appear in inferior or lateral leads.[24] Furthermore, ER is described to accompany BrS in 10% to 12% of cases[25–27] and up to 63% if repeated ECGs are examined.[28] In fact, these atypical electrocardiographic manifestations of BrS have been described as a bad prognostic sign in most[24,26–28] but not all[25] studies.

ERS

ERS is a very rare disorder characterized by the electrocardiographic manifestation of an ER pattern and the development of spontaneous VF/polymorphic VT. It is very important to make the distinction between ERS and ER pattern, as the vast majority of individuals with an ER pattern will remain asymptomatic for life. Furthermore, the high prevalence of ER pattern in the general population (3%–24%)[4,15,29–32] means that even in symptomatic patients, ER may be an innocent bystander. Therefore, the diagnosis of ERS should be made carefully and only after exclusion of all other arrhythmogenic etiologies.

Diagnosis

A joint consensus statement published by the Heart Rhythm Society, the European Heart Rhythm Association, and the Asian Pacific Heart Rhythm Association states that "ERS is diagnosed in the presence of J-point

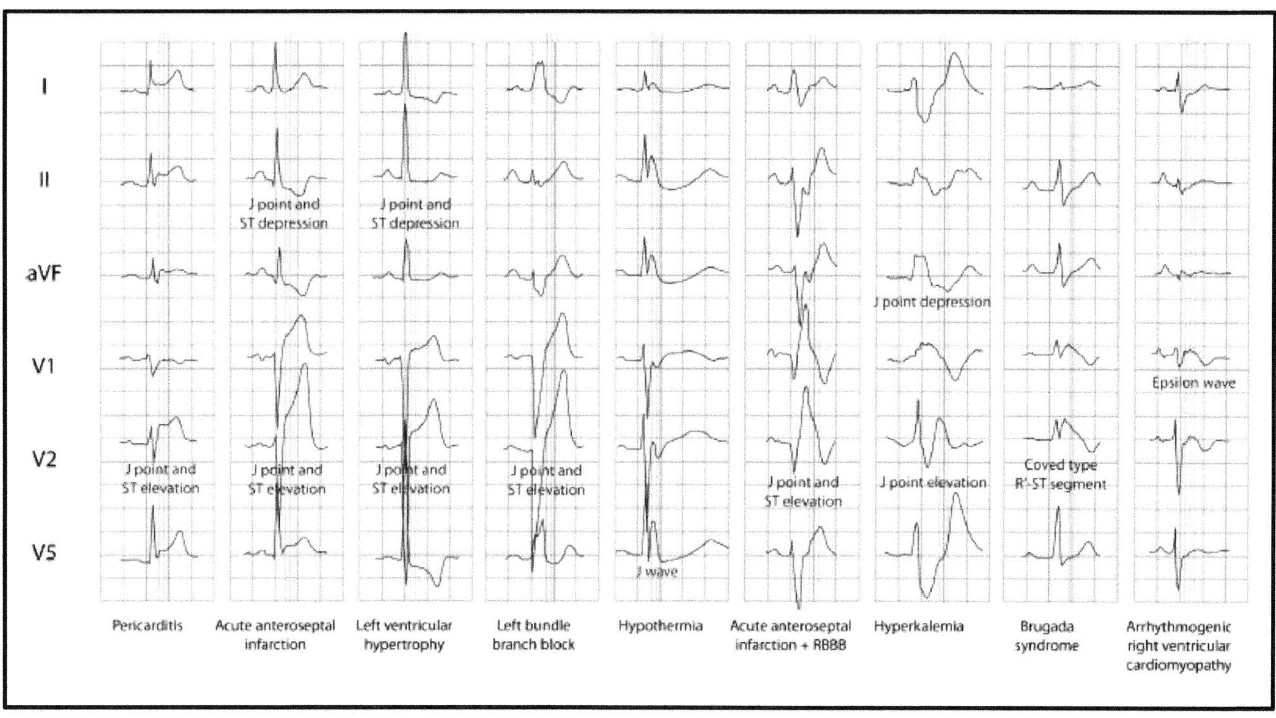

Figure 8.3. Differential diagnosis of J-point elevation. Several ECG examples of patients with spontaneous or intermittent aberrant terminal R waves or J–ST segments, J-point elevation, and J waves. RBBB, right bundle branch block. Modified with permission from Postema at al., J Electrocardiol 2013;46:461-5.

elevation ≥1 mm in ≥2 contiguous inferior and/or lateral leads of a standard 12-lead ECG in a patient resuscitated from *otherwise unexplained* VF/polymorphic VT."[33] Furthermore, it states that "ERS can be diagnosed in a sudden cardiac death (SCD) victim with a negative autopsy and medical chart review with a previous ECG demonstrating J-point elevation ≥1 mm in ≥2 contiguous inferior and/or lateral leads of a standard 12-lead ECG." As indicated, exclusion of all other etiologies is mandatory.

We have adopted a more restrictive definition and use the term *definitive ERS* when, in a patient fulfilling the clinical and ECG characteristics of ERS adopted by the consensus report, the onset of spontaneous VF is documented at least once (usually during a VF storm) and demonstrates the typical mode of onset of idiopathic VF (i.e., polymorphic VT initiated by a ventricular extrasystole with very short coupling interval),[34] often demonstrating augmentation of the J-wave amplitude immediately prior to the onset of VF.[10]

Unlike other arrhythmogenic syndromes, there are no accepted ancillary tests that aid in the diagnosis. Holter monitoring may be helpful for evaluation of ER appearance and characteristics during bradycardia.[33] The Valsalva maneuver has also been described to aid in the diagnosis by increasing the J-waves in patients with ERS and exposing ER in obligatory transmitters.[35] However, the diagnostic yield of this maneuver was only studied in big families with multiple symptomatic ERS patients. The yield of this test for the individual patient has not been examined and can be anticipated to be smaller.

Genetic testing may be useful in patients suspected of ERS. Mutations in genes encoding for the ATP-sensitive potassium channel (*KCNJ8*),[36,37] L-type calcium channels (*CACNA1C*, *CACNB2B*, and *CACNA2D1*),[38] and sodium channels (*SCN5A*)[39] have been associated with ERS. However, these mutations were found only in single cases and in a minority of ERS patients tested. It is, therefore, recommended that genetic testing for ERS be done in specialized centers experienced in genetic testing and interpretation.

Due to the limitations detailed above (lack of ancillary tests and limitations of genetic tests), there is no recommendation for family screening of patients with ERS.[33] Such screening may be considered in rare cases of strong family history and unique electrocardiographic features or positive genetic testing.

Management

The treatment of choice in patients diagnosed with ERS (i.e., patients resuscitated from CA) is the implantation of an ICD.[33] The decision to implant an ICD is more difficult in patients with syncope strongly suspected to be of arrhythmic origin who have an ER pattern but have no documented arrhythmias. This difficulty arises from the fact that our ability to correctly identify arrhythmic syncope based on symptoms is imperfect.[40]

Pharmacological treatment of ERS should be given to patients with arrhythmic storms and/or recurrent appropriate ICD shocks. Isoproterenol and quinidine have been shown to be very effective in case reports and small series.[11,41,42] These agents have also been shown to improve or even abolish the ER pattern in some cases.[41,42] Other agents, including amiodarone, mexiletine, verapamil, β-blockers, and class IC antiarrhythmics have shown no or very modest results in preventing arrhythmias in this patient population. Finally, rapid pacing has also been described to be effective in the termination of arrhythmic storms in ERS patients.[11] VF storms are not rare in ERS and may be fatal even for patients with implanted ICD. Therefore, prophylactic quinidine therapy should be considered after ICD implantation for ERS.

A proposed algorithm for treatment of ERS is shown in Figure 8.4.

EARLY REPOLARIZATION IN THE GENERAL POPULATION

The prevalence of the ER ECG pattern in the general population is estimated to be between 3% and 24%, depending on the population studied and the methods used for ECG interpretation (Table 8.2). Young individuals,[43] males,[14,43] African Americans,[31] and athletes[21,44] are subpopulations known to have a higher prevalence of ER. As reviewed above, the first evidence showing an association between ER and sudden death stemmed from case-control series of idiopathic VF. It was not until Tikkanen's population-based study, published in 2009,[14] that such an association in the general population was appreciated. This study showed a 1.3 adjusted relative risk of cardiac death in individuals with ER. As reviewed in detail elsewhere,[45] some other population studies,[15,29,32] but not all,[31] supported this finding. Importantly, the population studied by Tikkanen (and most other population studies to follow) was a middle-aged population (mean age 44, range 30–59) with a mean follow-up time of 30 years. When examining the Kaplan–Meier plot of that study, it becomes apparent that the survival curves of those with and those without ER began to diverge only after 20 years. In other words, the risk of cardiac death became evident only around the age of 60.[45] This is a very important point as idiopathic VF becomes overt (with cardiac arrest) most commonly before the age of 40. It is therefore difficult to believe that the increased arrhythmic mortality observed by Tikkanen in his adult population was due to idiopathic VF. Based on the above-mentioned observations, we

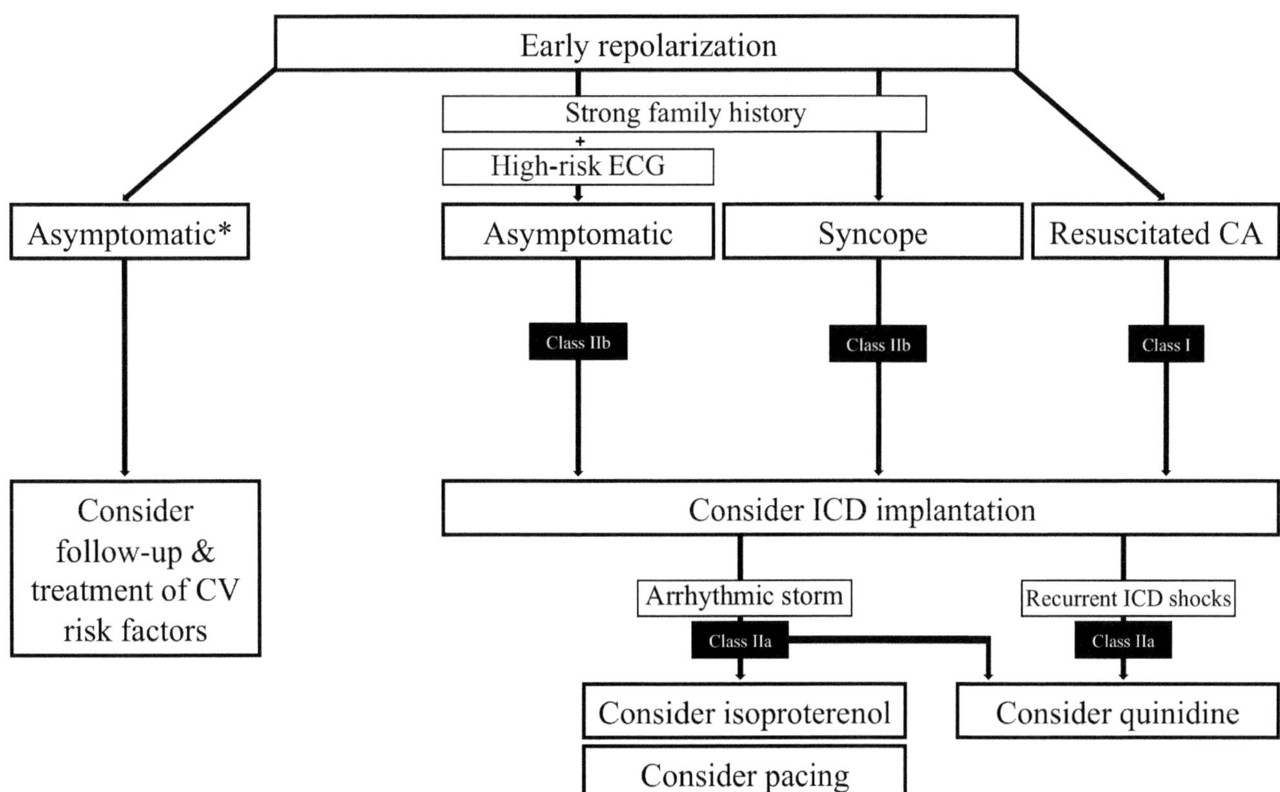

Figure 8.4. Proposed algorithm for management of ERS. Algorithm based on consensus report recommendation.[33] *Not defined as ERS but rather asymptomatic ER. CA, cardiac arrest; CV, cardiovascular; ICD, implantable cardioverter defibrillator.

Table 8.2. Mortality risk in population studies of ER in inferior leads.

	Tikkanen[‡14]	Sinner[§15]	Olson[§29]	Haruta[§30]	Uberoi[‡31]	Rollin[§32]
No. of subjects	10,864	6213	15,141	5976	29,281	1161
Follow-up (years)	30	19	17	24	8	14
% ER positive (all leads)	6	13	12	24	3	13
Location	Finland	Germany	USA	Japan	USA	France
Overall mortality						
Unadjusted	**1.25 (1.1 – 1.42)**		**1.52 (1.11 – 2.08)**			
Adjusted	1.1 (0.97 – 1.26)	**2.17 (1.11 – 4.23)**	**1.57 (1.12 – 2.20)**			**2.85 (1.62 – 5.02)**
Cardiac mortality						
Unadjusted	**1.47 (1.19 – 1.82)**				1.29 (0.72 – 2.18)	
Adjusted	**1.28 (1.04 – 1.59)**	**3.71 (1.44 – 9.53)**			1.73 (0.93 – 3.3)	**5.28 (1.96 – 14.2)**
Arrhythmic mortality						
Unadjusted	**1.79 (1.33 – 2.41)**		1.69 (0.54 – 5.27)			
Adjusted	**1.43 (1.06 – 1.94)**		1.88 (0.60 – 5.91)	1.91 (0.88 – 0.14)		
Variables adjusted for	Age, sex, BMI, smoking, BP, ECG evidence of LVH, or CAD	Age, sex, BMI, cholesterol, smoking, HTN, S/P MI, DM, HR, QTc	Age, sex , race, HR, BP, BMI, LDL, DM, major ECG abnormality, LVH ECG criteria, CAD, stroke, smoking, physical activity, serum potassium	Age, sex	Age, sex, BMI, HR, black race, ECG abnormalities	Age, sex, HTN, DM, GGT
Remarks		Complex case-cohort design	Computer-based ECG analysis with partial manual confirmation	Atomic bomb survivors cohort	Computer-based ECG analysis with partial manual confirmation	

Numbers in bold: statistically significant. ‡Relative risk; §Hazard ratio. Abbreviations: BMI, body mass index; BP, blood pressure; CAD, coronary artery disease; CAD, congenital heart defect/disorder; DM, diabetes mellitus; GGT, gamma-glutamyltransferase levels; HR, heart rate; HTN, hypertension; LDL, low density lipoprotein level; LVH, left ventricular hypertrophy; QTc, corrected QT interval; S/P MI, status post myocardial infarction.

hypothesized 3 years ago that ER is an electrocardiographic marker of a "vulnerable substrate" making these patients prone to the development of ventricular arrhythmias only when a certain trigger comes into play, the most common being myocardial ischemia. Recent case-control studies supported that hypothesis by showing an increased risk of VF during acute coronary syndromes in patients demonstrating ER on their baseline ECG (i.e., prior to the ischemic event).[46–48] Furthermore, a recent population study from Japan showed that J-point elevation confers increased risk of death from coronary artery disease in middle-aged individuals.[49] Whether other triggers play a role in the increased mortality risk of ER-positive patients is unknown at this time.

Mortality Risk and Risk Stratification

Table 8.2 summarizes the results of major population studies evaluating the prognostic value of ER in *inferior leads*. Direct comparison between the studies is difficult because of the major methodological differences (e.g., population characteristics, study design, end points, variables adjusted for, ECG evaluation methods). Nevertheless, most of these studies have found an increased mortality risk in patients with ER. When added to the accumulating data from basic research studies,[23] case reports,[6,36,50–53] and IVF cohorts,[10–12,54,55] these findings become difficult to ignore. However, implementing these data for the development of preventive measures is impeded by the high prevalence of ER in the general population. It is therefore crucial to find more specific characteristics of ER that could pinpoint a smaller population with a higher relative risk. To this date, several such characteristics have been found.

J-Wave Amplitude

Similar to the length of the QT interval in long QT syndrome and the magnitude of ST elevation in BrS,[56] higher J-wave amplitude has been shown to denote a greater risk in population studies. In Tikkanen's study, J-point elevation > 0.2 mV was associated with a risk about twice as high as those ≤ 0.2 mV (but ≥ 0.1 mV).[21] This finding, also noted for idiopathic VF by Haïssaguerre,[10] has not been confirmed in other population studies.[32] Moreover, although "giant" J-waves warrant special attention, minor differences above or below the 0.2 mV cutoff point probably have limited practical implications.

ER Location

The leads in which ER is demonstrated have been divided into inferior (II, III, aVF) and anterolateral (I, aVL, V_{4-6}) in most studies. As mentioned above, the right precordial leads have not been included in ER definitions in order to exclude BrS. In most studies,[14,30,32] but not all,[29,31] inferior ER location was associated with a greater risk than anterolateral. Anterolateral lead distribution was, in fact, not associated with increased risk at all in some studies.[14]

J-Point Elevation Morphology

J-point elevation has been divided into 2 morphologies: notching and slurring (see Figure 8.1). However, the attempt to find a greater risk associated with one of these morphologies resulted in equivocal results. This is not surprising taking into account the fact that, in some individuals, different morphologies are seen in different ECG recordings. Furthermore, different morphologies have been demonstrated in different leads on a single ECG recording (see Figure 8.1) and, in some cases, beat-to-beat variation in the J-point elevation morphology were noted.

ST-Segment Morphology

Perhaps, the most important observation regarding risk stratification of ER came from studies examining the ST-segment morphology.[21] It was observed that in athletes, a population ostensibly healthy but with a high prevalence of ER, an ascending ST segment comprises the vast majority of ER patterns noted.[12,21,44] In all but one study,[57] the overwhelming majority (>95%) of athletes with ER had the rapidly ascending pattern.[22] Revisiting his original cohort,[14] Tikkanen has shown that not only was ER with a horizontal/descending ST segment associated with a higher risk of sudden death, the ascending ST-segment variant was not associated with an increased risk at all.[21] This was supported by another study showing increased risk of cardiovascular death with a horizontal/descending ST-segment pattern.[32]

Furthermore, when examining the ratio of horizontal/descending to ascending patterns in different populations, it becomes evident that the horizontal/descending pattern is more common in populations at higher risk of sudden death (Figure 8.5). Thus, athletes have predominantly an ascending pattern while patients with idiopathic VF have a horizontal/descending one.[22]

Taking all the above ECG characteristics together, it is apparent that in contrast to the "classic ER" pattern long known to be benign (consisting primarily of rapidly ascending ST-segment elevation) the "potentially malignant" ER pattern consists of tall J waves with little or no ST-segment elevation. Having said that, it must be emphasized that the term "potentially malignant" denotes only a *relative risk*. In other words,

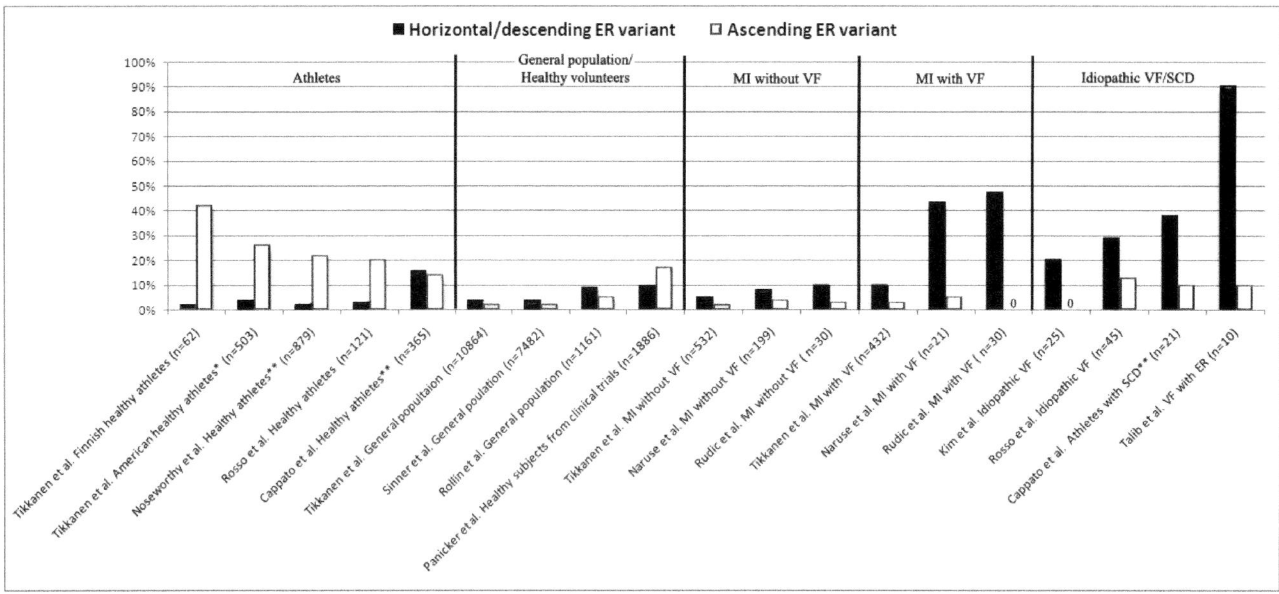

Figure 8.5. Incidence of ST-segment ER variants in different populations. Incidence of ER with rapidly ascending ST segment (blue bars) and with horizontal ST segment (red bars) in different populations. The numbers in parentheses represent the number of patients included in each study. *Only 107 of 151 ER-positive ECGs were available for ST-segment morphology evaluation, and values in the figure were estimated based on the available data. **Definition of ascending ST segment was in accordance with the Tikkanen et al[14] study (>0.1 mV elevation of the ST segment within 100 ms after the J point or a persistently elevated ST segment of 0.1 mV throughout the ST segment) for all studies in the figure except for Cappato et al (>0.05 mV above baseline)[57] and Noseworthy et al (visual analysis without cutoffs).[44] MI, myocardial infarction; SCD, sudden cardiac death; VF, ventricular fibrillation. Modified with permission.[22]

although the risk for individuals with tall J waves and horizontal ST segment in the inferior leads is higher that the risk for those with minor J waves and pronounced (ascending) ST elevation in the anterolateral leads, the majority of asymptomatic individuals with either form of ER will do well.

Management

Based on the above, physicians consulting asymptomatic individuals with ER ought to keep in mind 2 considerations: (1) the increased risk for "ischemic VF" in the event of an acute myocardial infarction and (2) the increased risk for sudden death from idiopathic VF.

Even when combining all the electrocardiographic characteristics of ER associated with higher risk, the relative risk for mortality is not high enough to justify specific preventive measures for the asymptomatic individual with ER. Furthermore, the high prevalence of ER in the general population and our current lack of understanding of the mechanisms putting these patients at risk make it impossible to devise additional diagnostic tests for risk assessment at the present time. Therefore, the only acceptable measures to prevent "ischemic VF" in individuals with ER are those with proven value for preventing coronary artery disease in the general population (i.e., aggressive treatment of arterial hypertension, dyslipidemia, etc., per accepted guidelines).[58] As to the risk of "dropping dead" from idiopathic VF with negative family history, one should emphasize that, according to present knowledge,[22] the risk for the asymptomatic individual with ER is only 1:3000 *even if all "high-risk" ECG characteristics are present.*

SUMMARY

When approaching a patient with ER, there are several key points that need to be remembered:

- ER includes 2 possibly distinct electrocardiographic phenomena: J-point elevation and ST-segment elevation. However, the association between ER and mortality has been restricted mainly to the appearance of J-point elevation with horizontal/descending ST segments in most studies.
- Symptomatic patients with ER (i.e., those with a history of CA) constitute a rare group with high risk of SCD. In these cases, the implantation of an ICD is indicated and quinidine therapy should be considered.
- Asymptomatic patients with ER constitute a large group with a low risk of SCD even if they have electrocardiographic "high-risk" criteria. Except for very unique and rare cases, no preventive measures can be recommended for these patients at this time.

REFERENCES

1. Grant RP, Estes EH, Jr., Doyle JT. Spatial vector electrocardiography; the clinical characteristics of S-T and T vectors. *Circulation.* 1951;3(2):182–197.
2. Shipley RA, Hallaran WR. The four lead electrocardiogram in 200 normal men and women. *Am Heart J.* 1936;11(3):325–345.
3. Myers GB, Kelin HA, Stofer BE, Hiratzka T. Normal variations in multiple precordial leads. *Am Heart J.* 1947;34(6):785–808.
4. Mehta M, Jain AC, Mehta A. Early repolarization. *Clin Cardiol.* 1999;22(2):59–65.
5. Otto CM, Tauxe RV, Cobb LA, et al. Ventricular fibrillation causes sudden death in Southeast Asian immigrants. *Ann Intern Med.* 1984;101(1):45–47.
6. Takagi M, Aihara N, Takaki H, et al. Clinical characteristics of patients with spontaneous or inducible ventricular fibrillation without apparent heart disease presenting with J wave and ST segment elevation in inferior leads. *J Cardiovasc Electrophysiol.* 2000;11(8):844–848.
7. Kalla H, Yan GX, Marinchak R. Ventricular fibrillation in a patient with prominent J (Osborn) waves and ST segment elevation in the inferior electrocardiographic leads: a Brugada syndrome variant? *J Cardiovasc Electrophysiol.* 2000;11(1):95–98.
8. Yan GX, Antzelevitch C. Cellular basis for the electrocardiographic J wave. *Circulation.* 1996;93(2):372–379.
9. Gussak I, Antzelevitch C. Early repolarization syndrome: clinical characteristics and possible cellular and ionic mechanisms. *J Electrocardiol.* 2000;33(4):299–309.
10. Haïssaguerre M, Derval N, Sacher F, et al. Sudden cardiac arrest associated with early repolarization. *N Engl J Med.* 2008;358(19):2016–2023.
11. Nam GB, Kim YH, Antzelevitch C. Augmentation of J waves and electrical storms in patients with early repolarization. *N Engl J Med.* 2008;358(19):2078–2079.
12. Rosso R, Kogan E, Belhassen B, et al. J-point elevation in survivors of primary ventricular fibrillation and matched control subjects: Incidence and clinical significance. *J Am Coll Cardiol.* 2008;52(15):1231–1238.
13. Nam GB, Ko KH, Kim J, et al. Mode of onset of ventricular fibrillation in patients with early repolarization pattern vs. Brugada syndrome. *Eur Heart J.* 2010;31(3):330–339.
14. Tikkanen JT, Anttonen O, Junttila MJ, et al. Long-term outcome associated with early repolarization on electrocardiography. *N Engl J Med.* 2009;361(26):2529–2537.
15. Sinner MF, Reinhard W, Muller M, et al. Association of early repolarization pattern on ECG with risk of cardiac and all-cause mortality: A population-based prospective cohort study (MONICA/KORA). *PLoS Med.* 2010;7(7):e1000314.
16. Viskin S, Rosso R, Halkin A. Making sense of early repolarization. *Heart Rhythm.* 2012;9(4):566–568.
17. Froelicher V, Wagner G. Symposium on the J wave patterns and a J wave syndrome. *J Electrocardiol.* 2013;46(5):381–382.
18. Kamakura T, Kawata H, Nakajima I, et al. Significance of non-type 1 anterior early repolarization in patients with inferolateral early repolarization syndrome. *J Am Coll Cardiol.* 2013;62(17):1610–1618.
19. Viskin S. Is there anyone left with a normal electrocardiogram? *J Am Coll Cardiol.* 2013;62(17):1619–1620.
20. Macfarlane PW, Clark EN. ECG measurements in end QRS notching and slurring. *J Electrocardiol.* 2013;46(5):385–389.
21. Tikkanen JT, Junttila MJ, Anttonen O, et al. Early repolarization: Electrocardiographic phenotypes associated with favorable long-term outcome. *Circulation.* 2011;123(23):2666–2673.
22. Adler A, Rosso R, Viskin D, Halkin A, Viskin S. What do we know about the "malignant form" of early repolarization? *J Am Coll Cardiol.* 2013;62(10):863–868.
23. Antzelevitch C, Yan GX. J wave syndromes. *Heart Rhythm.* 2010;7(4):549–558.
24. Rollin A, Sacher F, Gourraud JB, et al. Prevalence, characteristics, and prognosis role of type 1 ST elevation in the peripheral ECG leads in patients with Brugada syndrome. *Heart Rhythm.* 2013;10(7):1012–1018.
25. Letsas KP, Sacher F, Probst V, et al. Prevalence of early repolarization pattern in inferolateral leads in patients with Brugada syndrome. *Heart Rhythm.* 2008;5(12):1685–1689.
26. Sarkozy A, Chierchia GB, Paparella G, et al. Inferior and lateral electrocardiographic repolarization abnormalities in Brugada syndrome. *Circ Arrhythm Electrophysiol.* 2009;2(2):154–161.
27. Takagi M, Aonuma K, Sekiguchi Y, et al. The prognostic value of early repolarization (J wave) and ST-segment morphology after J wave in Brugada syndrome: Multicenter study in Japan. *Heart Rhythm.* 2013;10(4):533–539.
28. Kawata H, Morita H, Yamada Y, et al. Prognostic significance of early repolarization in inferolateral leads in Brugada patients with documented ventricular fibrillation: A novel risk factor for Brugada syndrome with ventricular fibrillation. *Heart Rhythm.* 2013;10(8):1161–1168.
29. Olson KA, Viera AJ, Soliman EZ, Crow RS, Rosamond WD. Long-term prognosis associated with J-point elevation in a large middle-aged biracial cohort: The ARIC study. *Eur Heart J.* 2011;32(24):3098–3106.
30. Haruta D, Matsuo K, Tsuneto A, et al. Incidence and prognostic value of early repolarization pattern in the 12-lead electrocardiogram. *Circulation.* 2011;123(25):2931–2937.
31. Uberoi A, Jain NA, Perez M, et al. Early repolarization in an ambulatory clinical population. *Circulation.* 2011;124(20):2208–2214.
32. Rollin A, Maury P, Bongard V, et al. Prevalence, prognosis, and identification of the malignant form of early repolarization pattern in a population-based study. *Am J Cardiol.* 2012;110(9):1302–1308.
33. Priori SG, Wilde AA, Horie M, et al. HRS/EHRA/APHRS expert consensus statement on the diagnosis and management of patients with inherited primary arrhythmia syndromes: Document endorsed by

HRS, EHRA, and APHRS in May 2013 and by ACCF, AHA, PACES, and AEPC in June 2013. *Heart Rhythm.* 2013;10(12):1932–1963.
34. Viskin S, Lesh MD, Eldar M, et al. Mode of onset of malignant ventricular arrhythmias in idiopathic ventricular fibrillation. *J Cardiovasc Electrophysiol.* 1997;8(10):1115–1120.
35. Gourraud JB, Le Scouarnec S, Sacher F, et al. Identification of large families in early repolarization syndrome. *J Am Coll Cardiol.* 2013;61(2):164–172.
36. Haïssaguerre M, Chatel S, Sacher F, et al. Ventricular fibrillation with prominent early repolarization associated with a rare variant of KCNJ8/KATP channel. *J Cardiovasc Electrophysiol.* 2009;20(1):93–98.
37. Medeiros-Domingo A, Tan BH, Crotti L, et al. Gain-of-function mutation S422L in the KCNJ8-encoded cardiac K(ATP) channel Kir6.1 as a pathogenic substrate for J-wave syndromes. *Heart Rhythm.* 2010;7(10):1466–1471.
38. Burashnikov E, Pfeiffer R, Barajas-Martinez H, et al. Mutations in the cardiac L-type calcium channel associated with inherited J-wave syndromes and sudden cardiac death. *Heart Rhythm.* 2010;7(12):1872–1882.
39. Watanabe H, Nogami A, Ohkubo K, et al. Electrocardiographic characteristics and SCN5A mutations in idiopathic ventricular fibrillation associated with early repolarization. *Circ Arrhythm Electrophysiol.* 2011;4(6):874–881.
40. Adler A, Viskin S. Syncope in hereditary arrhythmogenic syndromes. *Card Electrophysiol Clin.* 2013;5(4):479–486.
41. Haïssaguerre M, Sacher F, Nogami A, et al. Characteristics of recurrent ventricular fibrillation associated with inferolateral early repolarization role of drug therapy. *J Am Coll Cardiol.* 2009;53(7):612–619.
42. Sacher F, Derval N, Horlitz M, Haïssaguerre M. J wave elevation to monitor quinidine efficacy in early repolarization syndrome. *J Electrocardiol.* 2013;47(2):223–225.
43. Panicker GK, Manohar D, Karnad DR, et al. Early repolarization and short QT interval in healthy subjects. *Heart Rhythm.* 2012;9(8):1265–1271.
44. Noseworthy PA, Weiner R, Kim J, et al. Early repolarization pattern in competitive athletes: clinical correlates and the effects of exercise training. *Circ Arrhythm Electrophysiol.* 2011;4(4):432–440.
45. Rosso R, Adler A, Halkin A, Viskin S. Risk of sudden death among young individuals with J waves and early repolarization: Putting the evidence into perspective. *Heart Rhythm.* 2011;8(6):923–929.
46. Tikkanen JT, Wichmann V, Junttila MJ, et al. Association of early repolarization and sudden cardiac death during an acute coronary event. *Circ Arrhythm Electrophysiol.* 2012;5(4):714–718.
47. Naruse Y, Tada H, Harimura Y, et al. Early repolarization is an independent predictor of occurrences of ventricular fibrillation in the very early phase of acute myocardial infarction. *Circ Arrhythm Electrophysiol.* 2012;5(3):506–513.
48. Rudic B, Veltmann C, Kuntz E, et al. Early repolarization pattern is associated with ventricular fibrillation in patients with acute myocardial infarction. *Heart Rhythm.* 2012;9(8):1295–1300.
49. Hisamatsu T, Ohkubo T, Miura K, et al. Association between J-point elevation and death from coronary artery disease — 15-year follow up of the NIPPON DATA90. *Circ J.* 2013;77(5):1260–1266.
50. Sahara M, Sagara K, Yamashita T, et al. J wave and ST segment elevation in the inferior leads: a latent type of variant Brugada syndrome? *Jpn Heart J.* 2002;43(1):55–60.
51. Shinohara T, Takahashi N, Saikawa T, Yoshimatsu H. Characterization of J wave in a patient with idiopathic ventricular fibrillation. *Heart Rhythm.* 2006;3(9):1082–1084.
52. Takeuchi T, Sato N, Kawamura Y, et al. A case of a short-coupled variant of torsades de pointes with electrical storm. *Pacing Clin Electrophysiol.* 2003;26(2 Pt 1):632–636.
53. Tsunoda Y, Takeishi Y, Nozaki N, Kitahara T, Kubota I. Presence of intermittent J waves in multiple leads in relation to episode of atrial and ventricular fibrillation. *J Electrocardiol.* 2004;37(4):311–314.
54. Abe A, Ikeda T, Tsukada T, et al. Circadian variation of late potentials in idiopathic ventricular fibrillation associated with J waves: insights into alternative pathophysiology and risk stratification. *Heart Rhythm.* 2010;7(5):675–682.
55. Merchant FM, Noseworthy PA, Weiner RB, et al. Ability of terminal QRS notching to distinguish benign from malignant electrocardiographic forms of early repolarization. *Am J Cardiol.* 2009;104(10):1402–1406.
56. Viskin S, Adler A, Rosso R. Brugada burden in Brugada syndrome: The way to go in risk stratification? *Heart Rhythm.* 2013;10(7):1019–1020.
57. Cappato R, Furlanello F, Giovinazzo V, et al. J wave, QRS slurring, and ST elevation in athletes with cardiac arrest in the absence of heart disease: Marker of risk or innocent bystander? *Circ Arrhythm Electrophysiol.* 2010;3(4):305–311.
58. Perk J, De Backer G, Gohlke H, et al. European Guidelines on cardiovascular disease prevention in clinical practice (version 2012). The Fifth Joint Task Force of the European Society of Cardiology and Other Societies on Cardiovascular Disease Prevention in Clinical Practice (constituted by representatives of nine societies and by invited experts). *Eur Heart J.* 2012;33(13):1635–1701.

CHAPTER

9

Diagnostic Electrocardiographic Criteria of Early Repolarization and Idiopathic Ventricular Fibrillation

Méléze Hocini, MD, Ashok J. Shah, MD, Pierre Jaïs, MD, and Michel Haïssaguerre, MD

INTRODUCTION

Sudden cardiac death (SCD) occurs predominantly in patients with known or previously unrecognized underlying heart disease. Coronary artery disease is the leading cause for approximately 80% of patients who experience SCD. In 10% to 15%, structural cardiac abnormalities in idiopathic, hypertrophic, and arrhythmogenic ventricular cardiomyopathies account for the second largest number of SCD origin. Furthermore, in 5% to 10% of patients, there is no evidence of structural heart disease. The diagnosis of idiopathic ventricular fibrillation (IVF) and early abnormal repolarization syndrome is based mainly on exclusion of an underlying heart disease.

Early repolarization (ER) is a vague term which suggests premature repolarization of myocardial cells. ER was historically considered as a benign ECG variant until it emerged as a marker of risk for SCD, particularly when seen in the inferior and inferolateral ECG leads. In addition, this risk has been associated with IVF and has also been identified in the general population.[1–3] Although ER is a common ECG finding, the occurrence of SCD remains exceptional and determining risk for each individual is "the quest of Holy Grail." This chapter will describe the electrocardiographic criteria of ER and its relation with IVF.

DEFINITIONS OF ER

Slurring or notching of the terminal QRS, also referred to as an Osborn wave, is a deflection immediately following the QRS complex of the surface ECG. It has been described as a benign finding more prevalent in men, athletes, and individuals of black ethnicity. It was found predominantly in the anterolateral ECG leads and consisted of ST elevation from baseline by greater than 0.1 mV at the end of the QRS in 2 or more ECG leads (Figure 9.1) with the exclusion of leads V_1 to V_3 to avoid confusion with the Brugada syndrome (BrS). J-point elevation was noted to vary between different ECG recordings and generally decrease over time.[4] Additional ST-segment and T-wave morphology were furthermore identified and associated with SCD[5] such as rapidly ascending with >0.1 mV ST-segment

The ECG Handbook of Contemporary Challenges © 2015 Mohammad Shenasa, Mark E. Josephson, N.A. Mark Estes III
Cardiotext Publishing, ISBN: 978-1-935395-88-1

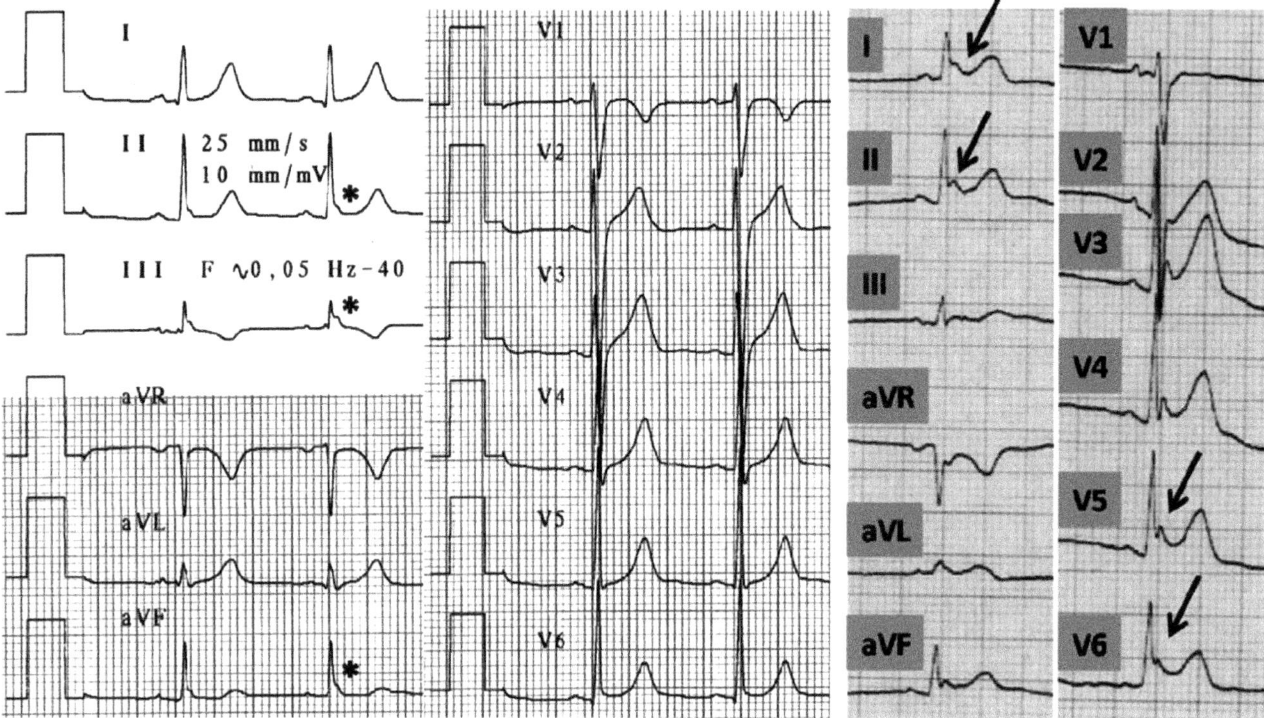

Figure 9.1. Different features of J-wave elevation as slurring (asterisks) or notching (arrows) in inferior (asterisks) or lateral (arrows) in patients with VF. Modified with permission.[18]

elevation within 100 ms after the J point or persisting through the ST segment; and horizontal/descending with ≤0.1 mV ST-segment elevation within 100 ms after the J point (Figure 9.2).

PREVALENCE OF ER IN THE GENERAL POPULATION

Its prevalence in the Caucasian general population ranges from 4.5% to 24% across different ethnic groups.[1,2,6,7] ER pattern has been described to be associated with a risk of VF, depending on the ER location, magnitude of J wave, and degree of ST elevation. The presence of inferior ER in white Europeans increased the risk of cardiac death by 2- to 4-fold. Similarly, inferior ER with J-point elevation ≥0.2 mV associated with a horizontal/descending ST-segment was independently associated with a 3-fold increased risk of SCD compare to lateral localization of ER and/or rapidly upsloping ST-segment.[1,5] Tikkanen et al systemically reported the long-term outcome of ER in the general population.[3] The authors assessed the prevalence and prognostic significance of ER on routine ECG performed during a community-based investigational coronary artery disease study involving 10,864 middle-aged subjects. The mean follow-up was 30 ± 11 years with the primary end point of cardiac death and secondary end points of all-cause mortality and arrhythmic death. The prevalence of ER was 5.8% in this cohort. Importantly, ER in the inferior leads was found to be associated with an increased risk of cardiac death (adjusted relative risk [RR], 1.28; 95% confidence interval [CI], 1.04e1.59; P_5, 0.03) in the general population. J-point elevation in the lateral leads was of borderline significance in predicting the cardiac death and all-cause death. Moreover, the survival curves started to diverge 15 years after the first ECG recording in the early 1980s and continued to diverge at a constant rate throughout the follow-up period, despite continued improvement in the treatment and prognosis of patients with cardiac disease during the past 2 decades. Although authors retrospectively classified cardiac deaths into arrhythmic and nonarrhythmic categories, the results strongly challenge the long-held benignancy of ER.

ER AND IVF

Among survivors of IVF, the prevalence of ER is higher than among healthy controls, with an estimate of 23% to 68%.[1,2,8] Our group compared 206 case subjects with IVF to 412 healthy control subjects and demonstrated that an ER pattern was more prevalent in subjects with IVF (31% vs. 5%, respectively). Furthermore, the amplitude of ER was greater in patients with IVF than in controls (2.15 ± 1.2 mm vs. 1.5 ± 0.2

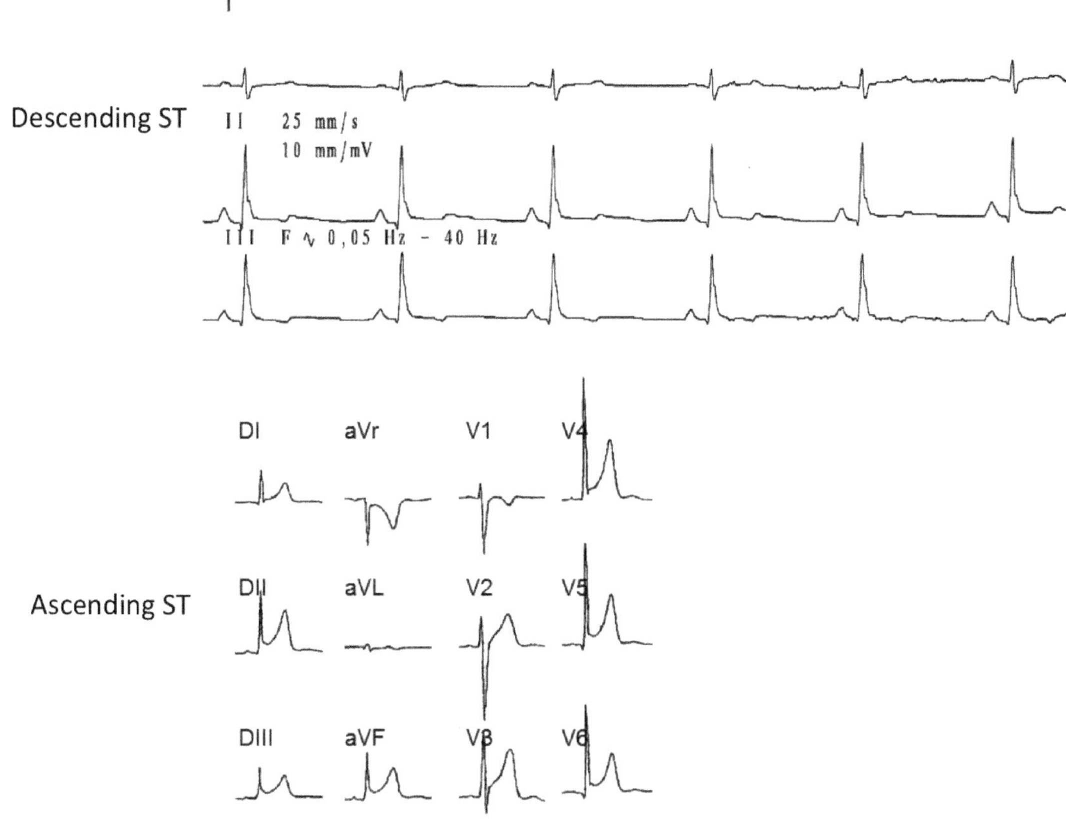

Figure 9.2. **Top panel:** Descending ST segments in inferior limb leads. **Bottom panel:** Ascending ST segments in inferolateral leads.

mm, respectively). In patients with IVF, the localization of ER pattern in the inferior leads was seen in 91% and 9% in lateral leads. Patients were more likely to be young and male and to experience syncope or cardiac arrest during sleep than those without the ER pattern.[1,9] In this series, all patients underwent implantation of a cardioverter defibrillator (ICD) and were monitored with an average follow-up of 5 years. It was remarkable to observe that patients with ER pattern had more recurrence of VF than those without ER pattern (42% vs. 23%, respectively), indicating that the ER pattern was not only a risk for primary SCD but also a risk factor for recurrence of VF. Of note, none of the arrhythmic event was ventricular tachycardia. Interestingly, the amplitude of J wave increased shortly prior to VF and returned to its baseline value thereafter. Other groups have also reported that J-point amplitude increases before an arrhythmic episode.[8,10] Additionally, our group mapped the site of origin of ventricular ectopic beat in 8 patients and found that the origin of ectopy was consistent with the location of the repolarization abnormality in ECG (Figure 9.3). When ER pattern was located in the inferior leads, the ectopy presented with a left axis, and the ectopy had variables morphologies when ER pattern was diffuse.

CHARACTERISTICS OF J-WAVE ELEVATION IN ER ASSOCIATED WITH VF

Amplitude of J Wave

Amplitude of J wave is more important in VF patients compared with controls (2.15 ± 1.2 mm in IVF vs. 1.05 ± 0.2 mm).[1] Tikkanen et al reported higher relative risk of cardiac death with a J-point elevation of 0.2 mV (RR 3.03; 95% CI: 1.88 – 4.90; $P = 0.001$) compared with 0.1 mV (RR 1.30; 95% CI: 1.05 – 1.61; $P = 0.02$).[3]

Spontaneous Dynamicity

Because most of the VF episodes cannot be predicted clinically in patients with sporadic episodes of VF, it is difficult to gain further insight into the role of ER in the mechanism of VF. However, some of the patients with VF experience electrical storm during hospitalization, unraveling the dynamics of ER in VF arrhythmogenesis. Haïssaguerre et al[11] performed serial ECGs during electrical storm (including frequent ventricular ectopy and episodes of VF) in 16 subjects and all patients showed consistent and marked increase in the amplitude of J wave during the period of storm when compared with baseline pattern (from 2.6 ± 1 mm to 4.1 ± 2 mm; $P < 0.001$). Besides

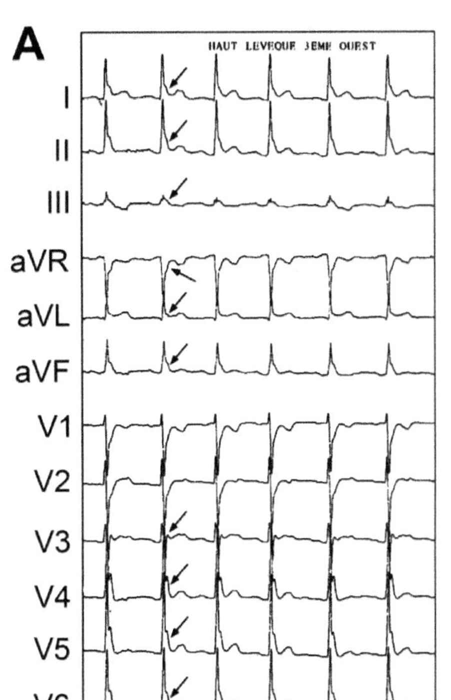

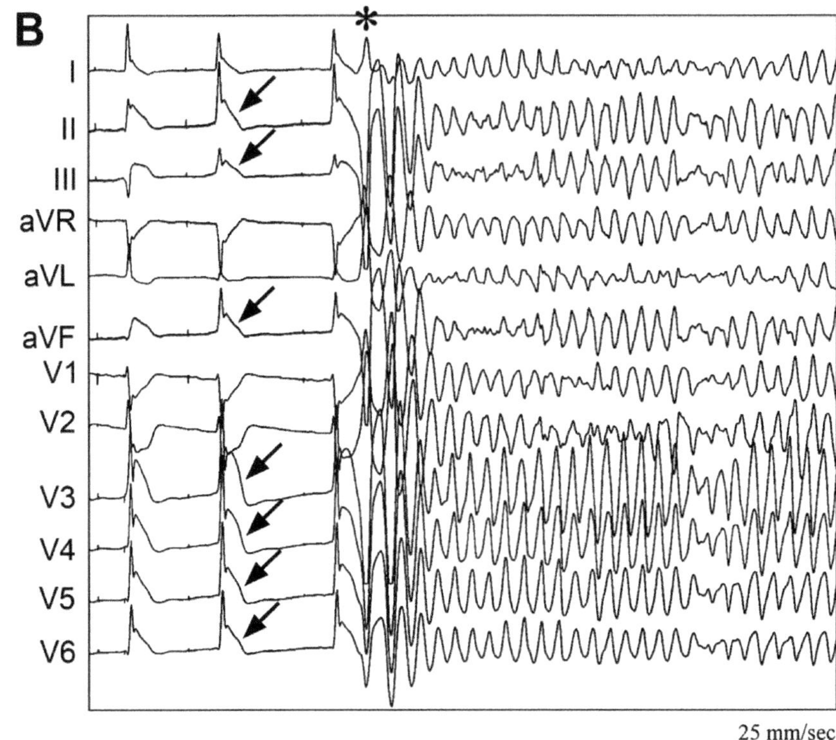

Figure 9.3. **A.** Baseline ECG of a survivor of sudden cardiac arrest (16-year-old girl). All known structural heart diseases and primary electrical diseases, including long/short-QT syndrome, BrS, and catecholamine-sensitive ventricular tachycardia were excluded in this patient. The only significant finding on the ECG was a prominent J wave (arrows) as can be seen in almost all the leads other than V_1 and V_2. **B.** During the electrophysiologic study, an episode of spontaneous ventricular fibrillation (VF) was triggered by a ventricular ectopy from the inferior posterior left ventricle with very short coupling interval (asterisk). Note the J wave in the inferior and precordial leads (arrows) gets significantly augmented before the occurrence VF than at the baseline. Sweep speed = 25 mm/s. Modified with permission.[18]

spontaneous accentuation of the J-wave amplitude preceding electrical storm, spontaneous beat-to-beat fluctuation in the morphologic pattern of ER was also observed.[1] Out of 11 patients with VF and ER reported by Nam et al,[12] 5 patients experienced VF storm during their stay in the intensive care unit. ECGs recorded within 30 minutes of the VF storm exhibited global appearance of J waves. These dynamic ECG features of ER appeared spontaneously for a transient period around the VF storm revealing the presence of functional “substrate” for arrhythmia.

J-Point Location and Site of Origin of Arrhythmia

As mentioned previously, the authors mapped patients with ER and VF targeting the ventricular ectopy initiating the VF (see Figure 9.3). In patients with ER recorded in inferior leads alone, all ectopies originated from the inferior left ventricular wall. In the subjects with widespread global ER, as recorded in both inferior and lateral leads, ectopy originated from multiple regions.[1,13] These findings prove that ER abnormality may be either limited to a single region in the ventricles or can extend beyond it to involve more than one region simultaneously. Whether or not J wave truly represents an abnormality of repolarization is still debated,[14] but these findings help towards localizing ER as an abnormality involving distal Purkinje tissue, its innervated myocardium, or the Purkinje-myocardial junctions.

RISK STRATIFICATION

As described previously, although ER is a common entity, unexplained sudden cardiac arrest in young adults is very rare. Some investigators addressed this issue by using the Bayes’ law of conditional probabilities. Rosso et al[2] claimed that the presence of J wave in a young adult would increase the probability of VF from 3.4:100,000 to 11:100,000, which is a negligible rise. They concluded that the incidental discovery of J wave on routine screening should not be interpreted as a marker of “high risk” because the odds for this fatal disease would still be approximately 1:10,000. Now, the question is: “how to differentiate subjects with ‘high risk’ ER from the so-called benign ER?”

Clinical History

In such a situation, we consider that close follow-up should be offered to patients with ER and unexplained syncope or a family history of unexplained sudden death. Abe et al[15] reported that the prevalence of ER in 222 patients with syncope and no organic disorder was 18.5%, which is almost 10 times that in 3915 healthy controls (2%). Therefore, the possibility of ER-associated syncopal episodes cannot be excluded in at least some of these patients. The genetic basis of ER is still largely unknown. Also, in patients with VF and ER, positive family history of sudden death was not significantly higher than in those without ER (16% vs. 9%; P_5 0.17).[1] Nevertheless, it does not imply that family history is not an important aspect of history-taking in ER patients.

Magnitude of J Wave

In the study by Tikkanen et al,[3] subjects with J-point elevation of more than 0.2 mV on inferior leads not only bore a higher risk of death from cardiac causes (adjusted RR, 2.98; 95% CI: 1.85 – 4.92; $P < 0.001$) as compared with J-point elevation of more than 0.1 mV, but also had a markedly elevated risk of death from arrhythmia (adjusted RR, 2.92; 95% CI:1.45-5.89; P = 0.01). This finding indicates that the magnitude of J-point elevation could be a discriminator of risk. However, this study did not provide the sensitivity and specificity of this measure in predicting the end point events. In accordance with this finding, Haïssaguerre et al[1] also found that the magnitude of J-wave elevation in case group was significantly higher than that in control subjects (2 ± 0.8 mV vs. 1.2 ± 0.4 mV; $P < 0.001$). It is noteworthy that the J-point elevation of more than 0.2 mV seems rare in the normal population. In 630 of 10,864 subjects with ER identified by Tikkanen et al,[3] 0.33% of the total population had J-wave elevation of more than 0.2 mV. However, it is also necessary to point out that the magnitude of J-wave elevation can fluctuate even without drug provocation or exercise (Figure 9.4). This means that low magnitude of J wave should not be considered as a static entity. It can potentially get augmented. Unfortunately, there is currently no reliable provocation test to augment ER in inferolateral leads.

Distribution of J Wave

In normal subjects, most of the ER is confined to inferior leads, lateral leads (I/aVL) or left precordial leads. As reported by Tikkanen et al,[3] out of 630 subjects with ER, only 16 subjects (2.5%) had ER[1] in both the inferior and lateral leads. Focusing on patients with VF, Haïssaguerre et al found that 46.9% of patients with VF and ER had ER in both inferior and lateral leads. Similarly, global presence of ER was observed in none of the 46 subjects with ER without VF (selected from among 1395 individuals from the general population) but in 45.5% of patients with ER who developed VF.[12]

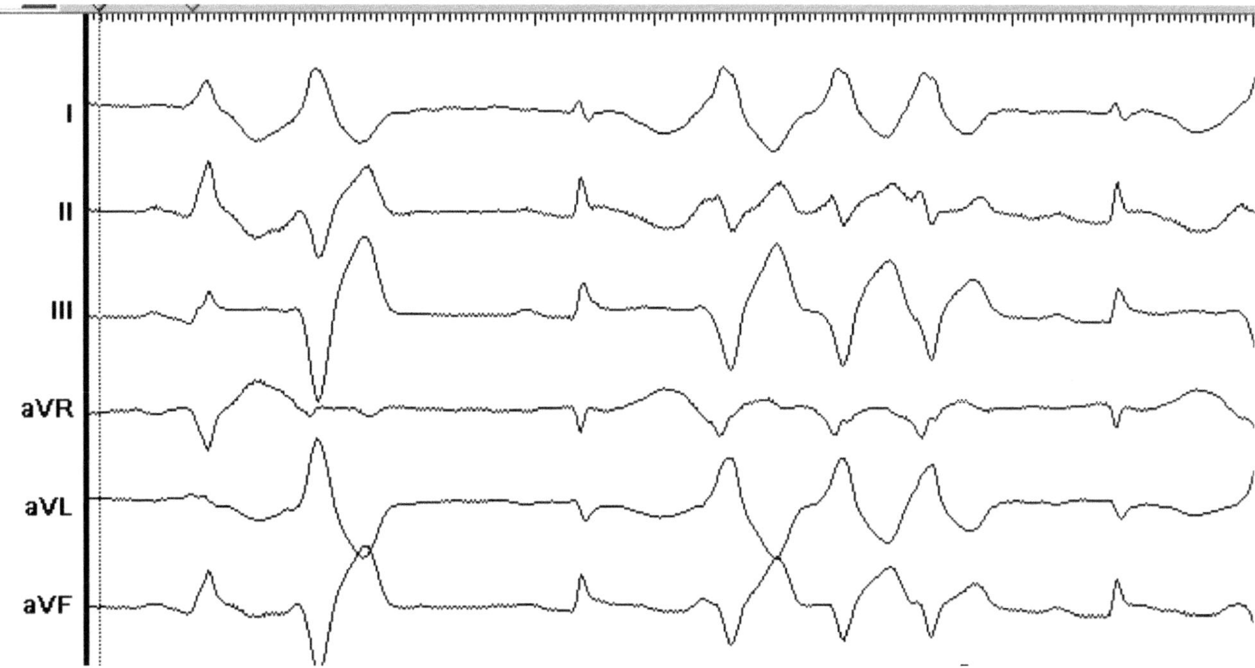

Figure 9.4. Limb leads of the surface ECG show beat-to-beat variation in the inferior ER in association with the occurrence of ventricular ectopics and salvos.

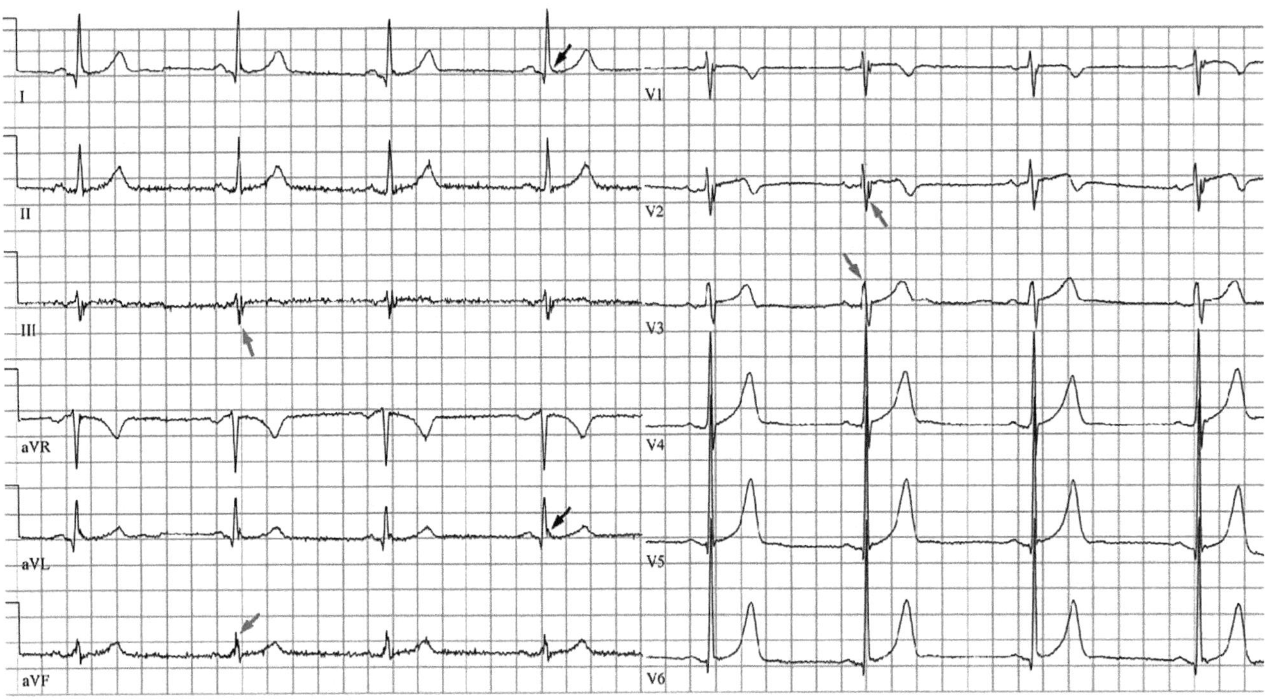

Figure 9.5. A representative electrocardiographic example of J-wave elevation in lateral leads (black arrows) and fragmentation of the QRS (red arrows) associated with recurrent ventricular fibrillation. Modified with permission.[18]

Morphology of J Wave

Recently, Merchant et al[16] compared the baseline ECGs between 9 patients with VF/VT and ER (so-called "malignant ER" group) and 61 age- and gender-matched controls with normal ER (so-called "benign ER" group). The results demonstrated that QRS notching was more prevalent among cases than controls in leads V_4 (44% vs. 5%; $P_5 = 0.001$); V_5 (44% vs. 8%; $P_5 = 0.006$); and V_6 (33% vs. 5%; $P_5 = 0.013$). They concluded that left precordial terminal QRS notching is more prevalent in malignant variants of ER than in benign cases and could be used as a tool for risk stratification of subjects with ER. However, the case number in this study is small, and it includes 3 patients with idiopathic monomorphic VT without VF.

Fragmented QRS (fQRS)

Liu et al[17] looked at fQRS (defined as presence of at least one additional deflection or notching within the QRS complex including top of R wave or nadir of S wave in at least 2 contiguous leads) of 16 ICD recipients with VF and ER. Seven patients (43.8%) had fQRS in 2 to 4 (mean: 2.7) leads and after a mean follow-up of 67 ± 66 months, 5 (71.4%) of 7 patients had recurrent VF (ICD shocks ranging from 1 to 8, mean 3.8) (Figure 9.5). None of the 9 patients lacking fQRS experienced appropriate ICD discharges ($P < 0.01$). The authors concluded that the presence of f-QRS, indicating depolarization disturbance, increases the risk of recurrent ventricular arrhythmias in patients with VF and ER.

Invasive Induction of VF

Induction of VF was attempted in 132 VF patients from 2 different ventricular sites and up to 3 extrastimuli with shortest coupling interval of 209 ± 30 ms. The patients with ER did not show significantly higher inducibility than those without ER (16 of 47 vs. 17 of 85; $P = 0.07$).[1] Moreover, a low rate of VF inducibility (34%) in the patients with ER on ECG makes electrophysiologic study less sensitive in risk stratification of asymptomatic patients.

SUMMARY

1. ER is a common ECG finding, particularly in young adults, men, individuals undertaking regular sporting activity, and/or individuals of black ethnicity.
2. The underlying pathophysiology of ER, depolarization versus repolarization is under debate.
3. ER was historically a benign finding in the general population and remains benign when found in

a typical lateral pattern with rapidly ascending ST-segment morphology and symmetrical T waves.

4. The definition of ER has evolved and inferior J-point elevation has been associated with risk of SCD in survivors of IVF and the general population.
5. Early repolarization syndrome (ERS), the presence of ER in the context of otherwise IVF is rare.
6. In an asymptomatic individual with ER, there is no indication to investigate unless an immediate blood relative has had a premature or sudden arrhythmic death syndrome death or has ERS.

REFERENCES

1. Haïssaguerre M, Derval N, Sacher F, et al. Sudden cardiac arrest associated with early repolarization. *N Engl J Med.* 2008;358:2016–2023.
2. Rosso R, Kogan E, Belhassen B, et al. J-Point elevation in survivors of primary ventricular fibrillation and matched control subjects: Incidence and clinical significance. *J Am Coll Cardiol.* 2008;52:1231–1248.
3. Tikkanen JT, Anttonen O, Junttila MJ, et al. Long-term outcome associated with early repolarization on electrocardiography. *N Engl J Med.* 2009;361:2529–2537.
4. Klatsky AL, Oehm R, Cooper RA, et al. The early repolarization normal variant electrocardiogram: Correlates and consequences. *Am J Med.* 2003;115:171–177.
5. Tikkanen JT, Junttila MJ, Anttonen O, et al. Early repolarization: Electrocardiographic phenotypes associated with favorable long-term outcome. *Circulation.* 2011;123:2666–2673.
6. Haruta D, Matsuo K, Tsuneto A, et al. Incidence and prognostic value of early repolarization pattern in the 12-lead electrocardiogram. *Circulation.* 2011;123:2931–2937.
7. Noseworthy PA, Tikkanen JT, Porthan K, et al. The early repolarization pattern in the general population: clinical correlates and heritability. *J Am Coll Cardiol.* 2011;57:2284–2289.
8. Nam GB, Kim YH, Antzelevitch C. Augmentation of J waves and electrical storms in patients with early repolarization. *N Engl J Med.* 2008;358:2078–2079.
9. Abe A, Ikeda T, Tsukada T, et al. Circadian variation of late potentials in idiopathic ventricular fibrillation associated with J waves: Insights into alternative pathophysiology and risk stratification. *Heart Rhythm.* 2010;7:675–682.
10. Derval N, Simpson CS, Birnie DH, et al. Prevalence and characteristics of early repolarization in the CASPER registry: Cardiac Arrest Survivors with Preserved Ejection Fraction registry. *J Am Coll Cardiol.* 2011;58:722–728.
11. Haïssaguerre M, Sacher F, Nogami A, et al. Characteristics of recurrent ventricular fibrillation associated with inferolateral early repolarization role of drug therapy. *J Am Coll Cardiol.* 2009;53:612–619.
12. Nam GB, Ko KH, Kim J, et al. Mode of onset of ventricular fibrillation in patients with early repolarization pattern vs Brugada syndrome. *Eur Heart J.* 2010;31(3):330–339.
13. Sacher F, Derval N, Jesel L, et al. Initiation of ventricular arrhythmia in idiopathic ventricular fibrillation associated with early repolarization syndrome. *Heart Rhythm.* 2008;5S:S150;PO1–PO136.
14. Borggrefe M, Schimpf R. J-wave syndromes caused by repolarization or depolarization mechanisms a debated issue among experimental and clinical electrophysiologists. *J Am Coll Cardiol.* 2010;55(8):798–800.
15. Abe A, Yoshino H, Ishiguro H, et al. Prevalence of J waves in 12-lead electrocardiogram in patients with syncope and no organic disorder. *J Cardiovasc Electrophysiol.* 2007;18(suppl 2):S88.
16. Merchant FM, Noseworthy PA, Weiner RB, et al. Ability of terminal QRS notching to distinguish benign from malignant electrocardiographic forms of early repolarization. *Am J Cardiol.* 2009;104:1402–1406.
17. Liu X, Hocini M, Derval N, et al. Fragmented QRS complexes as a predictor of ventricular arrhythmic events in patients with idiopathic ventricular fibrillation and early repolarization (abstract). *Heart Rhythm.* 2010;7(5):S175.
18. Shah AJ, Sacher F, Chatel S, et al. Early Repolarization Disease. *Card Electro Clinics.* 2010;2(4):559–569.

CHAPTER

10

Prevalence and Significance of Early Repolarization (a.k.a. Haïssaguerre or J-Wave Pattern/Syndrome)

Victor Froelicher, MD

INTRODUCTION

This contribution should begin with a clarification of the point of view that will be taken. The previous 2 chapters have been written by 2 of the most accomplished electrophysiologists of our time. In their clinical practice and research, they have seen a number of patients with rare condition of idiopathic ventricular fibrillation (VF). They were 2 of the first investigators of a new channelopathy, where the arrhythmic events in patients with idiopathic ventricular tachycardia/VF (IVT/VF) were often preceded by the dynamic appearance of large J waves[1] similar to the Osborne waves of hypothermia (Figure 10.1). Though their writings are hopeful in tone, neither has presented convincing data nor enthusiastic support that any ECG finding on the routine 10-second ECG taken at a stable period in the course of these patients' disease will identify them as having the channelopathy.

In contrast, in spite of extensive clinical contact with cardiology patients and screening of athletes for the risk of sudden cardiac death (SCD), this author has never diagnosed an individual with this new channelopathy. Furthermore, in spite of many years of interpreting ECGs from patients and athletes as well as reading Holter and event recorders, he has never observed dynamic J waves. This is not to say they do not exist, but to stress the point that they are rare, and most of us will only see the exciting examples of them in the literature. Hopefully, now that awareness is widespread, more cases will be recognized and patients helped.

My main interest in this new syndrome has been in analyzing the screening, at-rest 10-second ECG to demonstrate components of the downslope of the R wave or S-wave upslope that could identify individuals at a risk of sudden death. This unprecedented interest in phenomena occurring on the downslope of the R wave or S-wave upslope (i.e., the general area where ventricular depolarization and repolarization overlap) has highlighted other complicating issues. These include how should QRS end be measured when they are present (are current normal values for QRS duration correct?), what is the J point, where is the ST level set, and do the current automated ECG programs make these measurements correctly when slurring or J waves are present?

Interest peaked in this new channelopathy with the seminal paper in the *New England Journal of*

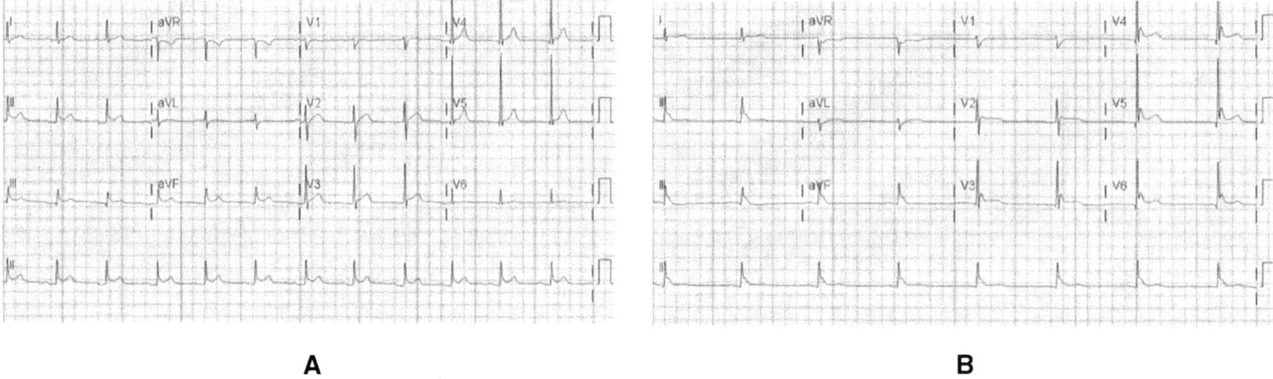

Figure 10.1. Example of Osborne waves. The 2 ECGs were obtained from a 56-year-old male with cerebral palsy admitted to a local hospital in pneumosepsis from a nearby long-term care facility. Cardiology called because of unusual ECG and the next day the patient's core temperature dropped to 33°C. The patient was treated with antibiotics and then the ECG returned to baseline. (Courtesy Dr. Bing Liem). **A.** Admission ECG. **B.** ECG from the next day (unfortunately serial ECGs are not available but Osborne waves disappeared while discharging).

Medicine (NEJM) from the French Multicenter study of patients with IVT/VF and interest sparked by the title inclusion of the term "Early Repolarization (ER)."[2] To most of the American physicians, that was a term associated with a benign ECG pattern of ST elevation (sometimes accompanied by J waves and slurring), often noted in healthy young athletes of African descent.[3] The only clinical concern with it was the similarity between it and the ST-elevation patterns of pericarditis, STEMI, variant angina, and acute transmural ischemia.[4] The implication that this ECG pattern could be predictive of arrhythmic death seemed unlikely, but any hope of confirming a new marker for sudden death in young athletes certainly was worth exploring. The possibility that the rest ECG could be used in population studies to predict arrhythmic death was supported by the unique Finnish study with a 30-year follow up published shortly after, also in the NEJM.[5] Subsequently, we hypothesized that this study and others supporting the routine rest ECG as a predictor of CV death were due to the association of J waves and slurs with Q waves, ST depression, and T-wave abnormalities, but that has yet to be resolved.[6]

Semantics were coming to the forefront of deciphering these new findings. ER had a definition long used by clinical electrocardiographers and clinicians (ST elevation on an otherwise normal ECG); to electrophysiologists and cellular physiologists, it was the first part of repolarization on the myocytes, action potential, and it was now being attached to J wave and slurs at the end of the QRS complex.[7] Figure 10.2 contrasts "classic" ER to the "new" ER on the surface ECG. While Viskin and Kukla first suggested the new channelopathy be called the Haïssaguerre syndrome,[8,9] Wagner suggested J-wave syndrome to be another option, but most electrophysiologists still (as the Editors of this book) use the confusing "ER."

Our research laboratory has a large, digital ECG database of veterans and athletes, and so when a group of young researchers coalesced in the summer of 2010, we began a series of investigations. The first step was to perform a careful literature review and determine the methodology of the ECG measurements in the new studies. The semantic confusion and lack of details became very evident. Terms such as "J-point," "QRS end," and "ST level," which had been

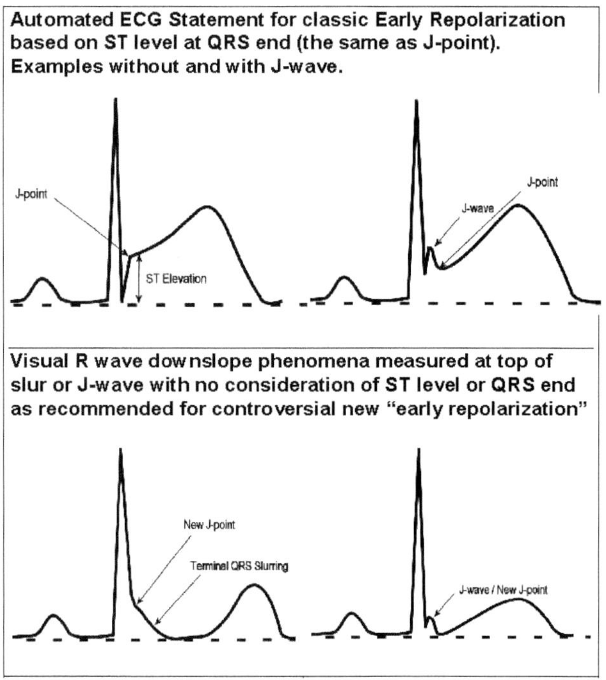

Figure 10.2. Contrasting surface ECG representations for "ER." Classic ER also required the ECG to not exhibit diagnostic Q waves, ST depression, or T-wave inversion, but not so for the "new" ER. Classic ECG interpretation considered the J point to be the end of the QRS complex, where the ST level for diagnosis of ischemia was set, while the "new" ER considered it to be the top of the J wave or slur.

clearly defined in guidelines and position papers were not being used consistently. Often the methods used could only be deciphered from the ECG examples provided. It appeared that the dynamic ECG waveforms of this new syndrome were causing confusion in the interpretation of the standard 10-second ECG. We initiated an email group of those working in this field to exchange ideas and found that experts no longer were agreeing on how to determine QRS duration or ST level. Furthermore, cellular physiologists were not in agreement regarding whether the J waves and slurs were late depolarization or ER phenomena. There was a concern that action potentials from isolated sections of dog hearts had less importance in the etiology of this channelopathy than studies of the electrical activity of the entire heart. This led to the collaboration with the Editor of the *Journal of Electrocardiography* and a special issue of the subject including many of the world experts.[10]

Most of the automated ECG programs used in U.S., including the GE MUSE 12-lead program used by all Veterans Affairs (VA) medical centers, make an interpretative statement of "ER" but this is based on ST elevation and normality of the Q and T waves (and certainly no ST depression). None of the commercially available programs code or measure terminal QRS J waves or slurs and in general they include them as a part of the QRS complex. Therefore, our ECGs had to be re-read and coded for J waves and slurs and QRS end confirmed. While facilitated using computerization for recall and display, this was still time-consuming. Having personally re-read and coded 4000 ECGs from veterans with a 10-year follow up for CV death, it was very disappointed to find no association. We are now in the process of validating our measurement techniques and expanding our coding to 20,000 ECGs with a 15-year follow up for CV death.

The databases we have, though, did have reliable measurements of ST level, and so we initiated a series of studies relating to ST elevation in athletes[11] and the Universal Definition of Myocardial Infarction (UDMI) for diagnosing ischemia.[12] Listed below are the causes of ST elevation (Table 10.1) and next the UDMI criteria (Table 10.2).

The UDMI criteria were empirical, too complex, and did not consider ethnicity, so we considered how many stable clinic patients fulfilled them and were false positives. These parallel efforts included studies of athletes and serial ECG studies in patients to demonstrate the natural history of ER. We demonstrated that the original ER based on ST elevation was related to age, gender, ethnicity, and heart rate as shown in Table 10.3. Figure 10.3 is an example of ST elevation due to pericarditis that can only be distinguished from classic ER by these features. We also noted that J waves and slurs were commonly associated with ST elevation in healthy and young individuals with normal ECGs, and were more common in elderly patients with Q waves or T-wave inversion with or without ST elevation than those with normal ECGs.

Table 10.1. **Causes of ST elevation on resting ECG.**

Acute (Dynamic)
1. Ischemia (localizes, arrhythmogenic).
2. Variant angina.
3. ST-elevation MI.
4. Before event in some patients with idiopathic VT/VF.
Chronic (Stable)
1. ER—changes with heart rate.
2. Pericarditis.
3. Over Q waves associated with LV aneurysm/wall motion abnormalities (WMA).
4. Spinal cord injury and mental patients—vagal tone?
5. Brugada patterns (V_{123})—but syndrome dynamic.
6. In 31% of idiopathic VT/VF (lateral, inferior).

NATURAL HISTORY OF THE J WAVE, SLURS, AND ST-ELEVATION PATTERNS

While ST elevation, J waves, and slurs are more common in the young, suggesting that it recedes with age, there have been limited studies of its prognosis and its natural history is uncertain. Demonstrating that these end-QRS phenomena can disappear naturally rather than its decreasing prevalence being due to death would supplement appropriate studies using survival analysis. Therefore, we published the natural history of lateral and inferior lead occurrences utilizing serial ECGs in an ambulatory clinical population.

Of the 250 patients selected with the greatest amplitude of ST elevation, J waves, or slurs in the lateral leads, after 6 were excluded for ECG abnormalities, 122 had another ECG at least 5 months later.[13] Their average age was 42 ± 10 years and average time between the first and second ECG was 10 years. Of the 122 patients, 47 (38%) retained the amplitude criteria while the majority (62%) no longer fulfilled

Table 10.2. **Criteria for ST elevation ischemia according to the third UDMI. New ST elevation at the J point in 2 contiguous leads (with V_1, III, and aVR excluded) using the lead gender and age cut-points.**

1. All leads, ages, and gender other than leads V_2–V_3 = ≥0.1 mV.
2. For leads V_2 to V_3:
   a. ≥0.2 mV in men ≥40 years
   b. ≥0.25 mV in men <40 years
   c. ≥0.15 mV in women

Table 10.3. **Features in otherwise-normal ECGs differentiating ST elevation that is physiological from pathological conditions.**

1. Heart rate (low, not high).
2. Age (young, not old).
3. Gender (male, not female).
4. ST level (<0.2 mV, not more).
5. Ethnicity (Afro-American, not other).
6. Athletic status (yes, not sedentary)

the amplitude criteria. This was not due to a higher heart rate, a longer time between the ECGs, death, acute disease, or alterations in ECG diagnostic characteristics. Figures 10.4 and 10.5 are the examples of ECGs from the serial lateral lead study.

We next studied the patients selected with the greatest amplitude of end QTS phenomena in the inferior leads, which became more important once some of the prognostic studies isolated mortality to them. Starting from the highest amplitude, we carefully reviewed the ECGs and medical records from the first 85%.[14] From this convenience sample, 36 were excluded for abnormal patterns (myocardial ischemia or infarction and pericarditis). The remaining 257 patients were searched for another ECG at least 5 months later, of whom 136 satisfied this criteria. All these ECGs were paired for comparison, printed, and coded by 4 interpreters. Their average age was 47 ± 13 years and average time between the first and second ECGs was 10 years. Of the 136 subjects, 64 (47%) retained the patterns while 72 (53%) no longer fulfilled the amplitude criteria. While no significant differences were found in initial heart rate or time interval between ECGs, those who lost the pattern had a greater difference in heart rate between the ECGs (ΔHR of 0.0 vs. 10 bpm) and higher percentage of cardiovascular events over the interval. In conclusion, the ECG pattern of ER was lost over 10 years in over half of this young clinical cohort. The change in heart rate and higher incidence of cardiovascular events partially explained the loss but it was not due to the time interval between the ECGs, association with lateral lead J waves/slurs, or alterations in other ECG diagnostic characteristics. The following are the examples of ECGs from the serial inferior lead study (Figures 10.6–10.8).

PREVALENCE OF END-QRS ECG PHENOMENA

To study the prevalence of all of the end-QRS components of interest (ST elevation, J waves, and slurs), we retrospectively studied 5085 ECGs obtained in a multiethnic clinical population from 1997 to 1999 at the Veterans Affairs Palo Alto Healthcare System, analyzing 4041 after excluding those with confounding ECG abnormalities. We also examined ECGs obtained from the preparticipation exams of 1114 Stanford University varsity athletes in 2007 and 2008.[15] Criteria for components of ER were as follows: ST elevation ≥1 mm from the end of the QRS complex; J wave as an upward deflection on the QRS downslope peaking ≥1 mm above the isoelectric line; and slur of the R-wave downslope as a decrease in the slope beginning at similar amplitude.

Components of ER were most prevalent in males, African Americans, and particularly in athletes, with the greatest variations demonstrated in the lateral

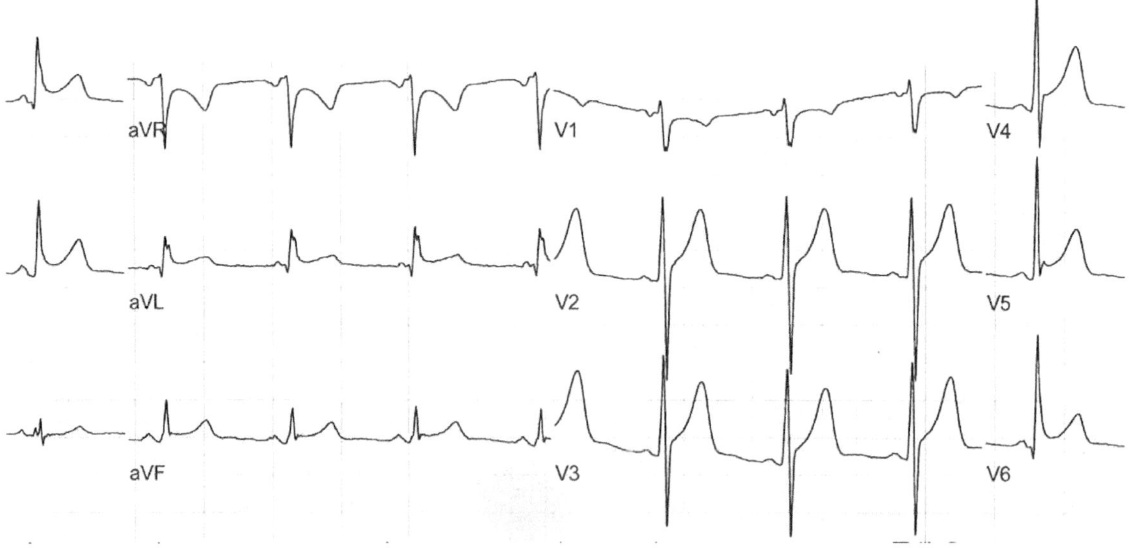

Figure 10.3. ECG in a 60-year-old white male with pericarditis (HR of 85 bpm due to β-blockers).

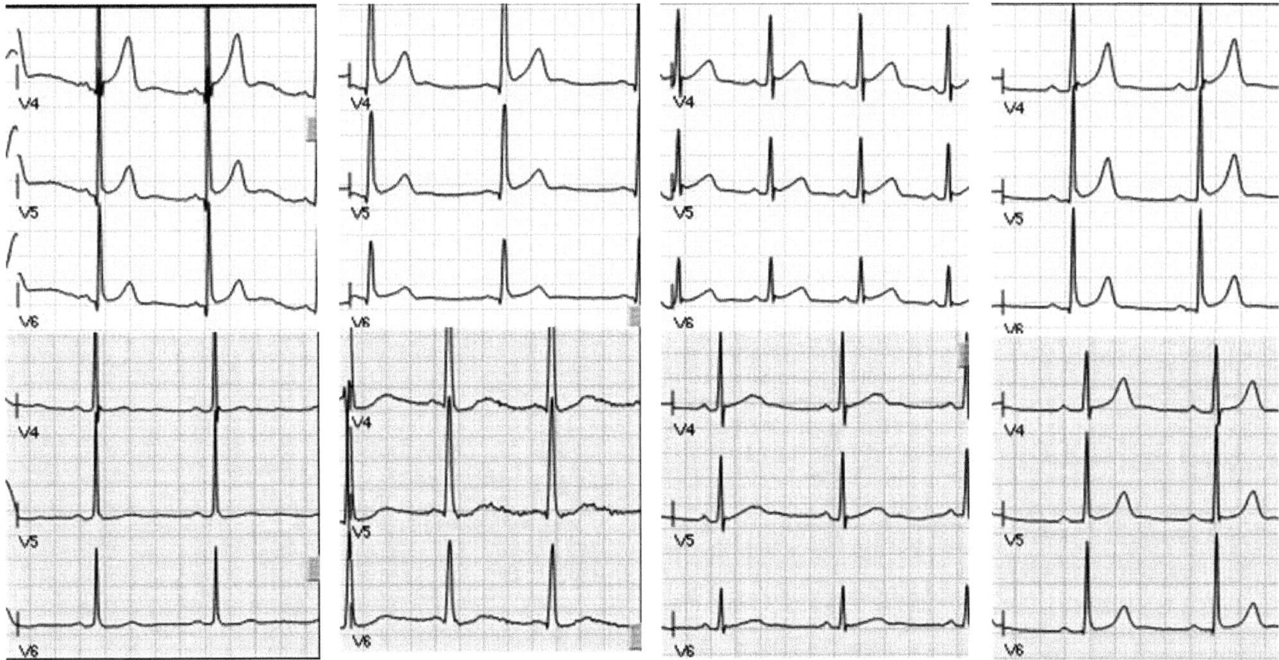

Figure 10.4. Four examples of paired ECGs with the greatest difference in amplitudes between ECGs consistent with loss of slurs and J waves in lateral leads (which occurred in 62%).

leads. ST elevation was most common, occurring in nearly one-third of male, African-American athletes in the lateral leads. Inferior J waves and slurs, previously linked to cardiovascular risk, were observed in 9.6% of clinical subjects and 12.3% of athletes. Figure 10.9 illustrates these findings.

PROGNOSTIC VALUE OF END-QRS ECG PHENOMENA

In those who manifest the Haïssaguerre pattern (R-wave downslope notching and slurring) on the stable, surface ECG, it will be necessary to identify

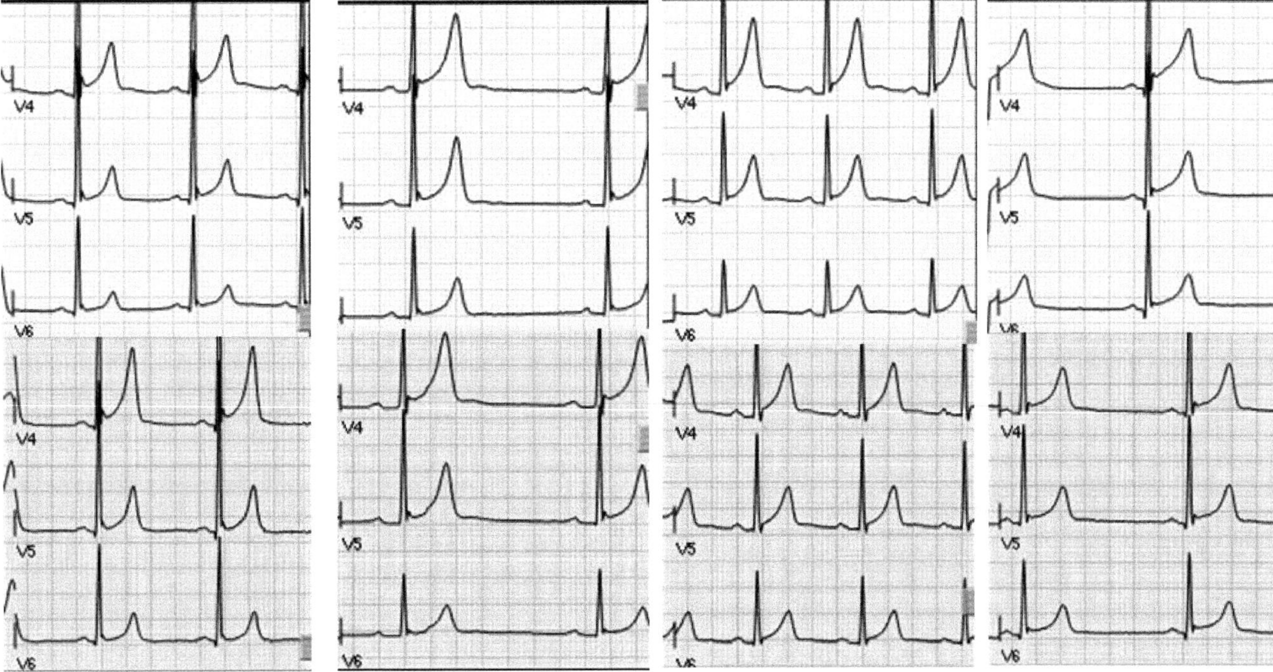

Figure 10.5. Four examples of paired ECGs with the least difference in amplitudes between ECGs consistent with retention of lateral slurs and J waves (which occurred in 38%).

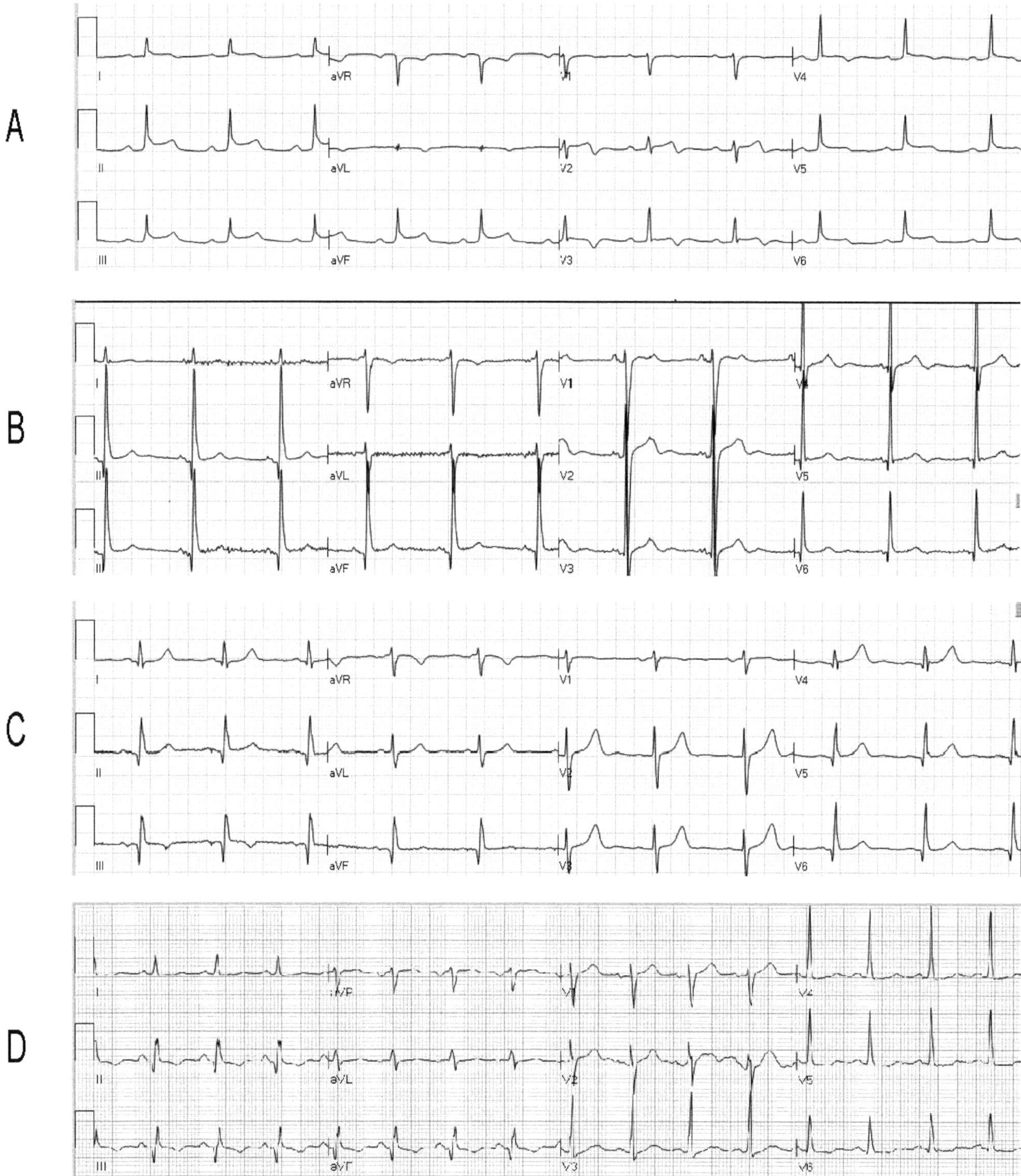

Figure 10.6. Examples of ECGs excluded from the inferior lead serial study. These were excluded because of (A) pericarditis, (B) HCM Q waves, (C and D) old inferior MIs. Such abnormalities were frequently associated with inferior J waves and slurs.

additional ECG markers that can predict risk of cardiovascular death and/or syncope, and thus develop the Haïssaguerre syndrome. This is of major importance, since we know that 50% of sudden deaths in young people occur with morphologically normal hearts.[16] Prognostic studies of this and similar ECG patterns have had differing results, but some suggest that end-QRS notching and slurring, particularly when occurring in the inferior leads and accompanied by downward-sloping ST segments, have associated risk of sudden or cardiovascular death. The differences in the studies appear to be due to terminology and

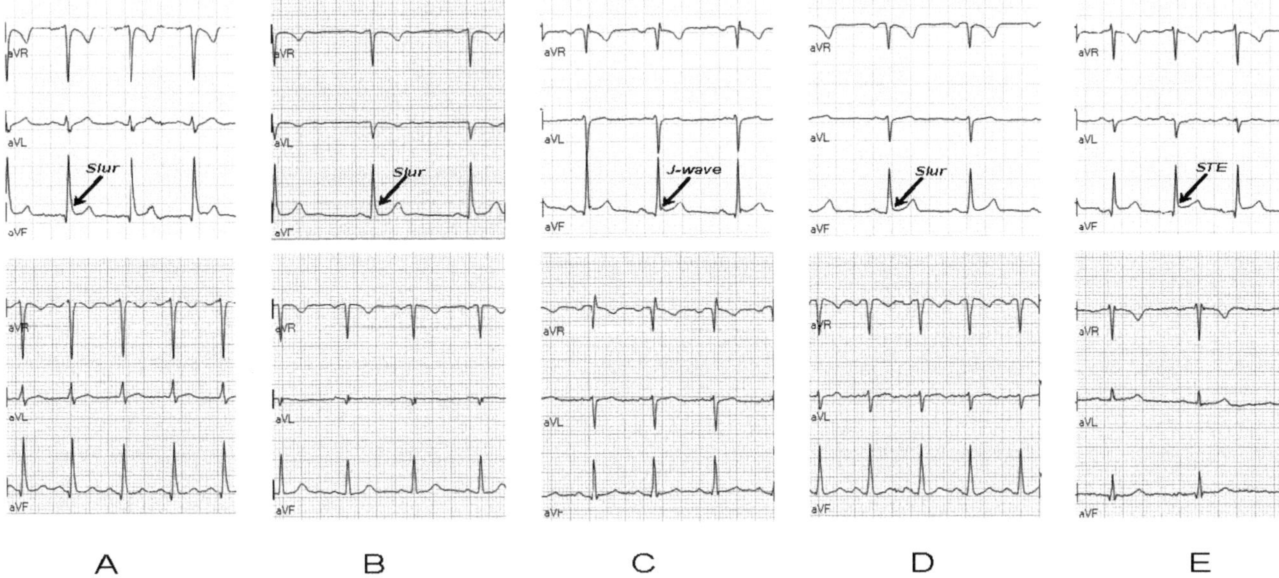

Figure 10.7. Five examples of paired ECGs with lost inferior J wave/slurs (which occurred in 53%).

methodology issues as well as design shortcomings.[17,18] A total of 8 prognostic studies were available as of February 2013 (Table 10.4).

Clearly, the best follow-up study and unlikely to be repeated is that by Tikkannen et al.[19] This classic study was only "limited" by noncomputerized ECG acquisition; the paper ECG recordings were gathered over 30 years ago (requiring the use of adjacent lead criteria for accuracy, unlike modern ECG analyses that rely on waveforms averaged over 10 seconds). Only inferior lead J waves or slurring were associated with CV or arrhythmic death risk. No risk was found for lateral lead slurring or J waves, and the anterior leads were not studied. The follow-up period of 30 years is important since the Kaplan–Meier survival curves only began to separate after 10 to 15 years. Furthermore, this study benefits from a national policy of standardized autopsies and investigations to determine the cause of death including arrhythmic deaths. Sinner et al[20] documented an increased hazard ratio for CV mortality associated with the Haïssaguerre pattern, especially in the inferior leads. However, they used a case-cohort design that only considered a younger subset of their community-based population. When

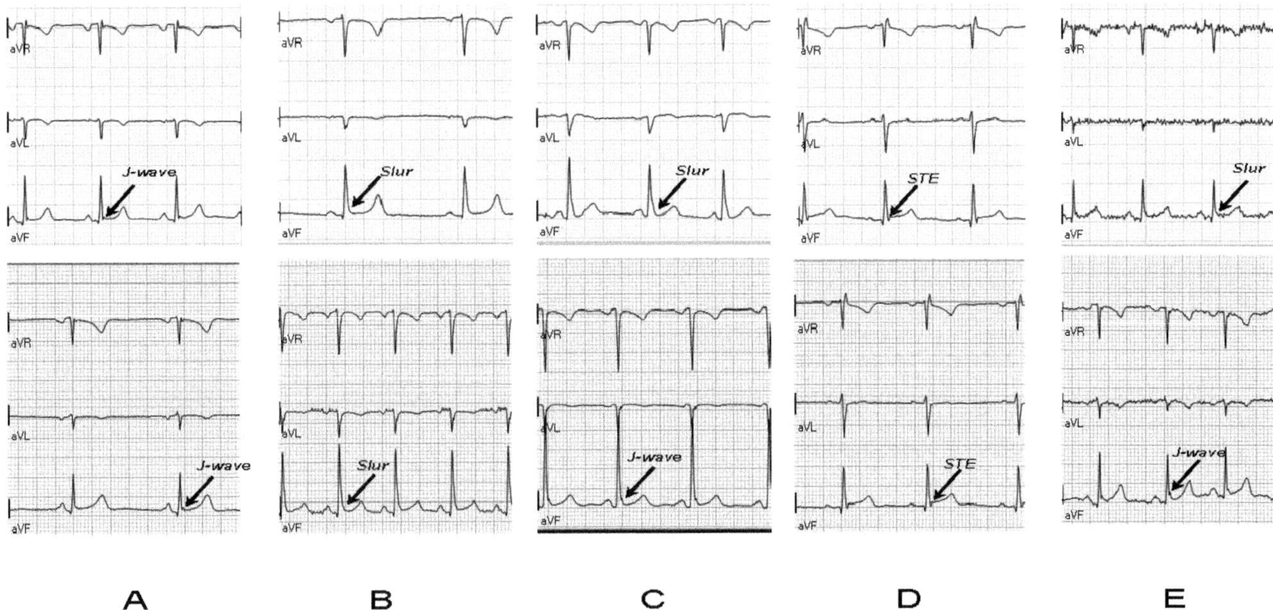

Figure 10.8. Five examples of paired ECGs with retained inferior J wave/slurs (which occurred in 47%).

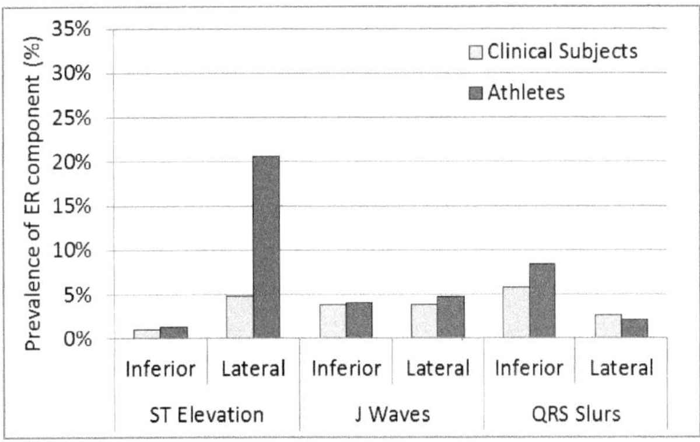

Figure 10.9. Prevalence of components of ER in clinical subjects and athletes.

analysis failed to demonstrate a risk in the younger subset, they were "enriched" by all those who died with J waves and slurs in the older segment of their population. This violated the Cox's model assumptions and results in age, not the Haïssaguerre pattern, being associated with death. The third outcome study, by Haruta et al[21] concluded that ER was only predictive of unexplained death. Although *unexplained death* was intended to be a surrogate for SCD, the main category included in this coding was unexplained accidental death.

The fourth study by Stavrakis et al[22] considered 852 consecutive patients with ST elevation ≥0.1 mV in the inferior or lateral leads from the VA ECG system and randomly selected 257 age-matched patients with normal ECGs as controls. They considered J waves or slurs and the ST elevation to be associated with a modest increased all-cause mortality compared to controls (hazard ratio of 1.5). Comparison to controls rather than the total population from the sampling period violates the assumptions of the Cox model. The fifth study was that of Rollins et al[23] with the French participants in the MONICA study. It was a retrospective study of 1161 southwestern French subjects aged 35 to 64 years. This relatively small study did not isolate the risk to the inferior leads and is therefore hard to reconcile with the larger Finnish study.

The sixth and seventh studies by Olson et al and Hisamatsu et al[24] were excellent population studies but did not consider R-wave downslope phenomena (Haïssaguerre/J-wave pattern) but only ST elevation and included the anterior leads. Uberoi et al[25] from the Veterans Affairs was one of the largest multiethnic population studies and considered R-wave downslope phenomena (Haïssaguerre/J-wave pattern) as well as ST elevation.

Two of the studies did not consider the Haïssaguerre/J-wave pattern but only reported ST elevation and should not be included. Six studies remain, but one had all-cause mortality as an end point, was really a case-control rather than a prospective study, and only reported a weak hazard ratio (1.5), leaving 5 studies for tabulation. Four of these 5 considered the Haïssaguerre pattern and found a hazard for CV and/or arrhythmic death. In tabulating the results of these studies, the impact of positive publication bias must be considered: authors and editors favor positive, exciting results over negativity. While

Table 10.4. **Descriptors of the prognostic studies of "ER."**

Lead Author	Year, Journal	Population Size	Female (%)	African Descent (%)	Mean Age (SD)	FU (yrs)	Nationality	Design
Tikkannen	2009, NEJM	10,864	48	0	44 ± 8	30	Finnish	community-based, prospective
Sinner	2010, PLOS	1945	51	0	35 - 45	18.9	German	MONICA, case-control, enhanced with deaths in older subjects*
Uberoi	2011, Circulation	29,281	13	13	55 ± 14	7.6	USA	clinic-based, prospective
Haruta	2011, Circulation	5976	56	0	45	24	Japan	atomic bomb survivors
Olson	2011, EHJ	15,141	56	27	54 ± 6	17	USA	ARIC population-based, prospective
Stavrakis	2012, ANEC	825 ER 255 controls	1	40	49 ± 12	6.4	USA	clinic-based, case-control
Rollin	2012, AJC	1161	48	0	50 ± 9	14.2	French	MONICA, prospective
Hisamatsu	2013, Circ Japan	7630	59	0	52 ± 4	15	Japan	National Circulatory Survey

shortcomings of these studies have been pointed out above, the majority favor a weak association of CV risk with the Haïssaguerre pattern. The average hazard ratio of approximately 3 is meaningful for a risk factor that can be modified (i.e., HBP, cigarette smoking), but does not provide adequate power for clinical decision-making, particularly when the risk may require 10 to 15 years before it manifests.

The strongest data supporting the prognostic risk of R-wave downslope phenomena (Haïssaguerre/J-wave pattern) is from the Finnish study. It demonstrates a risk only in the inferior leads and that there is no risk for the same ECG pattern in the lateral leads, where it is more common. The study suggests that the risk only is apparent after 10 to 15 years of follow-up and is an indicator of arrhythmic risk in older men with CAD. The hazard of up to 4 times has meaning for risk factors that can be modified but little value for a condition without a safe therapy.

When the Haïssaguerre study of idiopathic VT/VF is more closely examined, it becomes apparent that the Haïssaguerre pattern is only 33% sensitive for a condition with a high risk of sudden or cardiovascular death, and not very specific. The dynamic patterns with giant J waves are rare and may have different clinical implications. Provocative tools such as the Valsalva maneuver, drug challenges, further ambulatory monitoring, and exercise testing may help with further risk stratification. There may also be a better ECG marker of arrhythmic risk in phase 1 of repolarization. Certainly, the dream of identifying the cause of SCD in young individuals with normal hearts lies in this phase, but it appears that we are far from identifying it. The controversy regarding whether the Haïssaguerre/J-wave pattern is due to ER or late depolarization makes this ever more apparent.[26] Much research and careful epidemiological studies with modern ECG recording technology are very much needed.

ECG MEASUREMENT ISSUES

Before the prognostic significance of the Haïssaguerre pattern can be demonstrated, there must be agreement on precisely what measurements should be made. It appears that for stable ECG patterns with a QRS duration (including an end-QRS J wave/slur) less than 120 ms, we should follow the Computer Society of Electrocardiography (CSE) measurement statement (1985)[27] and consider the J point (also known as QRS end, J-junction, ST0 [0 ms], or ST beginning) to occur after the R-wave downslope notch/slur/or J wave as determined across all 12 leads. The measurement baseline should be set in an interval immediately preceding QRS onset as per the CSE measurement statement. Some of the bizarre and dynamic ECGs may require other rules for measurements but for now the CSE statement should be followed.

The major methodological issue in the studies is that ER and the J point is not consistently coded. Some defined ER as the presence of ST elevation (classic ER), while others defined it as the presence

Table 10.5. End points, results, and measurements used in the prognostic studies of "ER."

Lead Author	End Points	"ERP"	CVD Hazard	Measurement (1 mm)	Leads	J Waves/ Slurs	ST Elevation
Tikkannen	CV mortality, arrhythmic deaths	5.8%	2-3× inferior only	visual, 2 contig	Inf, Lat	yes	no
Sinner	CV mortality	13%	2-4×	visual, 2 contig	Inf, Lat	yes	no
Uberoi	CV mortality	14%	none	GE12SL, ST0/vis	Inf, Lat	yes	no
Haruta	CV mortality, unexpected and accidental deaths	24%	none, unexplained deaths only	visual, 2 contig	Inf, Lat	yes	no
Olson	Sudden Cardiac Death	STE 12.3%	1.2× (white females 2×)	GE 12SL ST0	Ant, Inf, Lat	no	yes
Stavrakis	all-cause mortality	NA	NA, 1.5× all cause	visual, 2 contig	Inf, Lat	yes	no
Rollin	CV mortality	13%	3 to 8× inf and lat	visual, 2 contig	Inf, Lat	yes	no*
Hisamatsu	CV mortality	STE 3.5%	2.5× anterior leads (>2 mm)	visual, any lead	Ant, Inf, Lat	no	yes

Vis, visual; contig, contiguous; GE12 L, General Electric MUSE program; ST0, ST at 0 ms; beginning of ST segment [J-point], Inf, inferior III, aVF, II; lat, lateral (V456,I,aVL); ant, anterior (V_{123}).

of R-wave downslope phenomena (J waves or slurs), which is most consistent with the definition used by Haïssaguerre (new ER). Is the resting ECG otherwise normal, as is the case for classic ER? Many subtle but important questions regarding appropriate use of the terminology remain: Is the J point the beginning of the ST segment (the classic J point) or is it the top of the J wave or slur (the new J point)? What is the QRS duration? Does it include J waves/slurs when they are present? Table 10.5 lists the definitions and measurements made by 8 studies. Even close reading of these studies does not always provide an answer to these questions.

CONCLUSIONS

The new channelopathy, preferably called the Haïssaguerre or J-wave syndrome, is a rare, new condition characterized by death during sleep and most notably the dynamic appearance of large J waves with or without ST elevation prior to idiopathic VT/VF. Unfortunately, it has been labeled "ER" by researchers, who have caused much confusion among clinicians, who have been taught that ER is physiological ST elevation occurring in an otherwise normal ECG. It is unlikely to cause SCD in athletes during exercise. Furthermore, it is unlikely that phenomena on the routine 10-second ECG will predict who will manifest idiopathic VT/VF. Cross-sectional studies suggesting a higher prevalence of J waves in patient groups is likely explained by their association with Q waves and other ECG abnormalities. All of the studies of ER, particularly the follow-up studies, are difficult to decipher because of confused semantics.[28] It is sad that the lack of consideration of established definitions used by all current automated ECG programs will probably cause more harm than good due to the "J wave- implantable cardioverter-defibrillator reflex."[29]

REFERENCES

1. Derval N, Lim H, Haïssaguerre M. Dynamic electrocardiographic recordings in patients with idiopathic ventricular fibrillation. *J Electrocardiol.* 2013;46(5):452–455.
2. Haïssaguerre M, Derval N, Sacher F, et al. Sudden cardiac arrest associated with early repolarization. *N Engl J Med.* 2008;358:2016–2023.
3. Kambara H, Phillips J. Long-term evaluation of early repolarization syndrome (normal variant RS-T segment elevation). *Am J Cardiol.* 1976;38:157–161.
4. Jayroe JB, Spodick DH, Nikus K, et al. Differentiating ST elevation myocardial infarction and nonischemic causes of ST elevation by analyzing the presenting electrocardiogram. *Am J Cardiol.* 2009;103(3):301–306.
5. Tikkanen JT, Anttonen O, Junttila MJ, et al. Long-term outcome associated with early repolarization on electrocardiography. *N Engl J Med.* 2009;361:2529–2537.
6. Uberoi A, Sallam K, Perez M, et al. Prognostic implications of Q waves and T-wave inversion associated with early repolarization. *Mayo Clin Proc.* 2012;87(7):614–619.
7. Perez MV, Friday K, Froelicher V. Semantic confusion: The case of early repolarization and the J point. *Am J Med.* 2012;125(9):843–844.
8. Viskin S. Idiopathic ventricular fibrillation "Le Syndrome d'Haïssaguerre" and the fear of J waves. *J Am Coll Cardiol.* 2009;53(7):620–622.
9. Kukla P, Jastrzebski M. Haïssaguerre syndrome – a new clinical entity in the spectrum of primary electrical diseases? *Kardiol Pol.* 2009;67(2):178–184.
10. Froelicher V, Wagner G. Co-editors of symposium issue on J wave patterns and a syndrome. *J Electrocardiol.* 2013;46:381–382.
11. Leo T, Uberoi A, Jain NA, et al. The impact of ST elevation on athletic screening. *Clin J Sport Med.* 2011;21(5):433–440.
12. Thygesen K, Alpert JS, Jaffe AS, et al. Joint ESC/ACCF/AHA/WHF task force for the universal definition of myocardial infarction. *Eur Heart J.* 2012;50(184):2173–2195.
13. Adhikarla C, Boga M, Wood AD, Froelicher VF. Natural history of the electrocardiographic pattern of early repolarization in ambulatory patients. *Am J Cardiol.* 2011;108(12):1831–1835.
14. Stein R, Sallam K, Adhikarla C, et al. Natural history of early repolarization in the inferior leads. *Ann Noninvasive Electrocardiol.* 2012;17(4):331–339.
15. Muramoto D, Singh N, Aggarwal S, et al. Spectrum of ST amplitude: athletes and an ambulatory clinical population. *J Electrocardiol.* 2013;46(5):427–433.
16. Perez M, Fonda H, Le VV, et al. Adding an electrocardiogram to the pre-participation examination in competitive athletes: A systematic review. *Curr Probl Cardiol.* 2009;34(12):586–662.
17. Perez MV, Friday K, Froelicher V. Semantic confusion: The case of early repolarization and the J point. *Am J Med.* 2012;125(9): 843–844.
18. Surawicz B, Macfarlane PW. Inappropriate and confusing electrocardiographic terms: J-wave syndromes and early repolarization. *J Am Coll Cardiol.* 2011;57(15):1584–1586.
19. Tikkanen JT, Anttonen O, Junttila MJ, et al. Long-term outcome associated with early repolarization on electrocardiography. *N Engl J Med.* 2009;361(26):2529–2537.
20. Sinner MF, Reinhard W, Müller M. Association of early repolarization pattern on ECG with risk of cardiac and all-cause mortality: a population-based prospective cohort study (MONICA/KORA). *PLoS Med.* 2010;7(7):e1000314.
21. Haruta D, Matsuo K, Tsuneto A. Incidence and prognostic value of early repolarization pattern in the 12-lead electrocardiogram. *Circulation.* 2011;123(25):2931–2937.

22. Stavrakis S, Patel N, Te C, et al. Development and validation of a prognostic index for risk stratification of patients with early repolarization. *Ann Noninvasive Electrocardiol.* 2012;17(4):361–371.
23. Rollin A, Maury P, Bongard V, et al. Prevalence, prognosis, and identification of the malignant form of early repolarization pattern in a population-based study. *Am J Cardiol.* 2012;110(9):1302–1308.
24. Hisamatsu T, Ohkubo T, Miura K, et al. Association between J-point elevation and death from coronary heart disease. *Circ J.* 2013;77(5):1260–1266.
25. Uberoi A, Jain NA, Perez M, et al. Early repolarization in an ambulatory clinical population. *Circulation.* 2011;124(20):2208–2214.
26. Borggrefe M, Schimpf R. J-wave syndromes caused by repolarization or depolarization mechanisms: A debated issue among experimental and clinical electrophysiologists. *J Am Coll Cardiol.* 2010;55(8):798–800.
27. The CSE Working Party. Recommendations for measurement standards in quantitative Electrocardiography. *Eur Heart J.* 1985;6:815–825.
28. Froelicher V. Early repolarization redux: the devil is in the methods. *Ann Noninvasive Electrocardiol.* 2012;17(1):63–64.
29. Martini B, Wu J, Nava A. A rare lethal syndrome in search of its identity: sudden death, right bundle branch block and ST segment elevation. In: Wu Y, Wu J, eds. *Sudden Death: Causes, Risk Factors and Prevention.* New York, NY: Nova Science Publishers Inc.; 2013:2–12.

CHAPTER

11

T-Wave Alternans: Electrocardiographic Characteristics and Clinical Value

Stefan H. Hohnloser, MD

ELECTRICAL ALTERNANS IN CLINICAL ELECTROCARDIOGRAPHY

Electrical alternans is defined as a repetitive beat-to-beat fluctuation of ECG amplitude affecting the QRS complex, the ST segment, or the T wave. The occurrence of visible electrical alternans (i.e., "macrovolt" alternans) has been first described by Hering in 1908 and was initially thought to be little more than an electrocardiographic curiosity.[1] Shortly thereafter, Lewis noted that alternans could occur in a normal heart following marked accelerations in heart rate and also in the diseased or intoxicated myocardium.[2] Electrical alternans can be classified as depolarization alternans, which affects predominantly the QRS complex. Such QRS alternans is often associated with supraventricular tachycardia; that is, AV-node reentrant tachycardia (AVNRT) or atrio-ventricular reentrant tachycardia (AVRT). The other form of electrical alternans affects the ST segment and the T wave and has been defined as repolarization alternans. Current evidence clearly points to the fact that the latter is much more strongly related to vulnerability to ventricular tachyarrhythmias, and hence repolarization alternans is the focus of this chapter.

Initially, several hundred cases of electrical alternans have been described associated with a diversity of clinical conditions. Again, the vast majority of these case reports focused on repolarization alternans primarily involving the ST segment and the T wave.

In 1948, Kalter and Schwartz set out to systematically examine ECG tracings as to the relationship of T-wave alternans (TWA) and malignant tachyarrhythmias.[3] They examined the ECGs from 6059 patients and described an association between macroscopic TWA (observed in 5 patients) and an increased mortality of the affected patients. The notion of a strong association of repolarization alternans and the occurrence of life-threatening ventricular tachyarrhythmias has been described in many apparently disparate clinical conditions. Repolarization alternans can precede ventricular fibrillation (VF), for instance, in patients with acute myocardial ischemia,[4] coronary artery spasm, electrolyte disturbances, or in the setting of the congenital[5,6] or acquired[7] long QT syndrome. A typical example of macroscopic TWA is shown in Figure 11.1 in a patient with the idiopathic long QT syndrome and in Figure 11.2 in a patient with antiarrhythmic drug-induced repolarization alternans.

This kind of observations later triggered the conduct of systematic experimental and clinical studies to evaluate whether repolarization alternans, which is not visible on the surface ECG (i.e., "microvolt" alternans)

The ECG Handbook of Contemporary Challenges © 2015 Mohammad Shenasa, Mark E. Josephson, N.A. Mark Estes III
Cardiotext Publishing, ISBN: 978-1-935395-88-1

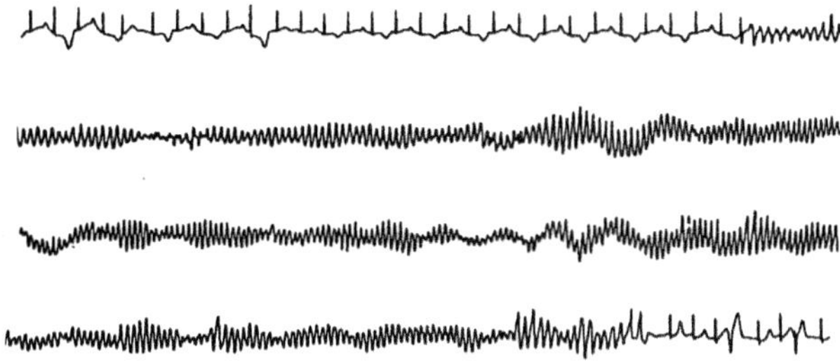

Figure 11.1. Macroscopic TWA in a patient with presumed congenital long QT syndrome. The tracing shows marked TWA prior to the onset of polymorphic VT. Adapted with permission.[6]

may be existing and may constitute a marker for intrinsic susceptibility to ventricular tachyarrhythmias.

Assessment of subtle microvolt TWA (MTWA) was first reported in 1982[8] by utilizing sophisticated computerized analysis. In the 1980s, Cohen et al established a close relationship between MTWA and vulnerability to VF in a dog model.[8,9] Similar findings were subsequently reported by Nearing et al, who used a different analysis method for measuring MTWA.[10] Since the inscription of the methods for assessment of MTWA, further compelling evidence for a mechanistic link between MTWA and the occurrence of ventricular tachyarrhythmias has been provided in a plethora of experimental and clinical studies. One of the most intriguing clinical examples of this has recently been reported by Shusterman et al.[11] They analyzed implantable cardioverter-defibrillator (ICD)-stored electrogram series and demonstrated that repolarization instability manifested by MTWA increased significantly shortly before the onset of ventricular tachyarrhythmias.

Over the last 3 decades, many important new findings on the mechanisms underlying MTWA, on implementation of this method in clinical practice, and on the prognostic value of this noninvasive ECG-derived risk marker have been reported. As this chapter focuses on the issue of MTWA assessment and its clinical yield as a risk prediction tool, the mechanisms and the cellular basis underlying MTWA will not be discussed here but are subject of several recent comprehensive review articles.[12,13]

METHODOLOGY OF TWA ASSESSMENT

Currently, MTWA is assessed either by the so-called spectral method[9] or the modified moving average (MMA) method.[10] Both of these techniques have been used in clinical studies on risk stratification in subjects deemed to be at risk for sudden death.

The Spectral Method

Correct assessment of MTWA depends heavily on the quality of the data collected since MTWA is a low-amplitude and relatively low-frequency phenomenon

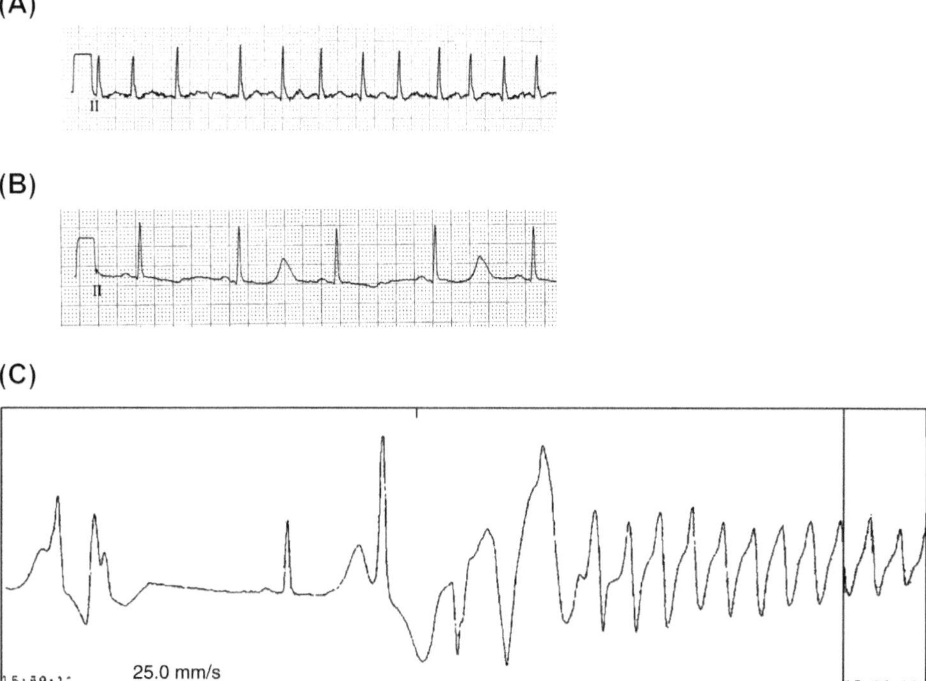

Figure 11.2. A. New-onset atrial fibrillation in a 62-year-old man. Following intravenous amiodarone administration, there is a conversion to SR. B. Marked QT prolongation. C. Macroscopic TWA preceding torsade de pointes tachycardia. Adapted with permission.[7]

that can be easily obscured by artifacts (i.e., baseline wander and muscle artifacts). Accordingly, measurement of MTWA requires careful skin preparation to minimize electrode-to-skin impedance. Specialized electrodes have been developed which record and process ECG signals, as well as impedance, from multiple segments of an electrode.

For MTWA assessment, an increase in heart rate is required and each individual patient shows a specific heart rate threshold above which MTWA will become apparent. In the initial clinical studies, heart rate was increased by means of atrial pacing but subsequently, techniques were developed to noninvasively elevate heart rate by means of treadmill or bicycle exercise testing. Currently, MTWA assessment is uniformly performed noninvasively.

The spectral method utilizes the vector magnitude ECG signal recorded from the 3 Frank orthogonal leads over at least 128 beats (Figure 11.3). Each T wave is measured at the same time relative to the QRS complex. Since this spectrum is created by measurements taken once per beat, its frequencies are in the units of cycles per beat. Accordingly, the point on the spectrum corresponding to 0.5 cycles per beat indicates the level of alteration of the T-wave wavefront (see Figure 11.3). The alternans power (μV_2) is defined as the difference between the power of the alternans frequency and the power at the noise

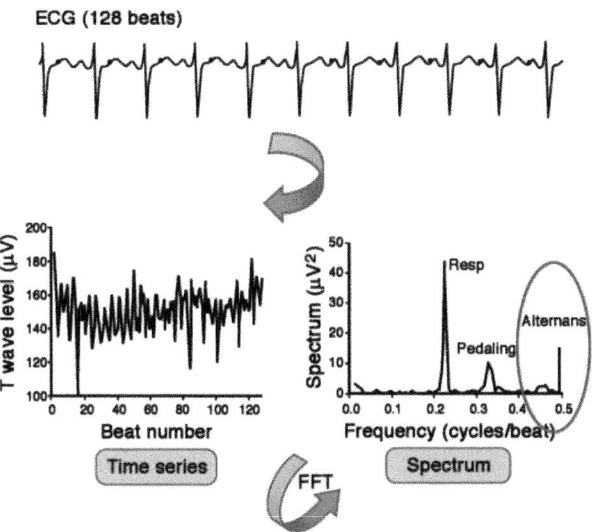

Figure 11.3. Schematic representation of MTWA assessment utilizing the spectral method. The amplitudes of the corresponding points on the T wave are measured for 128 beats. The power spectrum of this time series is computed using fast Fourier transform methods. In the power spectrum obtained from recordings during bicycle exercise, peaks corresponding to frequencies of respiration, pedaling, and alternans are illustrated. MTWA appears as a peak at exactly one-half of the beat frequency (0.5 cycles per beat). The amplitude of this peak is compared to the mean and standard deviation of the spectrum in a reference "noise band." FFT, fast Fourier transformation. Adapted with permission.[12]

frequency band (calculated over the reference frequency band between 0.44 and 0.49 cycles per beat). This is a measure of the true physiological alternans level. The alternans voltage (Valt) is simply the square root of alternans power and corresponds to the root mean square difference in the voltage (averaged over the T wave) between the overall mean beats and either the even-numbered or odd-numbered mean beats.

Based on the spectral analysis, MTWA tracings are classified as positive, negative, or indeterminate. The classification of a MTWA tracing as positive requires only the determination of whether sustained alternans is present and a determination of the onset heart rate. The distinction between tracings that are negative or indeterminate is made by the determination of the maximum negative heart rate as well as the maximum heart rate. Detailed definitions for indeterminacy or for negative test results have been described.[14]

The MMA Method

MMA-based MTWA can be assessed during exercise stress testing, during post exercise recovery, or from ambulatory ECG recordings.[15] MMA is based on the noise-rejection principle of recursive averaging. As shown in Figure 11.4, the algorithm continuously streams odd and even beats into separate bins and creates median complexes for each bin.[10] These complexes are then superimposed, and the maximum difference between the odd and even median complexes at any point within the JT segment is determined as the MTWA value, which is averaged every 10 to 15 seconds. The moving average allows control of the influence of new incoming beats on the median templates with an adjustable update factor, that is, the fraction of morphology change that an incoming beat can contribute. Respiration and motion artifacts are reduced by noise-reduction software. MMA-based MTWA can be assessed noninvasively from routine, symptom-limited exercise stress testing, and ambulatory ECG monitoring using precordial ECG leads. The algorithm excludes extrasystoles, noisy beats, and the beats preceding them. Risk stratification is based on the peak MTWA value throughout the 24 hours ECG recording or the exercise test; a cutoff of MTWA $\geq$ 60 µV during routine exercise testing or ambulatory ECG monitoring[15–17] was found in clinical studies to be associated with increased risk for sudden cardiac death and/or cardiovascular mortality. In patients during the early post-MI phase with or without heart failure, a lower cutpoint of $\geq$ 47 µV predicted sudden cardiac death.[18,19] Leino et al[20] demonstrated a 55% and 58% increase in risk of cardiovascular and sudden cardiac death, respectively, per 20 µV of MTWA.

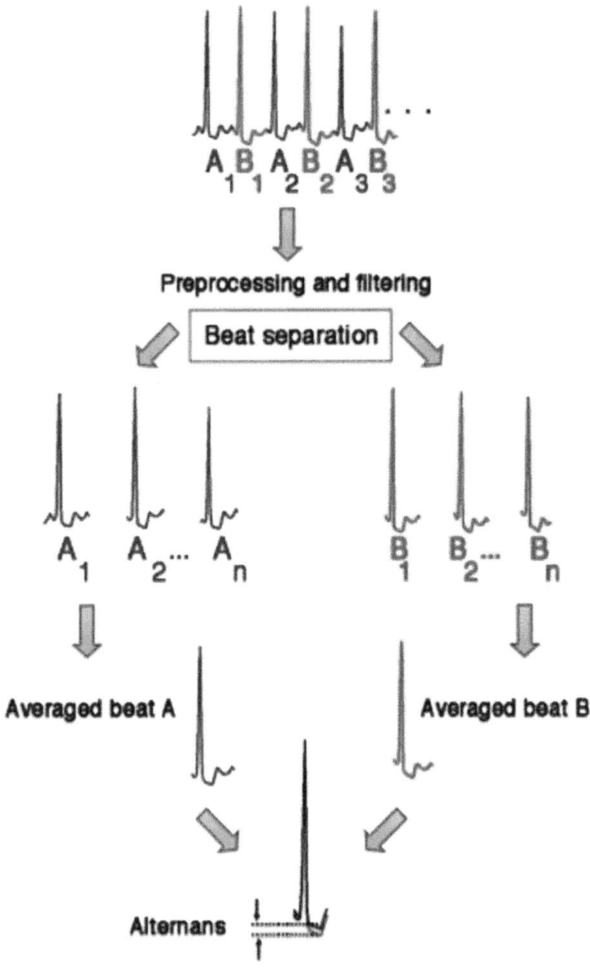

Figure 11.4. Schematic representation of MTWA assessment utilizing the MMA method. Adapted with permission.[15]

CLINICAL STUDIES ON MTWA

Initially, atrial pacing was used to achieve the critical increase in heart rate necessary to elicit MTWA, but after demonstrating reliable MTWA assessment during exercise stress testing this noninvasive measurement became standard technology for risk stratification for sudden death. The average heart rate at which alternans became positive was almost identical with exercise, and pacing induced alternans reemphasizing the patient-specific onset heart rate of MTWA.[21] Accordingly, MTWA assessment nowadays performed is completely noninvasive by using bicycle or treadmill exercise to increase heart rate.

A potential limitation of this methodology is the prevalence of indeterminate MTWA findings ranging from 12% to 40%. MTWA results can be indeterminate due to the inability of patients to increase their heart rate above 105 bpm (i.e., due to the presence of heart failure), or excessive ventricular ectopy, or excessive noise or an exercise protocol that causes an excessively rapid rise in heart rate (technical factors).

In terms of prognostic information, however, the current thinking is that an indeterminate test due to patient factors carries similar prognostic information as a positive MTWA test result.[22] Accordingly, newer studies have differentiated "nonnegative" tests (i.e., positive and indeterminate) from negative ones.

A major limitation of MTWA assessment for risk prediction of patients prone to ventricular tachyarrhythmias and sudden death is the fact that MTWA cannot be reliably determined in patients who are in atrial fibrillation.

MTWA ASSESSMENT FOR NONINVASIVE RISK STRATIFICATION

The prognostic power of noninvasively assessed MTWA for risk stratification of patients prone to sudden death has been scrutinized in a wealth of clinical studies.[12,15] Although the implantable defibrillator represents a highly efficacious tool for preventing arrhythmogenic death, its use carries its own risks due to the invasive character of this therapy, and its widespread applicability is limited by the high costs and the need for trained specialists to apply this therapy. Accordingly, better identification of the patient at highest risk for arrhythmogenic death is of paramount clinical importance.

As recently summarized by Verrier et al,[15] at least 29 studies comprising > 100 patients each have been published utilizing spectral MTWA analysis. These studies were carried out in subjects with dilative or ischemic cardiomyopathy (n = 8), congenital heart disease (n = 1), patients with impaired left ventricular ejection fraction (LVEF) (n = 6), heart failure (n = 3), survivors of myocardial infarction (MI) (n = 8), patients referred for EP testing (n = 2), and Brugada syndrome patients (n = 1). The majority of studies (22 out of 29) demonstrated significant predictivity of MTWA, i.e., patients with positive or indeterminate test results were found to be at significantly greater risk of sudden death/ventricular tachyarrhythmias than those who had negative test results. Several reasons for nonpredictability of MTWA have been discussed including its assessment too early after a cardiac event (MI), withholding β-blocker therapy, or the use of ICD therapy as a surrogate end point for sudden death (see below).

Utilizing the MMA method, at least 12 studies with more than 4800 individuals enrolled was published on the predictive capability of MTWA for cardiovascular or sudden death or serious ventricular arrhythmias.[15] In contrast to those utilizing the spectral MTWA assessment methodology, these studies used different test conditions for MTWA assessment such as measurement at peak exercise, during exercise recovery, or from ambulatory ECG monitoring. Accordingly, it is more difficult than in the case of the spectral MTWA studies to directly compare the predictive value of the method from one study to another study. In general, however, these studies have also reported encouraging predictive power of positive MTWA results. Of particular importance is the Finnish Cardiovascular Study trial, one of the largest MTWA study performed to date, since it enrolled unselected, low-risk subjects.[20] This study included 1972 individuals referred for routine exercise testing and followed them for 4 years. In multivariate Cox analysis after adjustment for common coronary risk factors, high exercise-based MTWA was associated with a relative risk of 12.3 (95% CI 0.2.1 – 12.2, $P < 0.01$) for cardiovascular mortality. High recovery-based MTWA carried a risk of 8.0 (95% CI 2.9 – 22.0, $P < 0.01$) for cardiovascular mortality.

MTWA-based Risk Assessment After MI or in Dilative Cardiomyopathy

More than a dozen studies utilizing both, the spectral and the time-domain measurement technique have been performed assessing the value of MTWA determination for risk stratification after MI.[15] Studies enrolled between 100 and 1000 patients and followed them for 1 to 2.5 years. In the majority of these investigations, MTWA was found to identify patients who were at increased risk for sudden or at least cardiovascular mortality or serious ventricular tachyarrhythmias.

Exner et al[23] conducted one of the most comprehensive studies in this area. They evaluated 322 infarct survivors with a LVEF < 0.50 in the initial week after MI and followed them for a mean of 47 months. Serial assessment of autonomic tone (heart rate turbulence, baroreflex sensitivity) and electrical substrate (MTWA) was performed. The primary end point was cardiac death or resuscitated cardiac arrest. Importantly, MTWA was assessed 2 to 4 weeks following the index infarct and again 10 to 14 weeks later. Of note, abnormal MTWA results after 2 to 4 weeks did not significantly predict end point events (HR 2.42, 95% CI 0.96 – 7.71). However, assessment 10 to 14 weeks after the index infarct yielded a HR of 2.91 (95% CI 1.13 – 7.48; $P = 0.026$). When abnormal autonomic function was combined with positive MTWA findings, predictive accuracy increased with a HR of 3.27 (95% CI 1.42 – 7.00).

Sudden death is common in patients with dilated cardiomyopathy. Conventional risk stratifiers, such as spontaneous ventricular arrhythmias, autonomic markers, or electrophysiologic testing do usually not predict future tachyarrhythmic events. Although prophylactic ICD therapy in such patients improves outcome, the absolute reduction in mortality was relatively small (i.e., 5.6% over 20 months in MADIT II). In U.S., approximately 400,000 patients are diagnosed every year with coronary disease and advanced left ventricular dysfunction. Thus, routinely implanting defibrillators in this population would be very expensive. These considerations have prompted several studies addressing the role of MTWA in guiding ICD therapy in patients with dilative cardiomyopathy. These studies comprised up to 750 patients with similar follow-up periods as the post infarction studies. A common feature of these studies was the observation that MTWA-negative patients had a very low mortality, particularly a low arrhythmic mortality (negative predictive values > 95%). In the largest of these trials,[24] 768 consecutive patients with ischemic cardiomyopathy (LVEF ≤ 0.35) were tested and followed for 18 months. Patients were classified as MTWA-negative or -nonnegative (including MTWA-positive and -indeterminate patients). After adjusting for important baseline variables, a nonnegative MTWA test was associated with a significantly higher risk for all-cause (HR 2.24; 95% CI 1.34 – 3.75; $P = 0.002$) and arrhythmic mortality (HR 2.29; 95% CI 1.0 – 5.25; $P = 0.049$). Nonarrhythmic mortality was not different in patients testing nonnegative or negative for MTWA.

Some studies in patients with ischemic or nonischemic cardiomyopathy, however, failed to show predictive value of MTWA.[25–27] On careful examination, there are important differences between these negative and the aforementioned positive studies, particularly as to whether β-blocker therapy was withheld prior to MTWA testing. There is evidence that β-blockers suppress MTWA amplitude and affect the presence of MTWA during testing.[28] This point of view is corroborated by a comprehensive meta-analysis of various MTWA studies. There was a significant predictive power of MTWA in those studies in which alternans was measured without interrupting β-blocker therapy[29] but not in those studies in which antiadrenergic treatment was interrupted. Thus, MTWA should be assessed in a pharmacological environment consistent with the patient's medical treatment to ensure that test results reflect the potential benefit of chronic drug therapy.

MTWA-based Risk Prediction for Sudden Death Versus Prediction of ICD Therapy

Some studies have yielded disappointing results on the predictive power of MTWA in high-risk patients. For instance, in a substudy of Sudden Cardiac Death Heart Failure Trial (SCDHeFT), MTWA was assessed in 490 patients at 37 sites.[26] There was a high rate of indeterminate tests (41%), and during a mean follow-up of 30 month, similar event rates of sudden death, VT/VF, or appropriate ICD therapy were found between MTWA-positive or -negative patients. Of note, the majority of end point events consisted of ICD therapies. Similarly, the MASTER study enrolled 575 MADIT-II like patients and followed them for 2.1 years[27] for the end point of sudden death or appropriate ICD discharge. A nonnegative MTWA test was associated with increased total mortality (HR 2.04, $P = 0.02$), but it did not predict a significant increase in the primary end point (HR 1.26, $P = 0.37$).

In an attempt to explain some of these controversial observations, we recently conducted a meta-analysis comprising 14 primary prevention trials. For this purpose, 9 trials in which few patients had implanted ICDs (and therefore in which ICD device therapies accounted for ≤ 15% of all end points) were compared with 5 trials in which many patients had implanted ICDs and thus device therapies comprised the majority of the end points.[30] In the "low ICD group" comprising 3682 patients, the hazard ratio for sudden death/cardiac arrest associated with a MTWA-nonnegative test versus an MTWA-negative test was 13.6 (95% CI 8.5 – 30.4) and the annualized event rate among the MTWA-negative patients was 0.3% (95% CI 0.1% – 0.5%). In contrast, in the "high ICD group" comprising 2234 patients, the hazard ratio was only 1.6 (95% CI 1.2% – 2.1%) and the annualized event rate among the MTWA-negative patients was elevated to 5.4% (95% CI 4.1% – 6.7%). These data suggest therefore that MTWA predominantly predicts lethal ventricular tachyarrhythmic events whereas more benign, often nonsustained ventricular tachyarrhythmias triggering ICD therapy is not as well predicted. This observation may be attributed to the fact that many "appropriate" device therapies treat arrhythmias that would have self-terminated or that ICDs may induce arrhythmias that they subsequently treat.

MTWA-based Risk Prediction in Depressed Versus Preserved LV Function Patients

The majority of sudden deaths occur in patients with preserved LV function. On the other hand, at present, LVEF ≤ 0.35 is used as the sole risk stratifier for primary preventive ICD therapy. Moreover, only a small percentage of patients undergoing primary prevention ICD implantation actually receive appropriate device therapy during long-term follow-up. These considerations led to a careful patient-level data-based analysis from 5 prospective studies of MTWA testing in patients with no history of previous ventricular tachyarrhythmias with further sub-classification of patients based on LVEF.[31] Among patients with LVEF ≤ 35%, the annual sudden death event rates for the positive, negative, and indeterminate groups were 4.0%, 0.9%, and 4.6%, respectively. Hence, MTWA carried similar prognostic information in patients with LVEF ≤ 35% who tested positive or indeterminate, but the incidence of sudden death was significantly lower among patients with a negative MTWA ($P < 0.001$ for both).

In the group of patients with LVEF > 35%, sudden death annual event rates stratified by MTWA test result were: positive (3.0%), negative (0.3%), and indeterminate (0.3%). Among patients in this category, survival free of sudden death was significantly worse for MTWA-positive patients than either the MTWA-negative ($P < 0.001$) or the MTWA-indeterminate ($P = 0.003$) groups, whereas event-free survival was not significantly different between the negative and indeterminate groups with LVEF > 35% ($P = 0.801$). These data therefore clearly indicate that a negative MTWA test result identifies a population of patients at very low risk of sudden death, irrespective of LV function. Hence, patients with a negative MTWA test, even with LVEF ≤ 35%, are unlikely to benefit from prophylactic ICD therapy.

A second important finding relates to patients with preserved LV function. Even among subjects with LVEF > 35%, a positive MTWA test identifies individuals at significantly increased risk of sudden death for whom device therapy may mitigate arrhythmic risk. Finally, the study shows that the risk of sudden death among patients with indeterminate MTWA results may dependent on left ventricular function. Among patients with LVEF ≤ 35%, an indeterminate MTWA test—particularly among those who are indeterminate due to excessive ectopy or inadequate heart rate—predicts an increased risk of sudden death (similar to that of a positive test). An indeterminate MTWA test in subjects with preserved LV function (LVEF > 35%) seems to be not associated with an increased risk, and therefore, these patients should not be grouped with patients who test positive.

Unresolved Issues

As indicated above, one of the most controversial issues regarding the usefulness of MTWA assessment for risk prediction confers to the issue of time dependence of MTWA test results. At present, it remains unknown if MTWA results in an individual patient are reflecting a time-dependent risk for sudden cardiac death or not. Studies are needed that address this issue by repeating MTWA assessment in regular time intervals, for instance in yearly or two-yearly intervals. Ultimately, a definitive, well-designed, randomized outcomes trial on the predictive power of MTWA is needed in which patients will be randomized to ICD or medical therapy based on results of MTWA testing. Given the accumulating data on predictivity of MTWA not only in patients with impaired left ventricular function but also in patients with preserved LVEF, a wide spectrum of patients could be considered for such a trial. Fortunately, such a trial has just begun patient enrollment (Risk Estimation Following Infarction Noninvasive Evaluation: REFINE-ICD; NCT 00673842).[32] Its results will show whether MTWA has a future as a risk predictor for ventricular tachyarrhythmias and sudden death.

REFERENCES

1. Hering HE. Das Wesen des Herzalternans. *Muenchner Med Wochenschr* 1908;4:1417–1421.
2. Lewis T. Notes upon alternation of the heart. *QJ Med.* 1910;4:141–144.
3. Kalter HH, Schwartz ML. Electrical alternans. *NY State J Med.* 1948;1:1164–1166.
4. Raeder EA, Rosenbaum DS, Cohen RJ. Alternating morphology of the QRST complex preceding sudden death. *N Engl J Med.* 1992;326:271–272.
5. Schwartz PJ, Malliani A. Electrical alternation of the T wave: clinical and experimental evidence of its relationship with the sympathetic nervous system and with the long-QT syndrome. *Am Heart J.* 1975;89:45–50.
6. Armoundas AA, Nanke T, Cohen RJ. T-wave alternans preceding torsade de pointes ventricular tachycardia. *Circulation.* 2000;101:25–50.
7. Wegener FT, Ehrlich JR, Hohnloser SH. Amiodarone-associated macroscopic T-wave alternans and torsade de pointes unmasking the inherited long QT syndrome. *Europace.* 2008;10:112–113.
8. Adam DR, Powell AO, Gordon H, Cohen RJ. Ventricular fibrillation and fluctuations in the magnitude of the repolarization vector. *IEEE Comp Cardiol.* 1982;8:241–244.
9. Smith JM, Clancy EA, Valeri CR, Ruskin JN, Cohen RJ. Electrical alternans and cardiac electrical instability. *Circulation.* 1988;77:110–121.
10. Nearing B, Huang HA, Verrier RL. Dynamic tracking of cardiac vulnerability by complex demodulation of the T wave. *Science.* 1991;252:437–440.
11. Shusterman V, Goldberg A, London B. Upsurge in T-wave alternans and nonalternating repolarization instability precedes spontaneous initiation of ventricular tachyarrhythmias in humans. *Circulation.* 2006;113:2880–2887.
12. Hohnloser SH. T wave alternans. In: Zipes D, Jalife J, eds. *Cardiac Electrophysiology.* 6th ed. Philadelphia, PA: Elsevier Inc.;2013:665–676.
13. Merchant FM, Armoundas AA. Role of substrate and triggers in the genesis of cardiac alternans, from myocyte to the whole heart. *Circulation.* 2012;125:539–549.
14. Bloomfield DM, Hohnloser SH, Cohen RJ. Interpretation and classification of microvolt T wave alternans tests. *J Cardiovasc Electrophysiol.* 2002;13:502–512.
15. Verrier RL, Klingenheben T, Malik M, et al. Microvolt T-wave alternans. *J Am Coll Cardiol.* 2011;58:1309–1324.
16. Nieminen T, Lehtimaki T, Viik J, et al. T-wave alternans predicts mortality in a population undergoing a clinically indicated exercise test. *Eur Heart J.* 2007;28:2332–2337.
17. Slawnych MP, Nieminen T, Kahonen M, et al. Post-exercise assessment of cardiac repolarization alternans in patients with coronary artery disease using the modified moving average method. *J Am Coll Cardiol.* 2009;53:1130–1137.
18. Verrier RL, Nearing BD, La Rovere MT, et al. Ambulatory electrocardiogram-based tracking of T wave alternans in post-myocardial infarction patients to assess risk of cardiac arrest or arrhythmic death. *J Cardiovasc Electrophysiol.* 2003;14:705–711.
19. Stein PK, Sanghavi D, Domitrovich PP, Mackey RA, Deedwania P. Ambulatory ECG-based T-wave alternans predicts sudden cardiac death in high-risk post-MI patients with left ventricular dysfunction in the EPHESUS study. *J Cardiovasc Electrophysiol.* 2008;19:1037–1042.
20. Leino J, Minkkinen M, Nieminen T, et al. Combined assessment of heart rate recovery and T-wave alternans during routine exercise testing improves prediction of total and cardiovascular mortality: The Finnish Cardiovascular Study. *Heart Rhythm.* 2009;6:1765–1771.
21. Hohnloser SH, Klingenheben T, Zabel M, et al. T wave alternans during exercise and atrial pacing in humans. *J Cardiovasc Electrophysiol.* 1997;8:987–993.
22. Kaufman E, Bloomfield D, Steinman R, et al. "Indeterminate" microvolt T-wave alternans tests predict high risk of death or sustained ventricular arrhythmias in patients with left ventricular dysfunction. *J Am Coll Cardiol.* 2006;48:1399–1404.
23. Exner DV, Kavanagh KM, Slawnych MP, et al. Noninvasive risk assessment early after a myocardial infarction: the REFINE study. *J Am Coll Cardiol.* 2007;50:2275–2284.
24. Chow T, Kereiakes DJ, Bartone C, et al. Microvolt T-wave alternans identifies patients with ischemic cardiomyopathy who benefit from implantable cardioverter-defibrillator therapy. *J Am Coll Cardiol.* 2007;49:50–58.
25. Grimm W, Christ M, Bach J, Muller HH, Maisch B. Noninvasive arrhythmia risk stratification in idiopathic dilated cardiomyopathy: results of the Marburg cardiomyopathy study. *Circulation.* 2003;108:2883–2891.
26. Gold MR, Ip JH, Costantini O, et al. Role of microvolt T-wave alternans in assessment of arrhythmia vulnerability among patients with heart failure and systolic dysfunction: primary results from the T-wave alternans sudden cardiac death in heart failure trial substudy. *Circulation.* 2008;118:2022–2028.
27. Chow T, Kereiakes DJ, Onufer J, et al. Does microvolt T-wave alternans testing predict ventricular tachyarrhythmias in patients with ischemic cardiomyopathy and prophylactic defibrillators? The MASTER (Microvolt T-wave Alternans Testing for Risk Stratification of Post-Myocardial Infarction Patients) trial. *J Am Coll Cardiol.* 2008;52:1607–1615.

28. Klingenheben T, Grönefeld G, Li YG, Hohnloser SH. Effect of metoprolol and d,l-sotalol on microvolt-level T-wave alternans. *J Am Coll Cardiol.* 2001;38:2013–2019.
29. Chan PS, Gold MR, Nallamothu BK. Do beta-blockers impact microvolt T-wave alternans testing in patients at risk for ventricular arrhythmias? A meta-analysis. *J Cardiovasc Electrophysiol.* 201;21:1009–1014.
30. Hohnloser SH, Ikeda T, Cohen RJ. Evidence regarding clinical use of microvolt T-wave alternans. *Heart Rhythm.* 2009;6:S36–S44.
31. Merchant FM, Ikeda T, Pedretti RFE, et al. Clinical utility of microvolt T-wave alternans testing in identifying patients at high or low risk of sudden cardiac death. *Heart Rhythm.* 2012;9:1256–1264.
32. http://www.ClinicalTrials.gov. Accessed October 10, 2012.

CHAPTER

12

Electrocardiographic Markers of Phase 3 and Phase 4 Atrioventricular Block and Progression to Complete Heart Block

John M. Miller, MD, Rahul Jain, MD, and Eric L. Krivitsky, MD

PREAMBLE

Phase 3 and 4 blocks refer to abnormalities of conduction [usually in reference to the His-Purkinje system (HPS)], due on the one hand to impingement of incoming wavefront of depolarization on refractoriness (phase 3) or on the other to a wavefront arriving at a time when spontaneous (phase 4) depolarization has begun and inhibits impulse propagation. These disorders of conduction may be physiologic or pathologic and, in the latter situation, may be the sole indication that investigation for structural heart disease is warranted.

INTRODUCTION

Transient functional bundle branch block (BBB), or aberration, occurs in a variety of settings. This aberrant interventricular conduction may be a manifestation of normal cardiac electrophysiology (EP) or be the result of some disease process affecting the HPS. In this chapter, we will explore 2 aspects of the mode of development of BBB as well as electrocardiographic (ECG) methods of distinguishing complexes that are abnormal due to aberrant conduction from those originating in the ventricles. Finally, the implications of transient BBB for the subsequent development of complete heart block will be discussed.

NORMAL HIS-PURKINJE PHYSIOLOGY

Normally, the cells of the HPS have the longest effective refractory periods (ERPs) in the entire conduction system. Within the HPS, the proximal portion of the right bundle branch (RBB) has the longest ERP, followed by the proximal left bundle branch (LBB) at relatively low heart rates. At faster heart rates, the ERPs of all HPS cells shorten progressively, but RBB refractoriness shortens more than does that of the LBB. Thus, at input cycle lengths <600 ms, the relationship reverses (i.e., LBB refractoriness exceeds that of the RBB). Further, at any particular moment, refractoriness in the HPS depends on the length of the preceding RR interval: the longer the RR interval,

The ECG Handbook of Contemporary Challenges © 2015 Mohammad Shenasa, Mark E. Josephson, N.A. Mark Estes III
Cardiotext Publishing, ISBN: 978-1-935395-88-1

the longer the ERP associated with that QRS complex. Repolarization currents return the action potential to its baseline, awaiting the next incoming depolarization wavefront; postrepolarization refractoriness, a property of the normal atrioventricular (AV) node is not present in normal HPS cells but can occur in the presence of HPS disease. Although HPS cells have the capability of spontaneous phase-4 depolarization, it results in a discharge rate around 40 beats per minute (bpm) and thus is generally not observed in the absence of significant sinus node dysfunction or AV block.

PHASE 3 BLOCK

Phase 3 block, sometimes referred to as "tachycardia-dependent" or "acceleration-dependent" block is due to the arrival of input to a portion of the HPS during phase 3 (repolarization) of the action potential before the cells in question have completely repolarized. As such, too few sodium channels are in the active state and available to participate in a normal phase 0 upstroke of the next action potential. This may result in a single complex showing BBB or fascicular or AV block, or block may persist for several cycles thereafter depending on the whether rapid input continues as well as the effect of rate-related accommodations of refractoriness in the affected cells. Phase 3 block may be a manifestation of normal physiology of the HPS disease.

Physiologic or functional phase 3 block occurs when supraventricular input occurs before repolarization is complete in normal, healthy HPS tissues (Figure 12.1, top). The most common manifestations of this are BBB following a relatively early premature atrial complex (PAC) as well as the Ashman phenomenon (short cycle following a long cycle; Figure 12.2).[1,2] Since the RBB has the longest refractory period at heart rates below 100 bpm, RBB block (RBBB) is most commonly observed in this setting (75%). At faster heart rates, PACs may produce left BBB (LBBB) due to the greater degree of shortening of ERP in the RBB than the LBB as the heart rate exceeds 100 bpm (as noted above). The Ashman phenomenon is most commonly observed during atrial fibrillation (AF), in which long–short sequences occur frequently. It can, however, also occur in second-degree AV block. As noted above, aberration due to phase 3 block may be limited to a single QRS complex (due to a PAC or long–short sequence) or may continue as long as the input cycle length to the affected bundle is shorter than the ERP (even with rate accommodation) or duc to concealed perpetuation of BBB related to repetitive transseptal conduction and retrograde penetration to into the anterogradely blocked bundle ("linking;" see elsewhere).

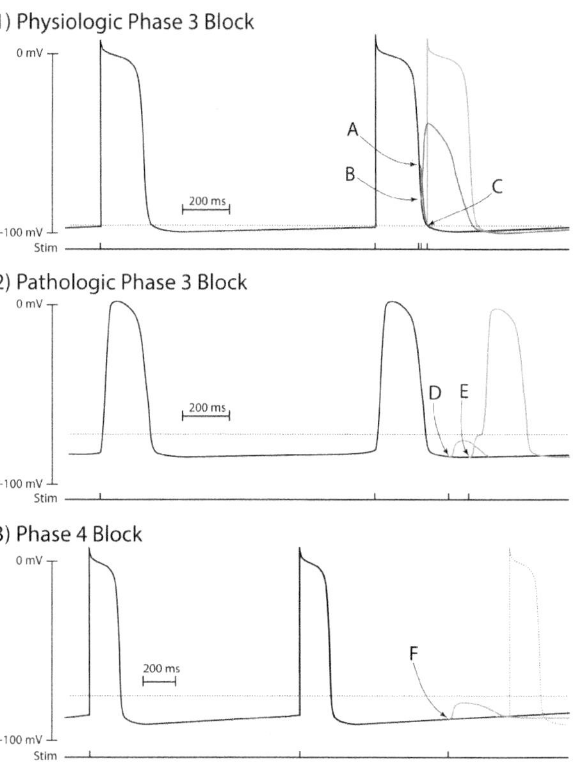

Figure 12.1. Diagrammatic representation of action potentials during phase 3 and 4 blocks. In each panel, a cell from the HPS is shown driven at 1000 ms (tick marks on "Stim" line indicate stimuli) under different conditions with voltage scale and time indicator; horizontal dashed line is threshold potential. **Top panel:** Normal action potential with premature stimulation at A, in absolute refractory period during repolarization, fails to generate any response (red line); at B, shortly thereafter during relative refractory period, generates an action potential with delayed upstroke (blue line); at C, after full repolarization, generates normal action potential (green line). **Middle panel:** HPS disease with elevated resting potential, delayed action potential upstroke at baseline and postrepolarization refractoriness; premature stimulation at D (after full repolarization) yields small response (orange line) that fails to reach threshold (that is itself elevated due to disease); at E, delayed response does reach threshold to generate action potential (green line). **Bottom panel:** Abnormally rapid phase 4 depolarization in diseased HPS. Premature stimulation at F yields subthreshold response (orange line) and prevents achievement of threshold when next complex would have been anticipated (dashed gray line).

Nonphysiologic phase 3 block occurs when refractoriness in a portion of the HPS is abnormally prolonged (due to prolongation of phase 3 repolarization or presence of postrepolarization refractoriness), or fails to accommodate normally to increases in heart rate, or both (see Figure 12.1, middle). This may be due to chronic ischemic heart disease, infiltrative disease, or degenerative disorders of the HPS. In this setting, LBBB is more common than RBBB, and its presence in this setting should raise the suspicion that some pathologic process is present (if not already evident). The typical clinical situation is development

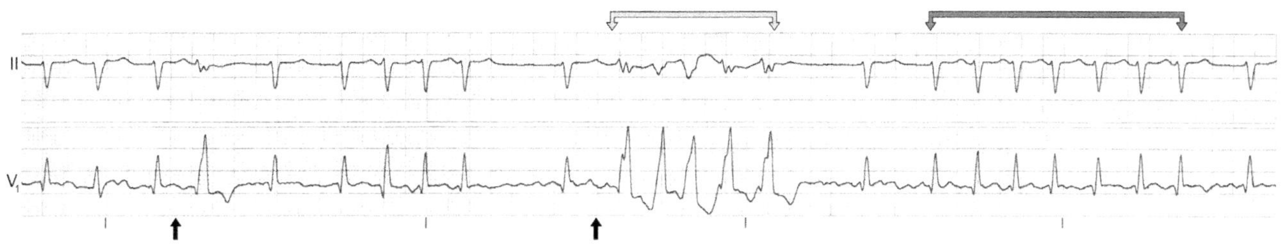

Figure 12.2. Phase 3 block (Ashman phenomenon) during AF. A long rhythm strip shows erratic AV conduction during AF with long–short sequences (dark arrows) ending with a RBBB complex; note the very different coupling intervals at the 2 dark arrows. The ventricular rate during a run of RBBB complexes (light gray upper bar) is similar to that during a subsequent run of narrow complexes (dark gray upper bar); finally, the run of RBBB complexes is quite irregular as are complexes in the narrow run. These are all features consistent with aberration.

of aberration with gradual increase in heart rate (which should shorten HPS refractoriness); other contexts in which this type of aberration is observed are development of aberration at relatively slow heart rates (<70 bpm; Figure 12.3) or within a few cycles after acceleration to a stable rate has occurred (but without further discernible rate change). Acceleration-dependent aberration may persist for as long as the heart rate remains elevated for reasons noted above, or may revert to a normal QRS if adequate rate adaptation of refractoriness eventually occurs.[3]

ECG clues to differentiate phase 3 block from premature ventricular complexes (PVCs) are listed in Table 12.1 and elaborated below.

1. When occurring as isolated wide complexes:
   a. Presence of preceding causal atrial activity—instances of phase 3 block due to supraventricular complexes impinging on HPS refractoriness are obviously preceded by atrial activity (a PAC or during AF). When a PAC is present prior to a wide QRS complex, if the PR interval in question is shorter than baseline, phase 3 block cannot be the cause (and thus the complex is a PVC).
   b. Pattern of occurrence (onset)—of necessity, phase 3 block requires that supraventricular input occurs before recovery of HPS refractoriness and thus a long–short sequence is typical (long RR interval followed by short RR interval; see Figure 12.2). Although this sequence is unnecessary with PVCs, they are by their nature "premature," such that they end a short cycle relative to a prior longer cycle. Thus, the long–short sequence is often of limited help in distinguishing aberration from ventricular ectopy.[4]
   c. Coupling interval of repeated sequences—PVCs arising from the same focus typically maintain a fixed coupling interval with the previous normal QRS, whereas when phase 3 block occurs on a repeated basis, the coupling intervals are variable (see Figure 12.2).[5]
   d. A pause that occurs after a PVC during sinus rhythm is typically fully compensatory (i.e., next sinus complex arrives at its expected interval), whereas a pause following a wide QRS due to phase 3 block following a PAC is less than fully compensatory. In addition, if the PR interval of the cycle following the wide QRS

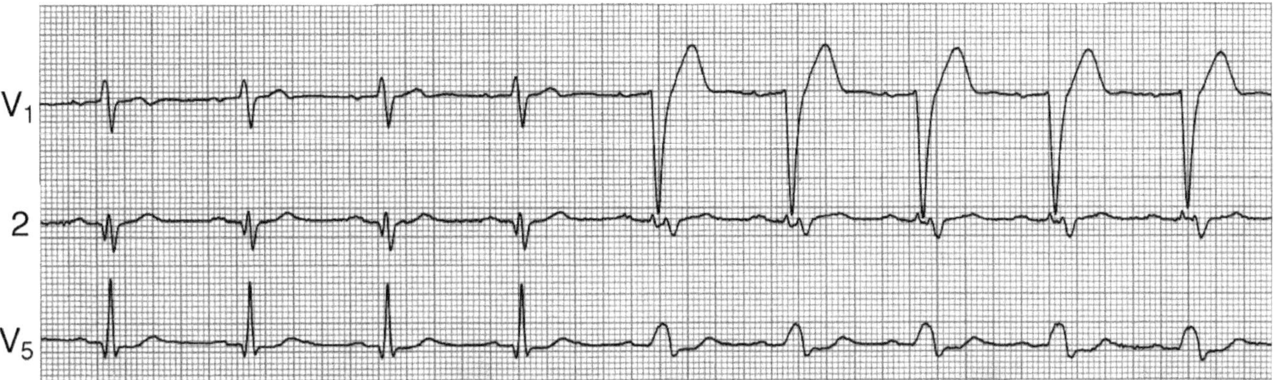

Figure 12.3. Development of aberration (LBBB type) with minimal heart rate change and at slow rate. The sinus rate is about 62 bpm and changes by <1 bpm over the course of the tracing. The lack of abrupt rate change and slow rate at which aberration develops, as well as being LBBB, all signify pathologic phase 3 block in a diseased HPS.

Table 12.1. **Electrocardiographic distinctions between phase 3 block and ventricular ectopic complexes.**

Criterion	Phase 3 Block	Ventricular Ectopic Complexes
Isolated complexes		
Preceding atrial activity	Essential	Absent or unrelated
Pattern of occurrence	Long-short sequence typical	Long-short sequence unnecessary
Coupling intervals of repeated occurrences	Random	Relatively fixed
Pause after wide QRS complex	Non-compensatory duration	Compensatory duration
Prevalence of bundle branch block pattern	RBBB >> LBBB	RBBB ≈ LBBB
QRS morphologic features	Consistent with aberrant conduction	Consistent with myocardial origin
Runs of wide complexes during AF		
Rate vs surrounding narrow complex runs	Similar rates of wide and narrow runs	Wide complex runs faster than narrow complex runs
Regularity vs surrounding narrow complex runs	Definitely irregular	Minimally irregular
Plausibility of conduction	Normal baseline PR interval	Long baseline PR interval (unlikely for SVT to conduct 1:1 to ventricle during rapid tachycardia)

RBBB, right bundle branch block; LBBB, left bundle branch block; AF, atrial fibrillation; SVT, supraventricular tachycardia.

complex is prolonged, concealed retrograde penetration of the AV node from a PVC is likely (this does not occur following wide QRSs due to phase 3 block).

e. BBB pattern—QRSs due to phase 3 block have patterns consistent with aberration whereas PVCs do not, being of myocardial origin.[6] In addition, wide QRSs due to phase 3 block are RBBB in 90% of cases whereas PVCs are roughly evenly distributed between RBB and LBB block-like patterns.

2. When occurring as a series (run) of wide complexes during AF:
   a. Rate parity—when a run of consecutive wide QRSs due to phase 3 block occurs during AF, the ventricular rate should be similar to that of contemporaneous conducted narrow-QRS complexes (see Figure 12.2). A run of ventricular tachycardia is typically significantly faster than surrounding normally conducted complexes.
   b. Irregularity—a run of wide QRSs due to phase 3 block during AF has irregular RR intervals that are readily evident, whereas VT is typically relatively regular (see Figure 12.2).
   c. Plausibility of AV conduction—if the conducted PR during sinus rhythm is long, it is unlikely that a rapid wide complex tachycardia is due to supraventricular tachycardia (SVT) with aberration (Figure 12.4).

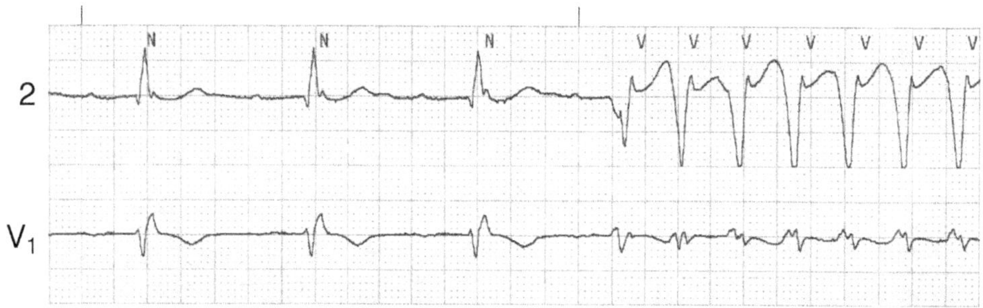

Figure 12.4. Wide QRS tachycardia, cycle length 320 ms, developing after a minimally premature complex. The baseline PR is long (320 ms), suggesting that SVT with aberration would very unlikely to conduct 1:1 at the rate of the tachycardia. In addition, conducted complexes have RBBB pattern while the wide QRS tachycardia (ventricular tachycardia) is more LBBB-type, suggesting it cannot be aberration. (N, normal complex; V, ventricular tachycardia complex).

PHASE 4 BLOCK

Phase 4 block, also referred to as "bradycardia-dependent" or "deceleration-dependent" block, is due to the arrival of input to the HPS during phase 4 (diastolic depolarization) of the action potential in affected cells, long after completion of repolarization (Figures 12.1 [bottom] and 12.5).[7,8] Spontaneous phase 4 depolarization is a normal feature of HPS cells and is the mechanism for escape rhythms during AV block once the membrane potential reaches threshold, but is not evident during sinus rhythm with heart rates > 40 bpm. However, in some pathologic conditions, phase 4 depolarization is accelerated such that it may be relevant at normal heart rates. When this occurs and the membrane potential becomes progressively less negative, too few sodium channels are available in the active state such that either slow conduction or block may occur. Of note, this membrane potential is about the same as the threshold potential for normal HPS cells (–70 mV); however, in diseased HPS, the threshold potential also becomes less negative,[8] creating a "window" of membrane potential during which it is high enough that incoming impulses cannot conduct (for reasons noted above), while at the same time it is too negative to result in spontaneous depolarization. Because some element of HPS dysfunction leads to the elevated (less negative) resting potential, enhanced rate of phase 4 depolarization, and decreased membrane responsiveness to stimuli, the presence of phase 4 block is practically always an indicator of a pathologic condition (degenerative disease, ischemia, infarction, infiltrative disease, etc.).

Phase 4 block thus occurs at low heart rates and, because of the greater propensity for pathologic conditions to affect the left HPS more than the right, as well as the tendency for the LBB to have a slightly more rapid rate of phase 4 depolarization than the RBB, phase 4 block is typically manifested with LBBB.

While accelerated spontaneous phase 4 depolarization definitely does occur in diseased HPS cells, it may not be necessary for development of block. Jalife et al[9] have shown in carefully controlled experimental preparations that: (1) conduction may persist via activation of slow calcium channels despite phase 4 depolarization to a membrane potential that inactivates practically all sodium channels; (2) bradycardia-dependent block may occur in the absence of phase 4 depolarization, and contrariwise; (3) phase 4 depolarization distal to a segment of depressed conduction may actually facilitate propagation through the area. Thus, although the experimental preparations may not be a perfect reflection of changes in human HPS physiology in the presence of a variety of disease states, the construct of phase 4 depolarization causing deceleration-related block of impulse propagation based on the previous discussion may be an oversimplification.

From the foregoing discussion, it should be clear that phase 3 and 4 blocks can occur in the same individual with structural heart disease, depending on the prevailing heart rate.[10]

PROGRESSION TO COMPLETE AV BLOCK

Since phase 3 block due to physiologic refractoriness is a normal phenomenon, it has no particular propensity to progress to complete AV block. However, in cases in which phase 3 block is a due to some form of structural pathology (and practically all cases of phase 4 block), progression to complete heart block can occur. Whether and how rapidly this progression will occur is more dependent on the underlying cardiac pathology than the presence of phase 3 or 4 blocks, however, LBBB, the most common manifestation of phase 4 block, has generally but not always been associated with a worse cardiovascular prognosis (particularly heart failure).[11,12] This is most likely related to the cause of the underlying abnormality rather than the block itself.

A particularly noteworthy condition is paroxysmal AV block (PAVB), in which sudden and persisting AV block occurs, most often after a premature complex leads to a pause (Figure 12.6). Phase 4 block, usually in the His bundle itself,[13] has been implicated as the primary mechanism[14]: a premature impulse during

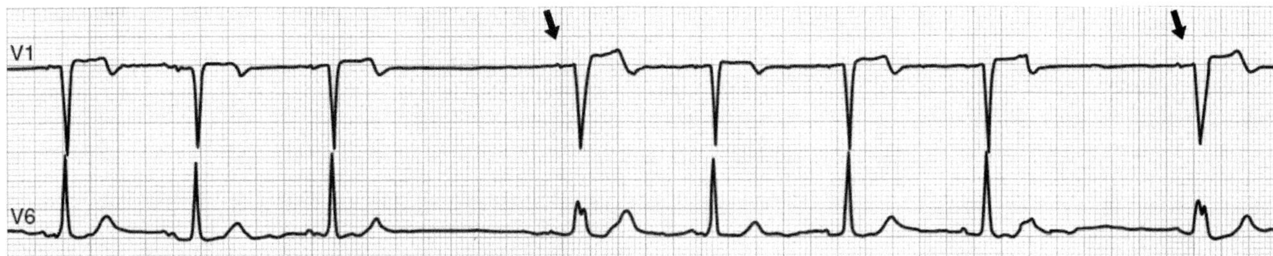

Figure 12.5. Phase 4 block in LBB. Sinus rhythm is present, until a sinus pause occurs; the sinus complexes ending the pause are conducted with LBBB aberration (arrows).

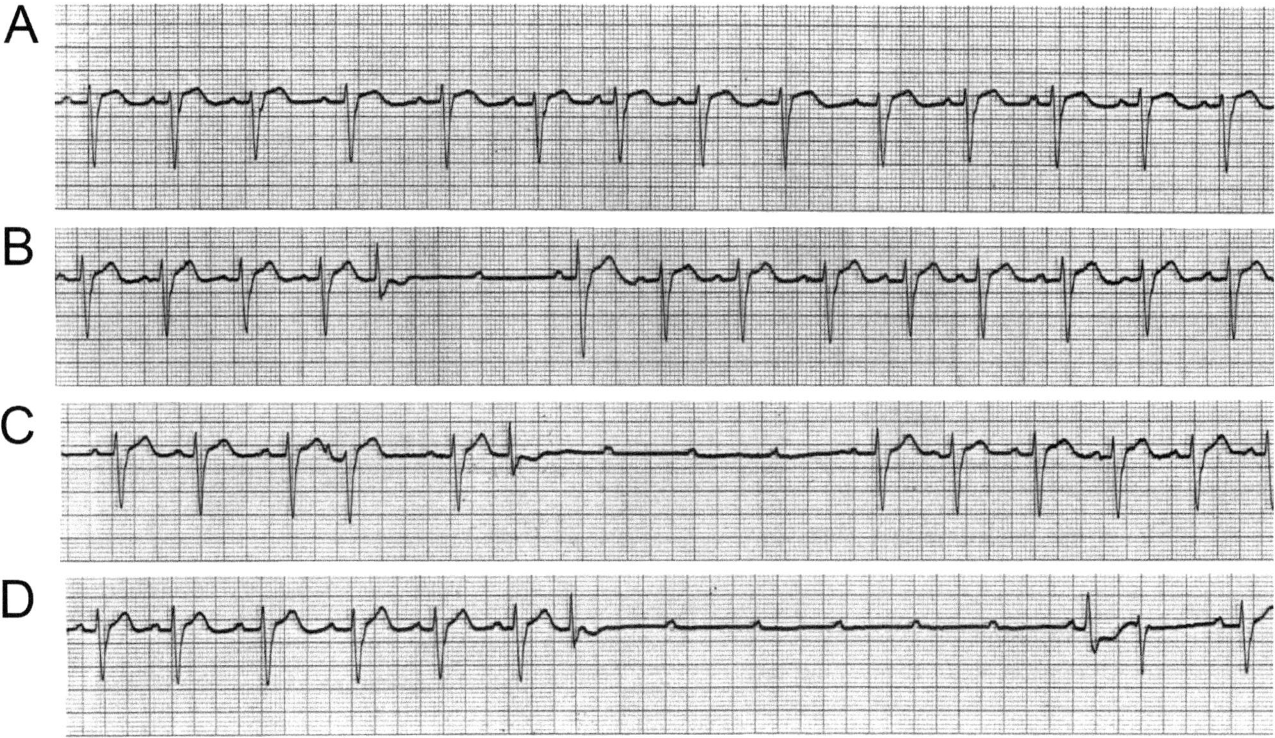

Figure 12.6. PAVB. **A.** Sinus rhythm with conduction is present baseline. **B.** PVC occurs triggering an episode of PAVB that ends spontaneously after one nonconducted P wave. **C.** Atrial premature complex precedes a sinus complex and then PVC that triggers a longer episode of AV block. **D.** PVC starts and ends a longer episode of AV block accompanied by dizziness. (Courtesy of M. Shenasa, MD).

a regular rhythm engenders a pause, and when the next on-time atrial activation wavefront propagates to the His bundle, the latter has already undergone enough phase 4 depolarization during the pause, with resultant sodium channel inactivation such that block occurs. However, since an action potential never results, repolarizing potassium channels are not activated, and thus the membrane potential remains at a level that prevents subsequent conduction until another premature complex interrupts the cycle. Many individuals with PAVB are relatively old and present with either syncope or cardiac arrest due to the sudden asystole. While many of these have some manifestation of HPS disease, such as RBBB, some do not. In the latter individuals, isolated disease of the His bundle seems likely. Some of the affected patients are relatively young and because of isolated His disease, may have normal PR intervals and QRS complexes (morphology and duration) and no abnormal findings on standard evaluation for syncope. As such, PAVB can be very insidious and result in recurrent syncope or cardiac arrest.

OTHER APPLICATIONS

By far, the most common clinical context for phase 3 and 4 block concerns cells of the HPS. However, the same physiology accounting for phase 3 and 4 conduction abnormalities in normal and diseased HPS should apply other analogous situations in which a narrow strand of myocardium is relatively insulated from surrounding cells; such is the case with AV accessory pathways (Figure 12.7) as well as pulmonary vein fascicles. Several reports of both types of conduction block have been reported in the former condition.[15,16] Although physiologic phase 3 block is common in pulmonary vein (PV) fascicles, phase 4 block has not as yet been reported.

SUMMARY

Episodic, temporary electrocardiographic BBB may have diverse mechanisms and clinical implications, depending on the nature and severity of the underlying cardiac disease responsible (if present). Phase 3, or loosely termed tachycardia-dependent, block may be a manifestation of normal physiology or be due to HPS disease; ECG clues have been identified that help make this distinction, while other ECG criteria help distinguish aberration from PVCs. In contrast, phase 4, or bradycardia-dependent block, is almost always associated with significant (albeit not always clinically evident) structural heart disease affecting the specialized conduction system. Progression to

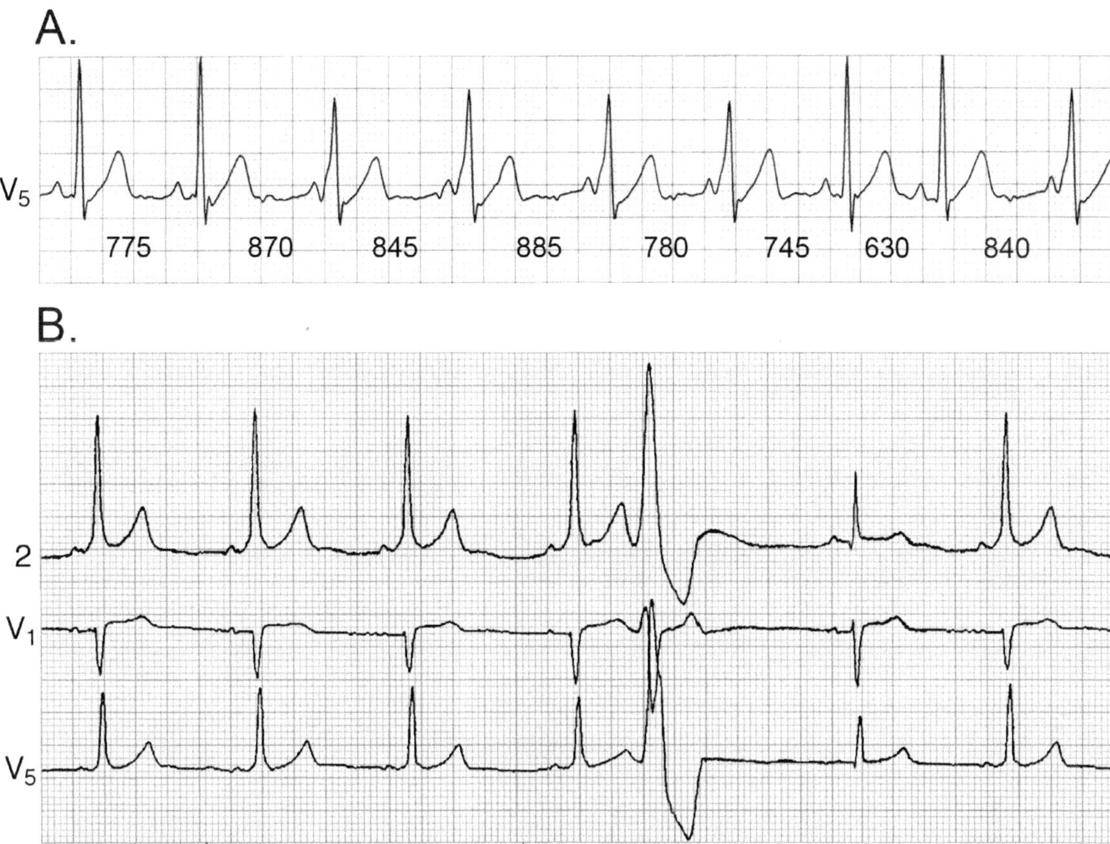

Figure 12.7. Phase 3 and 4 block in AV accessory pathways. **A.** Phase 3 block. Slight deceleration in sinus rate (PP intervals in milliseconds shown below) allows conduction over the AV accessory pathway (delta waves present) while acceleration to cycle length less than 760 ms results in phase 3 pathway block. **B.** Phase 4 block. Sinus rhythm with preexcitation is present until a PVC occurs and conducts retrogradely; this resets the sinus node, producing a pause. The sinus complex ending the pause fails to conduct over the accessory pathway for one complex due to phase 4 pathway block.

complete heart block is more likely in the presence of a significantly diseased HPS. As such, physiologic phase 3 block has little propensity for this, while it is substantially more common in cases in which phase 4 or nonphysiologic phase 3 block are present. PAVB, thought to be a relatively uncommon disorder, is most likely due to phase 4 block although complex mechanisms may be responsible.

SALIENT POINTS

- Phase 3 block, due to an impulse arriving at tissue before complete recovery of excitability, may be a normal phenomenon (RBBB aberration, occurring only at rapid rates) or an indicator of disease (LBBB, occurring at slower rates).
- Phase 4 block, due to diastolic depolarization to a membrane voltage at which most sodium channels are inactive and cannot form an action potential, almost always signifies the presence of heart disease.
- Phase 3 and 4 block may occur in the same individual at different times.
- The usual context of phase 3 and 4 block is the HPS, but they may occur in other situations in which bundles of conducting tissue are somewhat insulated from surrounding cells (i.e., AV accessory pathways).
- Phase 4 or and nonphysiologic phase 3 block may progress to complete heart block at varying rates and generally have a worse prognosis, based on the presence, type, and severity of associated structural heart disease.

REFERENCES

1. Lewis T. Paroxysmal tachycardia, the result of ectopic impulse formation. *Heart.* 1910;1:262–282.
2. Gouaux JL, Ashman R. Auricular fibrillation with aberration simulating ventricular paroxysmal tachycardia. *Am Heart J.* 1947;34(3):366–373.
3. Fisch C, Knoebel SB. Vagaries of acceleration dependent aberration. *Br Heart J.* 1992;67(1):16–24.

4. Gulamhusein S, Yee R, Ko PT, Klein GJ. Electrocardiographic criteria for differentiating aberrancy and ventricular extrasystole in chronic atrial fibrillation: validation by intracardiac recordings. *J Electrocardiol.* 1985;18(1):41–50.
5. Suyama AC, Sunagawa K, Sugimachi M, et al. Differentiation between aberrant ventricular conduction and ventricular ectopy in atrial fibrillation using RR interval scattergram. *Circulation.* 1993;88(5 Pt 1):2307–2314.
6. Miller JM, Das MK. Differential diagnosis of wide and narrow QRS complex tachycardia. In: Zipes DP, Jalife J, eds. *Cardiac Electrophysiology: From Cell to Bedside.* 6th ed. Philadelphia, PA: Elsevier; 2013:575–580.
7. Kretz A, Da Rous HO, Palumbo JR. Delay and block of cardiac impulse caused by enhanced phase-4 depolarization in the His-Purkinje system. *Br Heart J.* 1975;37(2):136–149.
8. Singer DH, Lazzara R, Hoffmna BF. Interrelationships between automaticity and conduction in Purkinje fibers. *Circulation Res.* 1967;12:537–558.
9. Jalife J, Antzelevitch C, Lamanna V, Moe GK. Rate-dependent changes in excitability of depressed cardiac Purkinje fibers as a mechanism of intermittent bundle branch block. *Circulation.* 1983;67(4):912–922.
10. Rosenbaum MB, Lazzari JO, Elizari MV. The role of phase 3 and phase 4 block in clinical electrocardiography. In: Wellens HJJ, Lie KI, Janse MJ, eds. *The Conduction System of the Heart. Structure, Function, and Clinical Implications.* Philadelphia, PA: Lea & Febiger; 1976:126–144.
11. Imanishi R, Seto S, Ichimaru S, et al. Prognostic significance of incident complete left bundle branch block observed over a 40-year period. *Am J Cardiol.* 2006;98(5):644–648.
12. Schneider JF, Thomas HE, Jr., Kreger BE, McNamara PM, Kannel WB. Newly acquired left bundle-branch block: The Framingham study. *Ann Intern Med.* 1979;90(3):303–310.
13. El-Sherif N, Jalife J. Paroxysmal atrioventricular block: Are phase 3 and phase 4 block mechanisms or misnomers? *Heart Rhythm.* 2009;6(10):1514–1521.
14. Lee S, Wellens HJ, Josephson ME. Paroxysmal atrioventricular block. *Heart Rhythm.* 2009;6(8):1229–1234.
15. Lerman BB, Josephson ME. Automaticity of the Kent bundle: Confirmation by phase 3 and phase 4 block. *J Am Coll Cardiol.* 1985;5(4):996–998.
16. Sauer WH, Lowery CM, Callans DJ, Lewkowiez L. Phase 4 conduction block of a right midseptal accessory pathway. *Heart Rhythm.* 2007;4(5):686–687.

CHAPTER

13

Myocardial Infarction in the Presence of Left Bundle Branch Block or Right Ventricular Pacing

Cory M. Tschabrunn, CEPS and Mark E. Josephson, MD

INTRODUCTION

Rapid and accurate diagnosis of acute coronary occlusion is critical in patients presenting with ischemic symptoms to facilitate timely initiation of reperfusion therapy.[1] Early identification and subsequent patient triage in individuals presenting with acute myocardial infarction (MI) is primarily reliant on the standard 12-lead ECG when ST-segment elevation criteria are observed. The 12-lead ECG is undoubtedly the most effective and inexpensive diagnostic test to determine the manifestation of a MI, the location of the culprit coronary lesion, and the severity of ongoing tissue injury.[2] However, recognition of ST-segment elevation myocardial infarction (STEMI) in the presence of left bundle branch block (LBBB) can be particularly difficult. Traditional electrocardiographic algorithms used to diagnose MI are ineffective in patients with LBBB, thus limiting the acute diagnostic value of the 12-lead ECG in these patients.[3–5]

In recognition of these diagnostic challenges, the 1996 and 2004 American College of Cardiology and American Heart Association (ACC/AHA) STEMI guidelines recommended emergent reperfusion therapy, including fibrinolytics or primary percutaneous coronary intervention, for patients with new or presumably new LBBB and clinical manifestation of symptoms compatible with STEMI within 12 hours.[6–8] It is often difficult for providers to determine new versus old LBBB when patients present to the emergency department, which has subsequently resulted in unnecessary urgent referral to the cardiac catheterization laboratory, exposing patients to a needless invasive procedure with increased risk of complication, prolonged hospital stay, and additional costs.[9] Furthermore, more recent and robust clinical trial data has indicated that the incidence of coronary occlusion requiring urgent coronary revascularization is low in patients with LBBB, and the development of a definitively new LBBB associated with ongoing MI is exceedingly rare.[10–13]

This chapter will review the LBB anatomy, mechanisms underlying LBBB, diagnostic challenges, and an overview of available ECG criteria that can be utilized to diagnose active MI in the setting of chronic LBBB and RV pacing. We will also discuss electrocardiographic clues to determine anatomical location of prior infarct in the setting of LBBB.

The ECG Handbook of Contemporary Challenges © 2015 Mohammad Shenasa, Mark E. Josephson, N.A. Mark Estes III
Cardiotext Publishing, ISBN: 978-1-935395-88-1

ANATOMY, PATHOPHYSIOLOGY, AND LBBB ECG CRITERIA

LBBB is observed when normal electrical activity in the His-Purkinje system is interrupted. The bundle of His divides at the junction of the fibrous and muscular boundaries of the interventricular septum (IVS) into the RBBs and LBBs. The main LBB penetrates the IVS under the aortic valve and then diverges into 3 to 4 fairly discrete subdivisions. These components include: (1) a predivisional segment; (2) anterior fascicle that crosses the left ventricular outflow tract (LVOT) and ends in the LV anterolateral wall Purkinje system; (3) posterior fascicle that extends into Purkinje fibers; and (4) a median fascicle that extends to the IVS in a subset of patients.[14–16]

There is only a limited data available evaluating the specific site of conduction disruption in patients with LBBB. Available data indicates that right ventricular activation continues without interruption and only left ventricular activation is altered.[17] Pathological studies in patients with LBBB have suggested that the site of conduction block is likely at the proximal level of the IVS (particularly in diffuse myocardial disease), but may also involve the distal subdivisions. It is hypothesized that the most vulnerable portion of the left bundle is located at the proximal junction of the His bundle and LBB.[15] This region may be more susceptible to fibrosis in the setting of structural heart disease. It is important to note that the manifestation of a LBBB pattern on ECG may be the result of marked conduction delay in the bundle branch structure and does not necessarily indicate complete conduction block in the left bundle or applicable subdivision(s).[14] Regardless, during LBBB, left ventricular activation propagates from the point of termination of the right bundle. The pathophysiological result from this conduction abnormality leads to asynchronous ventricular activation that can be distinctively recognized on the ECG. The LBBB configuration on ECG is represented by a series of common patterns that can be recognized in a majority of patients utilizing the following criteria.

1. QRS duration ≥ 120 ms.
2. Slurred R wave in leads I, aVL, V_5, and V_6
3. Absence of Q waves in leads I, V_5, and V_6.
4. R peak time > 60 ms in leads V_5 and V_6.
5. ST and T wave discordant to the QRS vector.

The complete AHA/ACCF/HRS electrocardiographic guidelines to diagnose LBBB are summarized in Table 13.1.[2] The ST and T wave discordance to the QRS vector represents the altered ventricular depolarization during LBBB that can conceal ST segment changes consistent with acute coronary occlusion that would ordinarily be identified during normal conduction.[4–6,18,19] This phenomenon is the source of difficulty in diagnosing acute MI in the setting of LBBB and why conventional ECG criteria cannot be utilized.

Table 13.1. **Complete LBBB ECG criteria.**

1. QRS duration ≥ 120 ms.
2. Broad, notched, or slurred R wave in leads I, aVL, V_5, and V_6 and occasional RS pattern in V_5 and V_6 attributed to displaced transition of QRS complex.
3. Absent Q waves in leads I, V_5, and V_6, but narrow Q wave may be present in lead aVL in the absence of structural heart disease.
4. R peak time > 60 ms in leads V_5 and V_6, but normal in leads V_1, V_2, and V_3, when small R waves can be discerned in the above leads.
5. ST and T waves usually opposite in direction to the QRS.
6. Positive T wave in leads with upright QRS may be normal (+ concordance).
7. The appearance of LBBB may change the mean QRS axis in the frontal plane to the right, to the left, or superior in a rate-dependent manner in some cases,

Modified with permission.[2]

ETIOLOGY

The development of LBBB can be the result of both structural and functional factors. Usually, LBBB is associated with a progressive degenerative disease involving the conduction system and is seldom the result of a single clinical event, including acute MI. As such, numerous chronic conditions such as hypertension, coronary artery disease, and/or other cardiomyopathies that contribute to myocardial hypertrophy, dilation, and subsequent fibrosis tend to be the typical culprits that lead to LBB conduction delay or block.[20,21] Occasionally, LBBB can be observed in a series of functional causes, such as hyperkalemia, drug toxicity, rate-related aberrancy, or in the presence of acute inflammatory changes.[22] Transient, rate-dependent LBBB can be seen in patients presenting with chest pain in the setting of physical exertion. This phenomenon, known as the "painful LBBB syndrome" has been occasionally reported in the literature and is often misconstrued as an acute coronary event that may result in unnecessary urgent cardiac catherization. Ellis et al have better illustrated this rare, but often mismanaged, syndrome that is characterized by the abrupt onset of exertional chest pain that coincides with the development of LBBB and subsequently resolves with the return of normal conduction.[23]

It is also important to note that a LBBB pattern can be seen in the setting of monomorphic ventricular tachycardia or during sinus rhythm with antegrade right-sided accessory pathway conduction (Figure 13.1). These patients may develop palpitations and chest pain secondary to the manifestation of an arrhythmia that is not related to an active coronary event. The ECG should always be carefully evaluated to determine the underlying rhythm, PR interval, and for the presence of a delta wave to avoid the possibility of misclassification.

PREVALENCE OF LBBB

The prevalence of LBBB in the general population is estimated to be approximately 1%, but with significantly higher predominance as individuals age. The frequency of LBBB may be seen in up to 5.7% of individuals at age 80. Rarely, LBBB with no identifiable underlying cause can be observed in young patients less than 30 years old and tends to be benign in nature.[24–27] Regardless, potential structural and functional etiologies should always be considered.

The prevalence of LBBB in patients presenting to the hospital with confirmed coronary occlusion was initially thought to be approximately 7% from early clinical trial data.[28] Concern began to develop as it became increasingly clear that patients with LBBB had significantly higher mortality following MI than those without LBBB. These findings were confirmed by multiple studies and were initially thought to be the result of inadequate recognition of ongoing ischemia and thus delayed referral to reperfusion therapy due to the difficulties associated with interpreting the LBBB ECG pattern.[20,28,29] This subsequently led to the current and problematic ACC/AHA guidelines that recommend coronary evaluation in the setting of new or presumed new LBBB. More recent data has appropriately suggested that this outcome disparity is likely the result of additional cardiac risk factors and underlying structural heart disease that is more often found in patients with LBBB.[30,31]

Larger and more robust clinical trials have concluded that the prevalence of LBBB (chronic or presumed new) is much lower than originally suggested. Results from the GUSTO-1 study concluded that the prevalence of LBBB in biomarker confirmed MI was only 0.5%.[18,32] These findings were corroborated from the Hero-2 trial, which concluded that the development of a confirmed, new LBBB in the setting of acute MI is 0.15%, indicating that a majority of patients considered to have "presumed new LBBB"

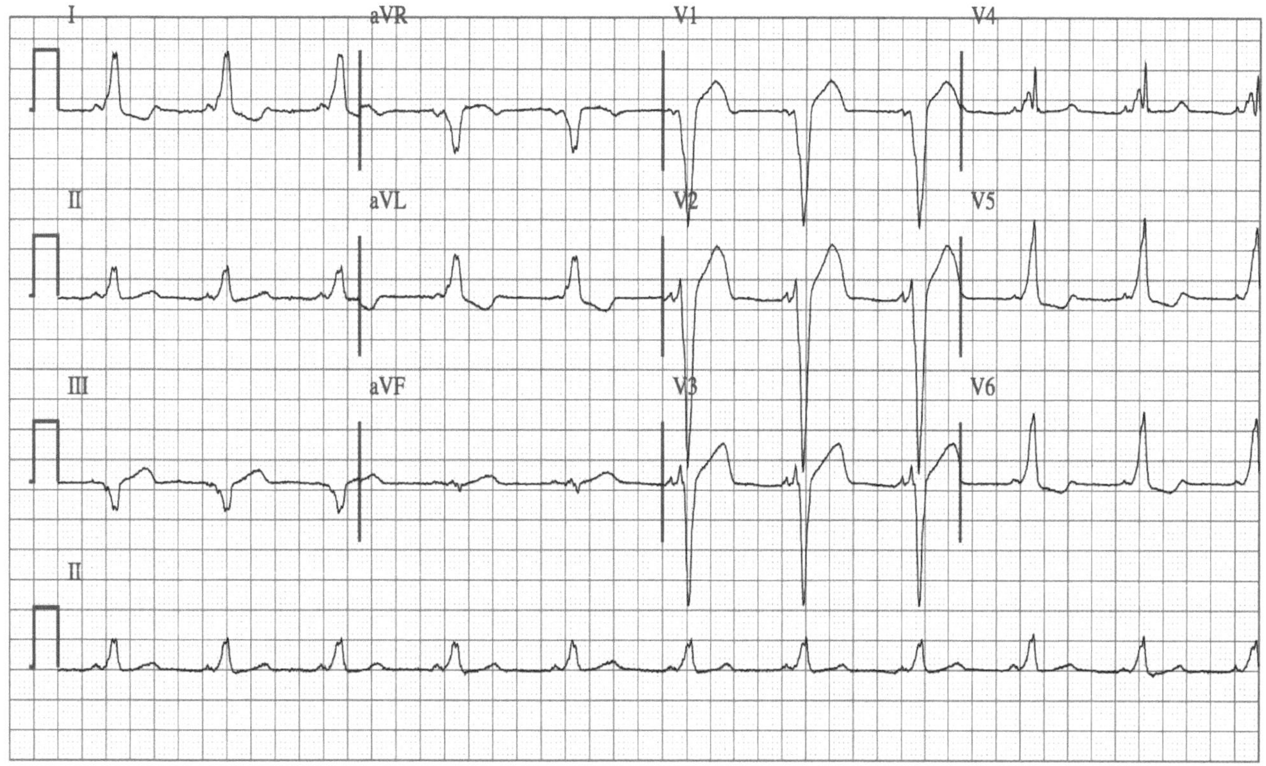

Figure 13.1. Twelve-lead ECG from a 45-year-old male presenting with chest pain referred for urgent cardiac catherization due to presumably new LBBB. ECG also demonstrates a short PR interval and preexcitation pattern consistent with a right free wall accessory pathway. Coronary angiography was normal and further workup demonstrated symptoms secondary to supraventricular tachycardia (SVT). Courtesy of Beth Israel Deaconess Medical Center.

are misclassified and likely represent patients with undiagnosed chronic LBBB.[10,33] The development of significant conduction delay or block in the left bundle as a result of acute MI is exceedingly rare.

DIAGNOSIS OF ACUTE MI IN THE SETTING OF LBBB

Although an abundance of evidence over the last several years has indicated a rare association between the development of new LBBB and acute MI, it is still important to develop appropriate ECG screening criteria that can be used to exclude or confirm active MI in patients with chronic LBBB. Significant efforts have been put forth over the last several decades to develop modified electrocardiographic criteria that can effectively and reproducibly determine active coronary occlusion in these patients.[5,18,19] Through this process, many ECG algorithms have been proposed but have consistently suffered from poor sensitivity and specificity upon further adjudication. The inability to accurately risk stratify this small but important patient population, in conjunction with unmodified ACC/AHA guidelines, has resulted in continued unnecessary coronary catherization procedures.

As discussed, the activation pattern associated with LBBB can conceal traditional STEMI ECG criteria, requiring proposed alternative algorithms to utilize surrogate markers to indicate tissue ischemia in the setting of abnormal ventricular activation. Many of these electrocardiographic algorithms sought to detect features that were not typically associated with LBBB such as the distribution of Q waves and/or patterns of S-wave notching. Although these patterns can be useful when attempting to determine the anatomical location of a prior infarct, they consistently proved to be unreliable for assessment of acute MI despite repeated attempts to modify grading scores and the addition of more criteria. In 1996, Sgarbossa et al described an improved methodology utilizing ST-segment concordance and discordance. The algorithm reports a specificity of at least 90% when a score of 3 or higher was observed. The Sgarbossa criteria, outlined in Table 13.2, have since undergone rigorous validation and continues to offer the highest specificity over any other 12-lead ECG algorithm. The criteria were created utilizing the expansive GUSTO-1 database, which included a large group of patients with chronic LBBB and MI.[10–12,34,35] The algorithm identified 3 specific metrics and the associated scoring system to determine the risk of active coronary occlusion in the setting of LBBB. An example of each criterion is demonstrated in Figure 13.2.

1. ST elevation ≥ 1 mm concordant (same direction) with QRS complex (Score 5).

Table 13.2. **ECG criteria to diagnose MI in LBBB: "Sgarbossa Criteria."**

Criteria	Odds Ratio (95% CI)	Score
ST elevation ≥ 1 mm concordant (same direction) with QRS complex	25.2 (11.6 – 54.7)	5
ST depression ≥ 1 mm in lead V_1, V_2, or V_3	6.0 (1.9 – 19.3)	3
*ST elevation ≥ 5 mm discordant (opposite direction) with QRS complex	4.3 (1.8 – 10.6)	2

A total score ≥ 3 associated with high specificity, but low sensitivity.
*Prominent J-point elevations may occur in V_1 – V_2 in the setting of left ventricular hypertrophy. Modified with permission.[32]

2. ST depression ≥ 1 mm in lead V_1, V_2, or V_3 (Score 3).
3. ST elevation ≥ 5 mm discordant (opposite direction) with QRS complex (Score 2).

Criterion 3 has been shown to be less helpful, as similar J-point elevations may be observed in patients with uncomplicated LBBB in the setting of left ventricular hypertrophy and thus adds little diagnostic value to the algorithm. Although this algorithm offers superior specificity to previous methodologies, serial trials have identified minimal sensitivity (20%–36%).[33,34] Performing serial ECGs and/or having access to previous ECGs for interpretation may increase this sensitivity further.

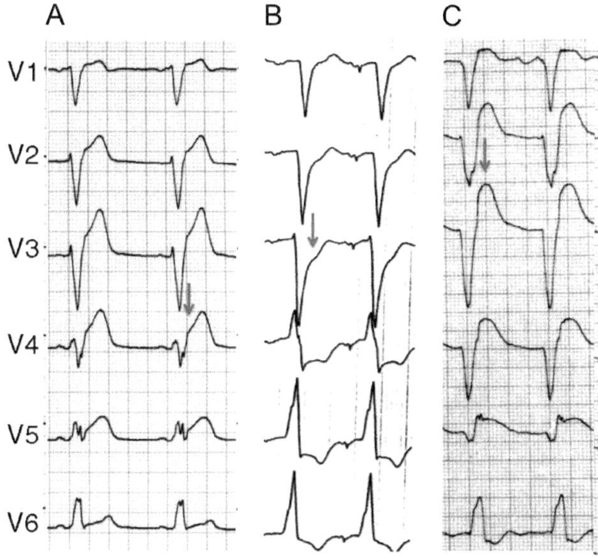

Figure 13.2. Precordial lead ECG tracings from 3 patients with LBBB and a component of the Sgarbossa criteria identified by the indicated arrow. **A.** ST elevation concordant with the QRS complex. **B.** ST depression in lead V_3. **C.** ST elevation discordant to QRS complex in lead V_3. Adapted with permission.[41]

Nonetheless, the Sgarbossa criteria continue to provide the most effective standard electrocardiographic technique available at this current time to evaluate patients with LBBB and symptoms consistent with MI.

There may still be cases where identification of new versus chronic LBBB may be helpful in the diagnosis process. Shvilkin et al described electrocardiographic criteria with assessment of the QRS/T and Max S/T ratio. This algorithm was associated with 100% sensitivity to differentiate new versus chronic LBBB when values were <2.25 mV and <2.5 mV, respectively (Figure 13.3).[36] This may be particularly useful in rare cases where acute MI does indeed involve the conduction system and results in the manifestation of a new LBBB or when evaluating a patient with possible painful LBBB syndrome. The algorithm to differentiate new versus chronic LBBB is described and demonstrated in greater detail in this chapter.

Although the use of imaging modalities such as cardiac magnetic resonance (CMR) imaging, computed tomography angiography (CTA), and/or transthoracic echocardiogram (TTE) may aid in the diagnosis of acute MI in the setting of LBBB, caution should be used when emphasizing the results of these less validated techniques, specifically in the case of CMR and CTA imaging. TTE is likely to be less useful in this particular context, as septal wall motion abnormalities and the high likelihood of underlying structural heart disease associated with LBBB will limit the imaging value of echocardiography.

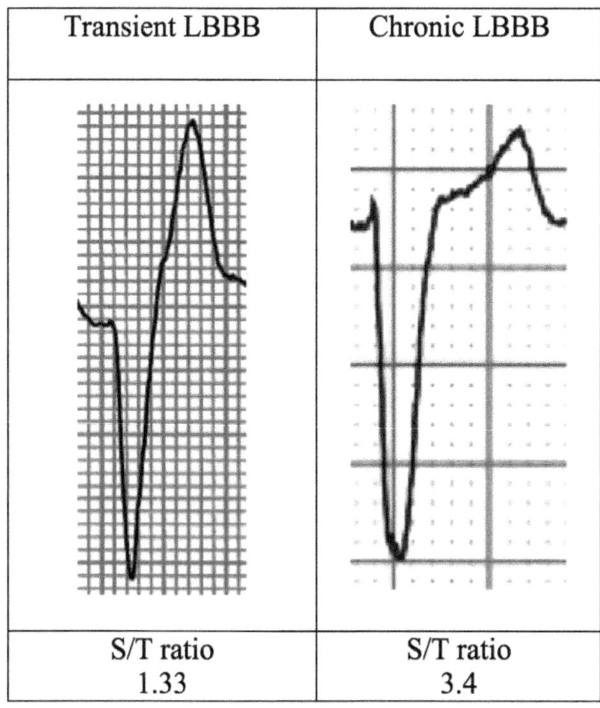

Figure 13.3. S/T wave ratio algorithm accurately identifies 2 patients with new and chronic LBBB as described by Shvilkin et al.[36]

ECG DIAGNOSIS OF MI IN THE PRESENCE OF RIGHT VENTRICULAR PACED RHYTHM

The diagnosis of MI during right ventricular pacing has major limitations. The problems of recognizing abnormal ST-segment deviation, abnormal T-wave polarity, and QRS abnormalities suggestive of MI in the presence of RV pacing rhythm are similar to those discussed in the setting of underlying LBBB.[37] Thirty-two patients in the GUSTO-1 trial (0.1 percent of enrolled patients) had a ventricular paced rhythm. The only ECG criterion with a high specificity for the diagnosis of an acute MI was ST segment elevation ≥5 mm in leads with a negative QRS complex. In addition, ST elevation ≥1 mm in leads with concordant QRS polarity and ST depression ≥1 mm in leads V_1, V_2, or, V_3 was associated with reasonable specificity, but has not been extensively validated.[19] If the patient is not pacemaker-dependent, it is also possible to inhibit the pacemaker to record the native ECG and assess for ischemic changes if significant T-wave memory does not preclude interpretation. Assessment of the T wave and determination of cardiac memory versus ischemia is discussed in this chapter.

While evaluating a patient with chest pain and chronic LBBB or RV pacing that does not fulfill Sgarbossa criteria, we recommend serial cardiac biomarker assessment with concurrent consideration of other differential diagnoses. It is essential to remember that the described ECG algorithms do not provide 100% sensitivity and specificity. We strongly advocate utilization of a detailed history and physical exam coupled with clinical intuition and consultation if necessary during potentially time-sensitive and diagnostically challenging cases.

PROGRESSION TO COMPLETE HEART BLOCK (CHB)

CHB is a known complication associated with ongoing MI and can be seen in both inferior and anterior infarctions. Patients with chronic LBBB are at a higher risk for the development of CHB. In addition to the heart block risk associated with the impending MI, the development of a new right bundle branch block (RBBB) would result in CHB in a patient with chronic LBBB. New RBBB in the setting of acute MI is rare (0.9%), but occurs more frequently than LBBB and is seen most often during anteroseptal infarcts.[33,38] Patients with acute MI and chronic LBBB should be carefully monitored as they have a higher likelihood of further conduction disturbances that may require immediate intervention (i.e., transcutaneous or transvenous pacing).

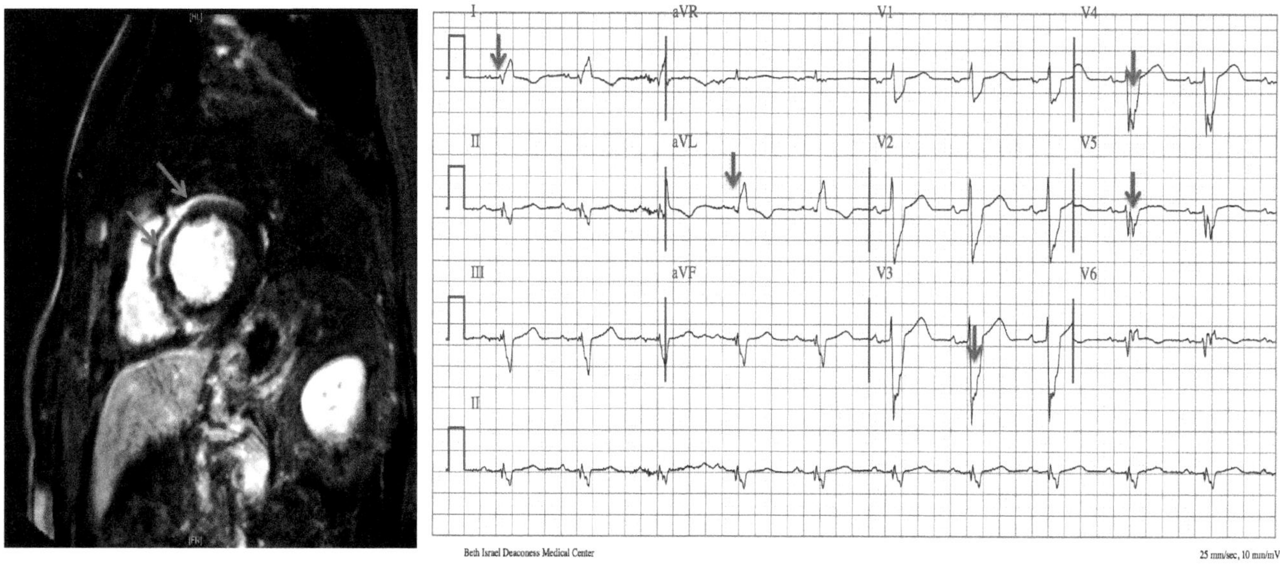

Figure 13.4. CMR imaging and 12-lead ECG in a patient with prior MI. CMR imaging demonstrates late gadolinium enhancement along the anterior-septal wall (arrow) consistent with scar and prior MI. Routine ECG is positive for Cabrera criteria with S-wave notching in leads V_3, V_4, and V_5 (arrow) consistent with prior complete left anterior descending artery occlusion. Courtesy of Beth Israel Deaconess Medical Center.

LBBB ECG ASSESSMENT IN PRIOR INFARCTION

The abnormal depolarization pattern associated with LBBB may also limit traditional ECG criteria utilized to evaluate prior transmural infarctions. Kindwall et al evaluated the predictive value of various ECG criteria by pacing the right ventricle at 2 sites in patients with various types of MI and also in patients without prior MI. This study demonstrated that although Cabrera's sign[39] (notching 0.04 second in duration in the ascending limb of the S wave of leads V_3, V_4, or V_5) is not a highly sensitive and specific algorithm for assessment of acute MI, it can provide reliable assessment of prior anterior wall infarct (Figure 13.4).[40] This study also demonstrated that Q waves in leads I, aVL, and aVF are useful for localizing the site of prior MI (inferior or anterior), but again not for the ongoing development of MI. In addition, the location of S-wave notching in lead II may indicate delayed conduction through scar (Figure 13.5). The LV activation pattern during LBBB may produce S-wave notching in lead II relatively early within the QRS representing delayed depolarization through scar from prior inferior

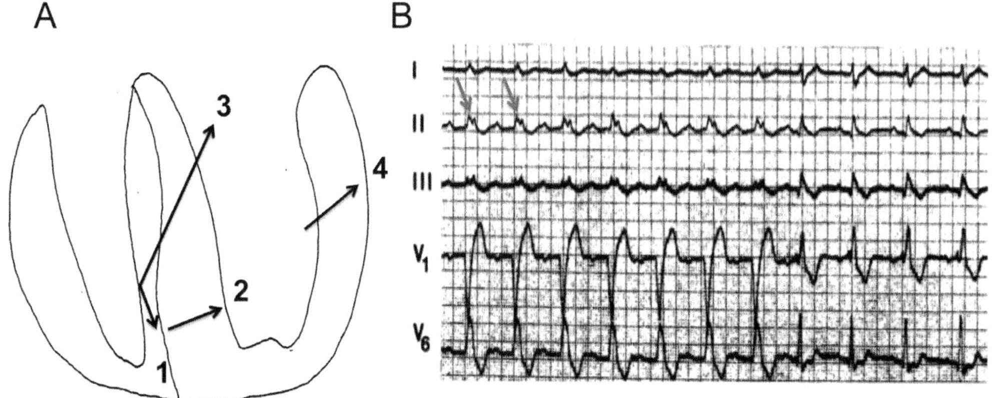

Figure 13.5. **A.** A schematic depicting the sequence of left ventricular activation in the setting of LBBB. The initial portion of the septum activated is the right side and spreads from the right mid-low septal region towards the apex (Vector 1). The lower septal mass towards the LV is then activated (Vector 2) and in conjunction with Vector 1, activates the remaining portion of the upper septum (Vector 3). Finally, Vector 4 represents terminal activation of the base and the remaining portions of the left ventricular free wall. **B.** ECG tracings from a patient with prior inferior infarction and intermittent LBBB. The red arrows depict S-wave notching in lead II that occurs relatively early within the tracing, consistent with the patients prior inferior wall infarct. This notching may occur later within the QRS in patients with prior anterior MI as this region of the LV is activated after the inferior wall as depicted in A during LBBB. Figure 13.5B adapted with permission.[41]

infarct. This notching will be seen towards the end of the QRS in patients with prior anterior infarction, as this region of the LV is activated after the inferior wall during LBBB.

CONCLUSIONS

1. The development of LBB conduction delay or block is a degenerative process and rarely the result of an acute event.
2. The development of LBBB is unlikely to be associated with acute MI.
3. LBBB results in abnormal left ventricular conduction, requiring alternative strategies to evaluate for myocardial ischemia in patients with chronic LBBB or RV pacing.
4. ST elevation ≥ 1 mm concordant with QRS complex and/or ST depression ≥ 1 mm in lead V_1, V_2, or V_3 of the Sgarbossa criteria offers at least 90% specificity for detection of acute MI in the setting of LBBB.
5. Evaluation of Cabrera's sign and the relative location of S-wave notching can indicate the presence and anatomical location of prior MI.

REFERENCES

1. Rude RE, Poole WK, Muller JE, et al. Electrocardiographic and clinical criteria for recognition of acute myocardial infarction based on analysis of 3,697 patients. *Am J Cardiol.* 1983;52:936–942.
2. Surawicz B, Childers R, Deal BJ, et al. AHA/ACCF/HRS recommendations for the standardization and interpretation of the electrocardiogram: Part III: Intraventricular conduction disturbances: a scientific statement from the American Heart Association Electrocardiography and Arrhythmias Committee, Council on Clinical Cardiology; the American College of Cardiology Foundation; and the Heart Rhythm Society. Endorsed by the International Society for Computerized Electrocardiology. *J Am Coll Cardiol.* 2009;53:976–981.
3. Kumar V, Venkataraman R, Aljaroudi W, et al. Implications of left bundle branch block in patient treatment. *Am J Cardiol.* 2013;111:291–300.
4. Wackers FJ. The diagnosis of myocardial infarction in the presence of left bundle branch block. *Cardiol Clinics* 1987;5:393–401.
5. Wellens HJ. Acute myocardial infarction and left bundle-branch block – can we lift the veil? *N Engl J Med.* 1996;334:528–529.
6. Antman EM, Anbe DT, Armstrong PW, et al. ACC/AHA guidelines for the management of patients with ST-elevation myocardial infarction – executive summary: A report of the American College of Cardiology/American Heart Association Task Force on Practice Guidelines (Writing Committee to Revise the 1999 Guidelines for the Management of Patients With Acute Myocardial Infarction). *Circulation.* 2004;110:588–636.
7. Group FC. Indications for fibrinolytic therapy in suspected acute myocardial infarction: collaborative overview of early mortality and major morbidity results from all randomised trials of more than 1000 patients. Fibrinolytic Therapy Trialists' (FTT) Collaborative Group. *Lancet.* 1994;343:311–322.
8. Hindman MC, Wagner GS, JaRo M et al. The clinical significance of bundle branch block complicating acute myocardial infarction. 1. Clinical characteristics, hospital mortality, and one-year follow-up. *Circulation.* 1978;58:679–688.
9. Larson DM, Menssen KM, Sharkey SW et al. "False-positive" cardiac catheterization laboratory activation among patients with suspected ST-segment elevation myocardial infarction. *JAMA.* 2007;298:2754–2760.
10. McMahon R, Siow W, Bhindi R, et al. Left bundle branch block without concordant ST changes is rarely associated with acute coronary occlusion. *Int J Cardiol.* 2013;167:1339–1342.
11. Liakopoulos V, Kellerth T, Christensen K. Left bundle branch block and suspected myocardial infarction: Does chronicity of the branch block matter? *Eur Heart J Acute Cardiovasc Care.* 2013;2:182–189.
12. Chang AM, Shofer FS, Tabas JA, et al. Lack of association between left bundle-branch block and acute myocardial infarction in symptomatic ED patients. *Am J Emerg Med.* 2009;27:916–921.
13. Wong CK, French JK, Aylward PE, et al. Patients with prolonged ischemic chest pain and presumed-new left bundle branch block have heterogeneous outcomes depending on the presence of ST-segment changes. *J Am Coll Cardiol.* 2005;46:29–38.
14. Josephson M. *Clinical Cardiac Electrophysiology: Techniques and Interpretations.* Philadelphia, PA: Lea & Febiger; 2003.
15. Hecht HH, Kossmann CE, Childers RW, et al. Atrioventricular and intraventricular conduction. Revised nomenclature and concepts. *Am J Cardiol.* 1973;31:232–244.
16. Demoulin JC, Kulbertus HE. Histopathological examination of concept of left hemiblock. *Br Heart J.* 1972;34:807–814.
17. Vassallo JA, Cassidy DM, Miller JM, et al. Left ventricular endocardial activation during right ventricular pacing: Effect of underlying heart disease. *J Am Coll Cardiol.* 1986;7:1228–1233.
18. Sgarbossa EB. Value of the ECG in suspected acute myocardial infarction with left bundle branch block. *J Electrocardiol.* 2000;33(suppl.):87–92.
19. Sgarbossa EB, Pinski SL, Gates KB, Wagner GS. Early electrocardiographic diagnosis of acute myocardial infarction in the presence of ventricular paced rhythm. GUSTO-I investigators. *Am J Cardiol.* 1996;77:423–424.
20. Hesse B, Diaz LA, Snader CE, Blackstone EH, Lauer MS. Complete bundle branch block as an independent predictor of all-cause mortality: report of 7,073 patients referred for nuclear exercise testing. *Am J Med.* 2001;110:253–259.

21. Grines CL, Bashore TM, Boudoulas H, et al. Functional abnormalities in isolated left bundle branch block. The effect of interventricular asynchrony. *Circulation.* 1989;79:845–853.
22. Ohmae M, Rabkin SW. Hyperkalemia-induced bundle branch block and complete heart block. *Clinical Cardiol.* 1981;4:43–46.
23. Ellis E, Gervino E, Litvak A, Josephson M, Shvilkin A. The painful LBBB syndrome. 2014.
24. Siegman-Igra Y, Yahini JH, Goldbourt U, Neufeld HN. Intraventricular conduction disturbances: a review of prevalence, etiology, and progression for ten years within a stable population of Israeli adult males. *Am Heart J.* 1978;96:669–679.
25. Ostrander LD, Jr., Brandt RL, Kjelsberg MO, Epstein FH. Electrocardiographic findings among the Adult Population of a Total Natural Community, Tecumseh, Michigan. *Circulation.* 1965;31:888–898.
26. Hiss RG, Lamb LE. Electrocardiographic findings in 122,043 individuals. *Circulation.* 1962;25:947–961.
27. Lamb LE, Kable KD, Averill KH. Electrocardiographic findings in 67,375 asymptomatic subjects. V. Left bundle branch block. *Am J Cardiol.* 1960;6:130–142.
28. Go AS, Barron HV, Rundle AC, Ornato JP, Avins AL. Bundle-branch block and in-hospital mortality in acute myocardial infarction. National Registry of Myocardial Infarction 2 Investigators. *Ann Intern. Med.* 1998;129:690–697.
29. Newby KH, Pisano E, Krucoff MW, Green C, Natale A. Incidence and clinical relevance of the occurrence of bundle-branch block in patients treated with thrombolytic therapy. *Circulation.* 1996;94:2424–2428.
30. Badheka AO, Singh V, Patel NJ, et al. QRS duration on electrocardiography and cardiovascular mortality (from the National Health and Nutrition Examination Survey-III). *Am J Cardiol.* 2013;112:671–677.
31. Lewinter C, Torp-Pedersen C, Cleland JG, Kober L. Right and left bundle branch block as predictors of long-term mortality following myocardial infarction. *Eur J Heart Failure* 2011;13:1349–1354.
32. Sgarbossa EB, Pinski SL, Barbagelata A, et al. Electrocardiographic diagnosis of evolving acute myocardial infarction in the presence of left bundle-branch block. GUSTO-1 (Global Utilization of Streptokinase and Tissue Plasminogen Activator for Occluded Coronary Arteries) Investigators. *New Engl J Med.* 1996;334:481–487.
33. Wong CK, Stewart RA, Gao W, et al. Prognostic differences between different types of bundle branch block during the early phase of acute myocardial infarction: insights from the Hirulog and Early Reperfusion or Occlusion (HERO)-2 trial. *Eur Heart J.* 2006;27:21–28.
34. Tabas JA, Rodriguez RM, Seligman HK, Goldschlager NF. Electrocardiographic criteria for detecting acute myocardial infarction in patients with left bundle branch block: a meta-analysis. *Ann Emerg Med.* 2008;52:329e1–336e1.
35. Smith SW, Dodd KW, Henry TD, Dvorak DM, Pearce LA. Diagnosis of ST-elevation myocardial infarction in the presence of left bundle branch block with the ST-elevation to S-wave ratio in a modified Sgarbossa rule. *Ann Emerg Med.* 2012;60:766–776.
36. Shvilkin A, Bojovic B, Vajdic B, et al. Vectorcardiographic and electrocardiographic criteria to distinguish new and old left bundle branch block. *Heart Rhythm.* 2010;7:1085–1092.
37. Shvilkin A, Ho KK, Rosen MR, Josephson ME. T-vector direction differentiates postpacing from ischemic T-wave inversion in precordial leads. *Circulation.* 2005;111:969–974.
38. Al-Faleh H, Fu Y, Wagner G, et al. Unraveling the spectrum of left bundle branch block in acute myocardial infarction: insights from the Assessment of the Safety and Efficacy of a New Thrombolytic (ASSENT 2 and 3) trials. *Am Heart J.* 2006;151:10–15.
39. Cabrera E, Friedland C. [Wave of ventricular activation in left bundle branch block with infarct; a new electrocardiographic sign]. *Gaceta Med Mexico.* 1953;83:273–280.
40. Kindwall KE, Brown JP, Josephson ME. Predictive accuracy of criteria for chronic myocardial infarction in pacing-induced left bundle branch block. *Am J Cardiol.* 1986;57:1255–1260.
41. Josephson M, Wellens HJJ. "Josephson and Wellens: How to Approach Complex Arrhythmias." Medtronic EP Fellows Training and Transition Program, 2013.

CHAPTER

14

T-Wave Memory

Henry D. Huang, MD, Mark E. Josephson, MD, and Alexei Shvilkin, MD

INTRODUCTION

Cardiac memory (CM) is a term used to describe lasting changes in myocardial repolarization, which are evident once sinus rhythm returns following a period of abnormal ventricular activation. In clinical practice, CM is usually encountered in the setting of intermittent ventricular pacing, ventricular arrhythmia, or ventricular conduction abnormalities, most often presenting as T-wave inversions (TWI). While the development of CM itself is not believed to be of intrinsic pathologic consequence, CM may be confused with other clinically relevant conditions manifesting with TWI such as myocardial ischemia; therefore, identification of CM may help to avoid unnecessary coronary interventions. Although originally CM was described in the narrow QRS rhythms, later it was detected during continuous abnormal activation, which has important diagnostic implications, for example in the age determination of the left bundle branch block (LBBB). CM is closely related to the broader phenomenon of "electrical remodeling" and may provide insight into its mechanisms.

DEFINITION OF CM AND ITS PROPERTIES

In 1915, P. D. White was the first to observe the phenomenon of transient TWI following single ventricular premature beats.[1] Later in the 1940s, TWI following conversion to sinus rhythm was described after paroxysmal tachycardias.[2–4] Among the explanations of these transient T-wave abnormalities at the time were "anoxia" and "exhaustion" of the cardiac muscle, as well as changes in ventricular filling due to a sudden prolongation of diastole following the cessation of tachycardia. Later, abnormal T waves of various duration have been documented following intermittent Wolff-Parkinson-White syndrome,[5–10] transient ventricular pacing,[11,12] LBBB,[13–16] and even sodium-channel blocker toxicity associated QRS widening.[17]

It was not until 1982 that Rosenbaum et al[18] finally introduced the term "heart memory" and presented a unified hypothesis of how abnormal ventricular activation could lead to the development of T-wave abnormalities by a process known as "electrotonic modulation." In this seminal paper, he summarized 3 principles of CM: (1) the spatial direction of T waves in sinus rhythm should follow the direction of the QRS complex during abnormal activation; (2) the amplitude of abnormal T wave should increase the longer abnormal conduction continues; and (3) repeated disruption in the activation sequence should result in more rapid and intense accumulation of T-wave changes analogous to memory formation due to synaptic plasticity in the central nervous system.

The ECG Handbook of Contemporary Challenges © 2015 Mohammad Shenasa, Mark E. Josephson, N.A. Mark Estes III
Cardiotext Publishing, ISBN: 978-1-935395-88-1

Later observations by Costard-Jackle et al[19] in an isolated rabbit heart confirmed the gradual development of an inverse relationship between local activation and repolarization times upon initiation of ventricular pacing, suggesting CM is a part of the adaptation to the new activation sequence to achieve optimal repolarization. The adaptive nature of this process is further evidenced by the fact that CM development during ventricular pacing results in QT interval shortening, while QT prolongs when normal conduction is restored.[20]

Figure 14.1A illustrates properties of CM in a chronic canine model of ventricular pacing.

Leads I and aVF are shown on the top. At baseline (left column) T waves during sinus rhythm are positive in both leads. Left ventricular pacing (column 2) results in wide QRS with secondary T-wave abnormalities and discordant T waves. Pacing interruption after 7 and 21 days results in the development of progressive (accumulation) TWI during sinus rhythm that persists during day 3 of recovery. The polarity of T waves corresponds to the polarity of paced QRS complex.

At the bottom, the corresponding frontal plane vectorcardiograms are displayed demonstrating the gradual alignment of the T-vector loop during sinus rhythm with the QRS loop during ventricular pacing.

Vectorcardiogram has proved to be extremely useful in studying CM allowing T-wave changes to be expressed quantitatively as the 3-dimensional distance between T-vector loop peaks during sinus rhythm at baseline and after the period of abnormal activation (T-vector displacement, measured in mV,[21] Figure 14.1B).

MOLECULAR MECHANISMS OF THE 2 PHASES: SHORT-TERM AND LONG-TERM CM

The ST segment and T waves on 12-lead surface ECG are concurrent with the repolarization phase of the cardiac action potential and reflect the summation of transmural (endocardial to epicardial surface) and regional (apical-basal and right-to-left) ventricular gradients although relative contributions of these gradients remain controversial.[22] It is believed that regional modification of the repolarizing currents affecting these gradients is the primary mechanism of T-wave changes caused by CM. In the setting of CM, there is a prolongation of the epicardial action potential resulting in the decrease or disappearance of the endo-epicardial transmural gradient normally present at baseline[23] (Figure 14.2).

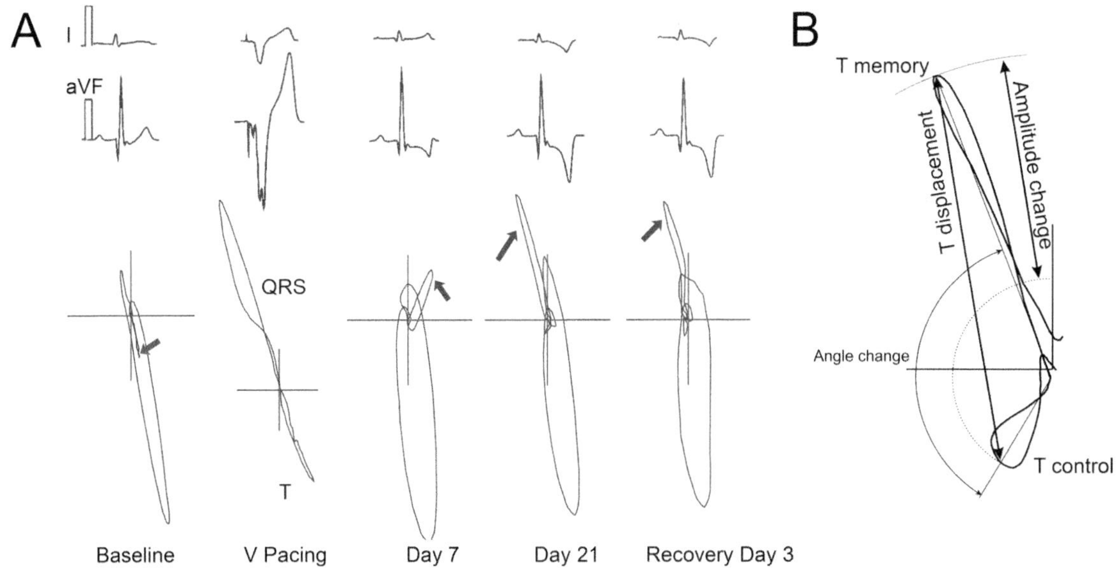

Figure 14.1. A: Development and resolution of CM in a chronic canine model of epicardial left ventricular pacing. Leads I, aVF, and frontal plane VCG are shown at baseline during ventricular pacing. One hour after interruption of ventricular pacing for 7, 21 days, and 3 days after cessation of ventricular pacing. Note the increase in T-vector amplitude and rotation towards the direction of the paced QRS complex (*arrows*). Cross-hair represents calibration at 1 mV. (From Yu et al.[44] Reprinted with permission from Wolters Kluwer Health.) B: Quantitative assessment of CM. The baseline and memory T-vector loops superimposed. CM can be measured by the change in T vector direction, amplitude, and 3-dimensional distance (T-peak displacement, TPD measured in mV) between T-vector peaks ("T control" represents the baseline T-vector loop, "T memory" represents T-vector loop after CM induction). TPD is the preferred method of CM measurement. (From Plotnikov et al.[21] Reprinted with permission from Oxford University Press.)

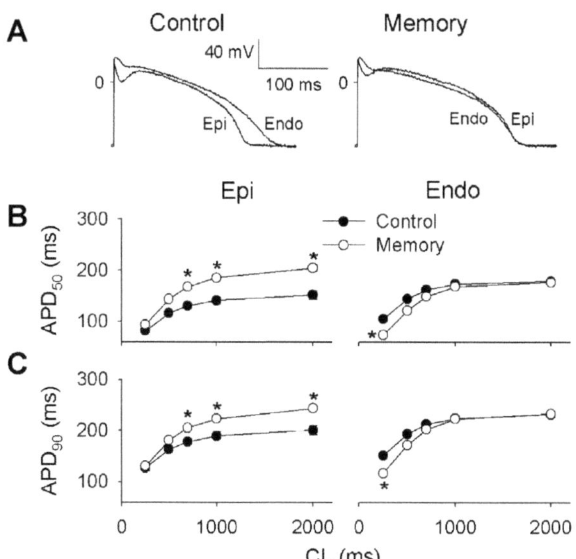

Figure 14.2. CM-induced changes in the action potential shape and duration. A. Representative experiments showing superimposed epicardial and endocardial action potential in a control dog and a dog with CM at cycle length = 1000 ms. B, C. Effects of CM on APD50 (B) and APD 90 (C) in epicardium and endocardium. *P < 0.05 versus respective control at the same cycle length. (From Obreztchikova et al.[23] Reprinted with permission from Elsevier.)

Action potential changes observed in CM are caused by alterations of multiple ion channels, receptors, and cell coupling. Originally, the epicardial action potential prolongation with the loss of the characteristic Phase 1 notch was attributed to the decrease in the transient outward current, Ito. Since then, multiple other channels including IKr[23] and ICa[26] were also implicated in CM development. In addition, AT1 angiotensin receptors[27] and stretch-activated receptors[28] were shown to be involved. Gap junction redistribution, potentially further affecting electrophysiological properties of the myocardium, has also been observed in the setting of CM.[29]

It is now clear that CM comprises a spectrum of two distinct but overlapping phenomena, which differ in the molecular mechanisms of initiation and perpetuation: short-term and long-term CM.[30] Short-term CM is observed within minutes of ventricular pacing and is thought to occur from modulation and/or modification of existing proteins and channel trafficking. Therefore, it is relatively short-lived and dissipates within minutes. Long-term CM is seen following longer periods of abnormal activation. There is an evidence that T-wave changes in long-term CM may peak and plateau after a few weeks of ventricular pacing in humans. In the laboratory, it has been confirmed that long intervals of abnormal activation allow time for *de novo* protein synthesis and changes in cell coupling, which are not seen in short-term CM.[33]

These molecular mechanisms explain the "accumulation" property of CM by increasing duration of abnormal activation, summarized by Rosenbaum as "... the longer the teaching lasts, the better the cells will learn the lesson."[18]

The unified concept of CM mechanisms was developed by the work of Rosen et al and postulate the changes in the local mechanical ventricular wall stress as the primary initiating event (as opposed to "electrotonic modulation" originally proposed by Rosenbaum).[30] Altered contractility pattern induces the local angiotensin II release which in turn affects the repolarization currents. For example, internalization of the angiotensin AT1 receptor/Kv4.3/KchIP2 complex results in the decrease of Ito1 current in short-term CM, while the reduction in the transcription factor CREB diminishes its protein synthesis and Ito1 current in the long-term CM.

For detailed discussion of molecular mechanisms of short and long-term CM, see comprehensive reviews.[30,34]

CM IN NARROW QRS RHYTHMS

Traditionally, clinical presentation of CM has been associated with TWI during sinus rhythm with narrow QRS for several reasons.

First, normal T waves during sinus rhythm are positive in the majority of the leads and TWI is usually associated with pathologic conditions (strain, ischemia). Therefore, T-wave changes are more likely to be noticed when TWI is present. Second, in the majority of scenarios leading to CM development (LBBB, right ventricular apical pacing) major QRS deflections are negative in most of the leads and therefore produce TWI.

Third, large secondary repolarization changes during wide QRS rhythms mask CM until the QRS becomes narrow (Figure 14.3).

However, it is important to keep in mind that CM can produce not only TWI but also tall, positive T waves if the wide QRS causing CM is positive (such as in manifest left-sided accessory bypass tracts, either intermittent or after ablation, or left ventricular tachycardias). In these cases, CM can be confused with hyperkalemia, transmural ischemia, or pericarditis.

Figure 14.4 demonstrates CM after ablation of a left posteroseptal bypass tract. Panel A shows tall, positive delta waves in precordial leads. ECG in panel B obtained 30 minutes after the bypass tract ablation demonstrates tall, peaked T waves across the precordium as well as inferior TWI corresponding to the vector of delta wave. ECG in panel C obtained 1 week after ablation has decrease in the amplitude of both positive and negative T-wave deflections. It took

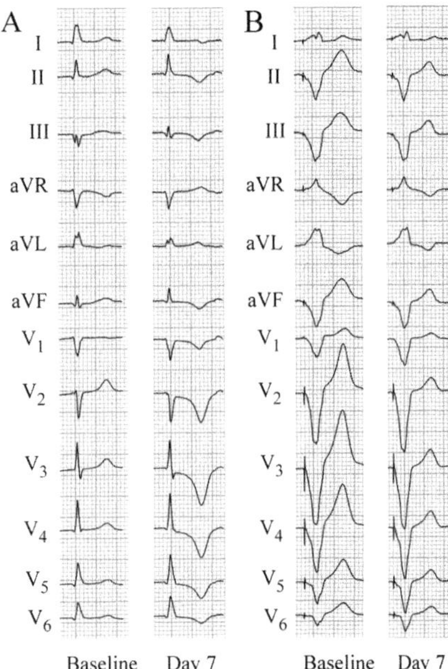

Figure 14.3. 12-lead ECG during AAI (A) and DDD (B) pacing before (baseline) and after induction of CM (Day 7). On Day 7 during AAI pacing, T waves in multiple leads become inverted assuming the polarity of the paced QRS complex. During DDD pacing, CM manifests as a decrease in the T-wave amplitude with no change in polarity. Subtle changes in QRS axis and amplitude between baseline and Day 7 are most likely positional. (From Shvilkin et al.[20] Reproduced with permission from Elsevier.)

6 months for the ECG to normalize completely (not shown). A year later, the patient was again noted to have T-wave abnormalities and his Holter monitor showed the evidence of intermittent preexcitation although without symptomatic arrhythmias. Therefore, sometimes CM can be used to monitor the recurrence of abnormal antegrade conduction over the bypass.

Recurrent monomorphic ventricular tachycardia can also produce CM. In this case, T-wave polarity in sinus rhythm, which follows the QRS polarity during arrhythmia, provides a rough estimate of its axis and origin. ECG tracings of a patient with structurally normal heart and frequent episodes of verapamil-sensitive ventricular tachycardia are presented on Figure 14.5. Based on the presence of inferior TWI and tall peaked T waves in the right precordial leads, one can estimate its origin in the inferior portion of the left ventricle relatively close to the septum (left precordial TWI are not pronounced, excluding left lateral origin).

As becomes evident from the case presentations above, CM always produces a mixture of positive and negative T-wave changes based on the "offending" QRS vector polarity although positive changes are often overlooked. Nevertheless, it is the positive T-wave changes that are critically important in some clinical applications of CM (see below).

CLINICAL APPLICATIONS OF CM IN NARROW QRS: DISTINGUISHING BETWEEN TWI FROM CM AND ISCHEMIA

Since the time CM was first recognized, its similarity to ischemic TWI has made it a significant cofounder in the diagnosis of myocardial ischemia. In particular, precordial TWI due to intermittent right ventricular pacing or LBBB (by far the most commonly encountered presentations of CM in clinical practice) can be easily confused with the Wellens' syndrome characteristic of ischemia due to the transient proximal left anterior descending artery occlusion, a condition requiring prompt coronary intervention to avoid extensive infarction.

A set of criteria was developed to differentiate CM due to the right ventricular pacing from the ischemic TWI[37] based on the following considerations.

Generally, the direction of the ischemic T waves points away from the area of ischemia. Since the ischemic region usually involves the left ventricle, the ischemic TWI has a rightward axis in the frontal plane and is characterized by TWI in leads I and aVL (Figure 14.6A).

On the other hand, right ventricular apical pacing and LBBB have QRS vectors positive in leads I and aVL resulting in positive T waves in these leads upon resumption of normal conduction (Figure 14.6C).

There is a rare pattern of infero lateral ischemia due to right coronary artery (RCA) lesions that produces positive T waves in leads I and aVL (Figure 14.6B). However, in the RCA ischemia, TWI is deeper in magnitude in the inferior leads (II, III, and aVF) than the deepest TWI in the precordial leads, whereas the reverse is true for CM-induced TWI. The following combination of criteria was found to be highly accurate in discriminating CM-induced TWI from ischemia.[37]

- Positive T in lead aVL.
- Positive/isoelectric in lead I.
- Precordial TWI> inferior TWI.

Although not confirmed in larger prospective trials, these easily applicable criteria have been used successfully in clinical practice to distinguish between CM and ischemia.[38] Since the axis during RV pacing and LBBB is similar with positive QRS complex in leads I and aVL, the criteria can also be extended to cases of TWI due to intermittent LBBB.[39] One possible limitation in using this diagnostic tool is that T-wave changes due to CM can counter balance or obscure ischemic TWI when CM and ischemia occur simultaneously in the same patient. No published data are available in patients with T-wave abnormalities due to coronary artery disease, but our preliminary results in this population indicate that CM does not "override"

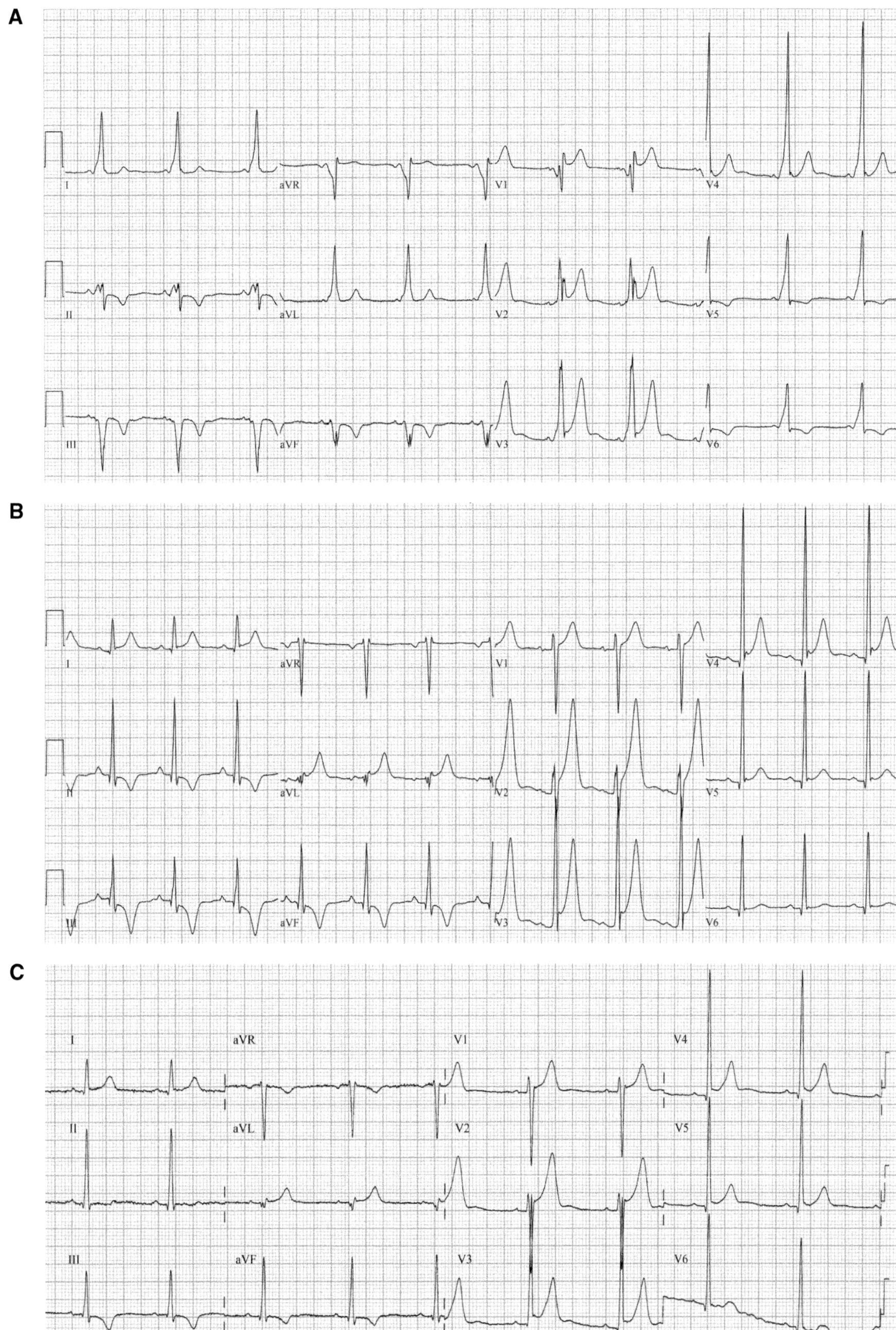

Figure 14.4. CM after ablation of a left posteroseptal accessory bypass tract. **A**. Before ablation. Left posteroseptal bypass tract is present. **B**. Thirty minutes after ablation. Note tall, positive-peaked T waves in the right precordial leads as well as inferior TWI. **C**. One week after ablation. Both positive and negative T waves decreased in amplitude but have not normalized completely.

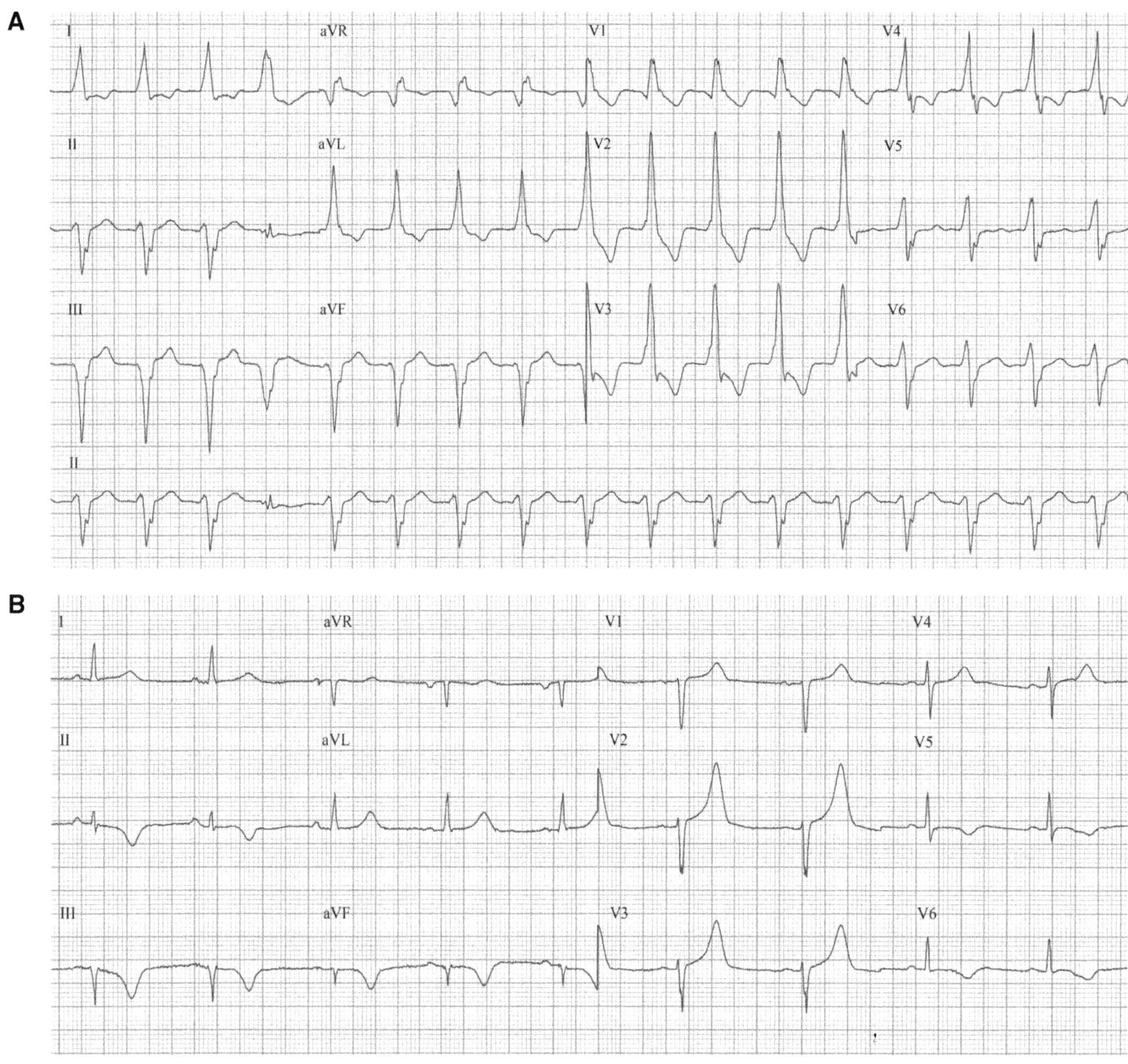

Figure 14.5. CM in a setting of recurrent monomorphic ventricular tachycardia. **A.** Exercise-induced, verapamil-sensitive ventricular tachycardia in a patient with structurally normal heart. **B.** Sinus rhythm after spontaneous termination of arrhythmia. Note tall, positive T waves in the right precordial leads corresponding to the right bundle branch block (RBBB) QRS configuration during VT.

ischemic TWI lessening the possibility of missing myocardial ischemia. Notable though is that when TWI in leads I and aVL are present at baseline as the result of the structural heart disease, T waves stay inverted despite the development of CM (T vector never fully aligns with the paced QRS vector), which can result in over-diagnosis of ischemia. Regardless, clinical history or presence of markedly positive biomarkers should take precedence over decisions made from ECG findings alone.

CM IN WIDE QRS RHYTHMS WITH SECONDARY REPOLARIZATION CHANGES

Despite the fact that processes underlying CM do not develop suddenly upon disappearance of abnormal ventricular activation but rather progress gradually, for a long time it was thought that CM cannot be detected until QRS becomes narrow. Though the concept of simultaneous repolarization changes due to the LBBB or ventricular pacing and from CM might be hard to grasp, one may view secondary T-wave changes due to the LBBB or ventricular pacing as early and dominant, whereas CM-induced T-wave changes are delayed and nondominant, but gradually increasing in time as progressive alterations at the molecular level take hold. The assessment of CM by surface ECG in the setting of wide QRS is limited due to the dominance of secondary T-wave changes, and repolarization changes due to CM in this situation have been largely overlooked being masked by the large discordant T waves. CM, in this situation, can be readily detected using vectorcardiogram. Figure 14.7

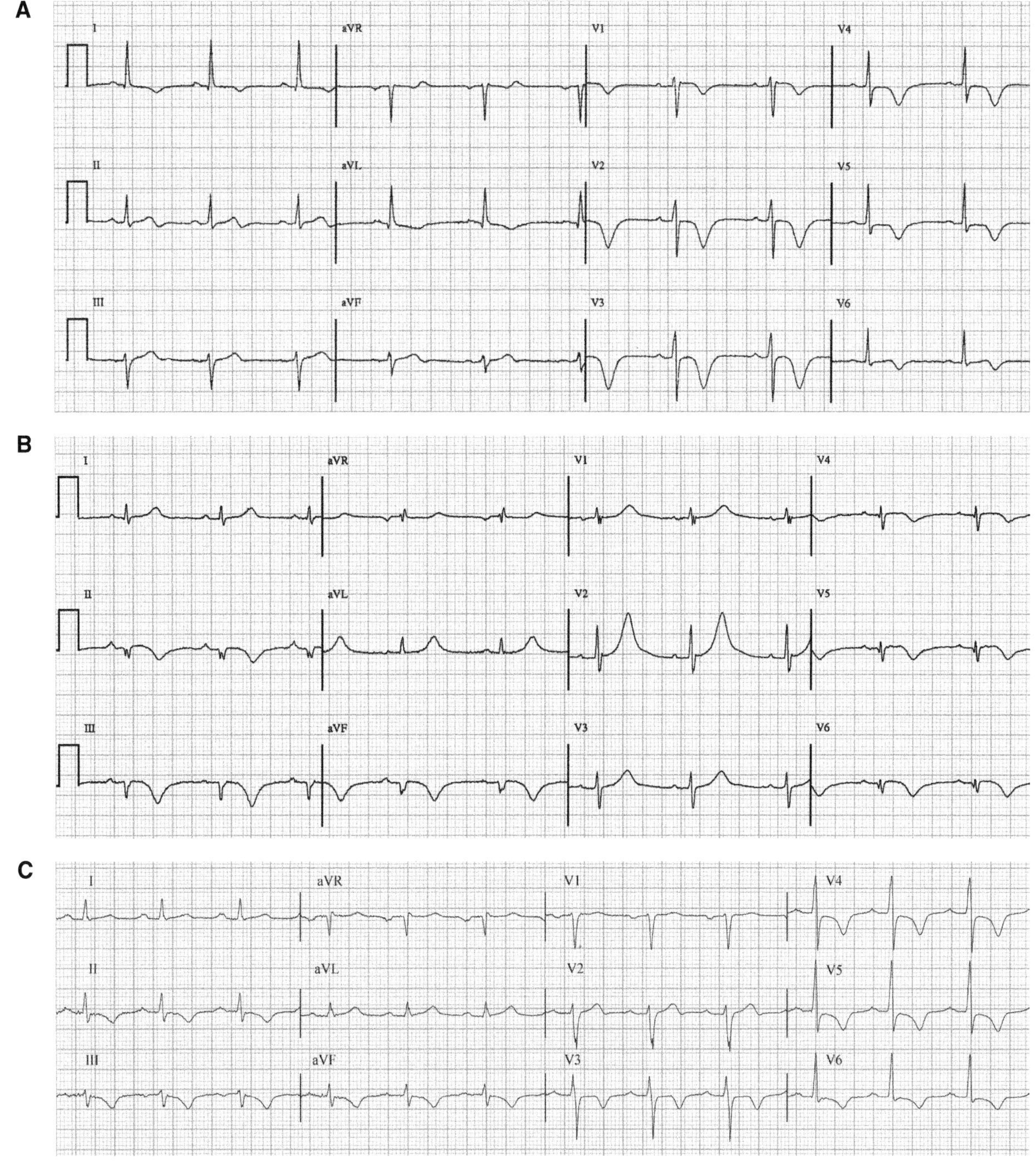

Figure 14.6. TWI due to ischemia and CM. **A.** LAD ischemia. Note TWI in leads I, aVL. **B.** Dominant RCA ischemia. Although the TWI pattern is similar to CM due to the right ventricular pacing (positive T waves in leads I, aVL), the ratio of inferior to precordial TWI is different (maximal inferior TWI > maximal precordial TWI). **C.** TWI due to CM. T waves in leads I, aVL are positive; precordial TWI > inferior TWI.

presents the vectorcardiogram of the patient shown in Figure 14.3 demonstrating the 3-dimensional T-vector displacement after 7 days of right ventricular pacing during narrow (AAI pacing) and wide (DDD pacing) QRS. The actual T vector change in narrow and wide QRS is nearly identical in both magnitude and direction. As seen on both Figures 14.3 and 14.7, CM in wide QRS rhythms presents as a decrease in T-vector magnitude without directional change in contrast to the narrow QRS rhythm where T vector becomes larger and rotates towards the paced QRS.

CLINICAL APPLICATION OF CM IN WIDE QRS: AGE DETERMINATION OF LBBB

The feature of CM to decrease discordant T-wave amplitude in wide QRS rhythms has important clinical

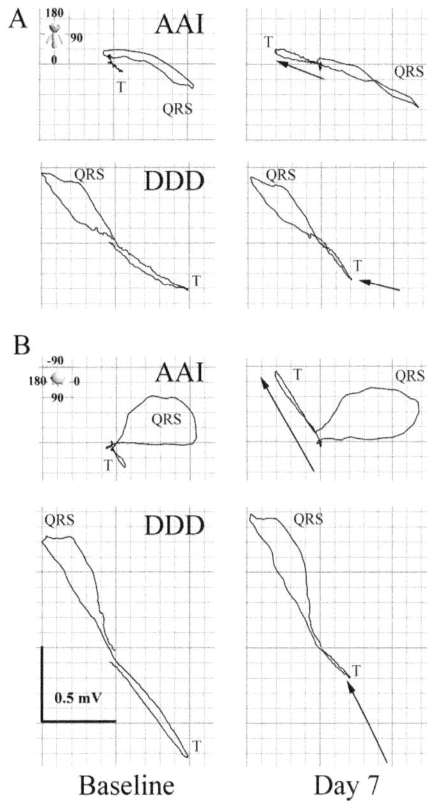

Figure 14.7. Vectorcardiogram of the patient in Figure 14.3 during AAI and DDD pacing in frontal (A) and transverse (B) projections before (baseline) and after induction of CM (Day 7). On Day 7 during AAI pacing, the T vector assumes the direction of the paced QRS complex while increasing in magnitude. At the same time in DDD mode, the T-vector magnitude decreases without significant change in direction. Black arrows indicate the direction and magnitude of the projection of T-peak displacement (TPD) as the result of CM and are very similar in AAI and DDD modes. Sagittal plane (not shown) showed similar changes. (From Shvilkin et al.[20] Reproduced with permission from Elsevier.)

implications. For example, it can be used to determine whether LBBB is old or new, which becomes extremely valuable in the setting of chest pain.

Current American College of Cardiology/American Heart Association Guidelines for the management of patients with ST elevation myocardial infarction consider new or presumed new LBBB a class I indication for reperfusion therapy when associated with symptoms suggestive of ischemia[40] creating a decision-making dilemma.

In addition, recent attention has been brought to a condition called "Painful LBBB Syndrome" which is characterized by chest pain, onset, and resolution of which is simultaneous with the onset and resolution of intermittent LBBB, often rate-dependent (and therefore exercise-induced).[41] Patients with painful LBBB have no evidence of myocardial ischemia but often undergo urgent cardiac catheterization since they fall into the abovementioned guidelines.

In clinical practice, determining whether LBBB is actually "new" is virtually impossible as prior ECGs for comparison even if available are usually dated well beyond the relevant period of time (from the onset of symptoms which ranges from minutes to a few hours). LBBB in the vast majority of patients presenting with chest pain is old.

The criterion for LBBB age determination was developed[42] on the premise that new LBBB would have larger T vector (and taller T waves on a 12-lead ECG) compared to the old one. As the duration of LBBB increases, discordant secondary T waves become smaller (Figure 14.8A). A retrospective analysis over 1700 LBBB ECGs showed that indeed the new onset LBBB (defined as less than 24 hours duration) had significantly larger T waves as well as smaller QRS vector magnitude compared to the chronic LBBB. The 12-lead ECG criterion for LBBB age determination uses the ratio of the maximal precordial S wave to the maximal precordial T wave (used as approximations of the QRS and T vectors, respectively). A conservative cutoff of $S/T < 2.5$ allows to detect 100% of the new LBBBs. In reality, the T-vector magnitude in LBBB changes significantly over the first 24 hours. In cases of painful LBBB when ECG is recorded within seconds/minutes of symptom onset (often during an exercise stress test), S/T ratio can be as low as 1.4. The majority of T-wave changes occur within the first 24 hours of LBBB persistence when it assumes "chronic" QRST configuration. In the true chronic LBBB, the S/T ratio is close to 3.0 or greater (Figure 14.8A–D). It is important to recognize that LBBB is often a dynamic phenomenon and can be intermittent or rate-dependent. Repeated episodes of intermittent LBBB can cause accumulation of CM-related T-wave changes, sometimes making the distinction between new and old LBBB difficult.

The "new" LBBB S/T criterion held true in a small subgroup of patients with acute coronary syndrome (Figure 14.8D) but needs to be confirmed in larger clinical trials.

Using this criterion in low risk patients can help justify conservative management and avoid unnecessary coronary interventions.

CM IN THE SETTING OF BIVENTRICULAR PACING

Dynamic T-wave changes have been reported in the setting of biventricular pacing.[43] This situation is of a particular interest as it demonstrates that the CM can develop on top of already existing CM-induced repolarization changes and the heart is capable of "re-learning". Whether the new T waves follow the biventricular or left ventricular paced QRS direction

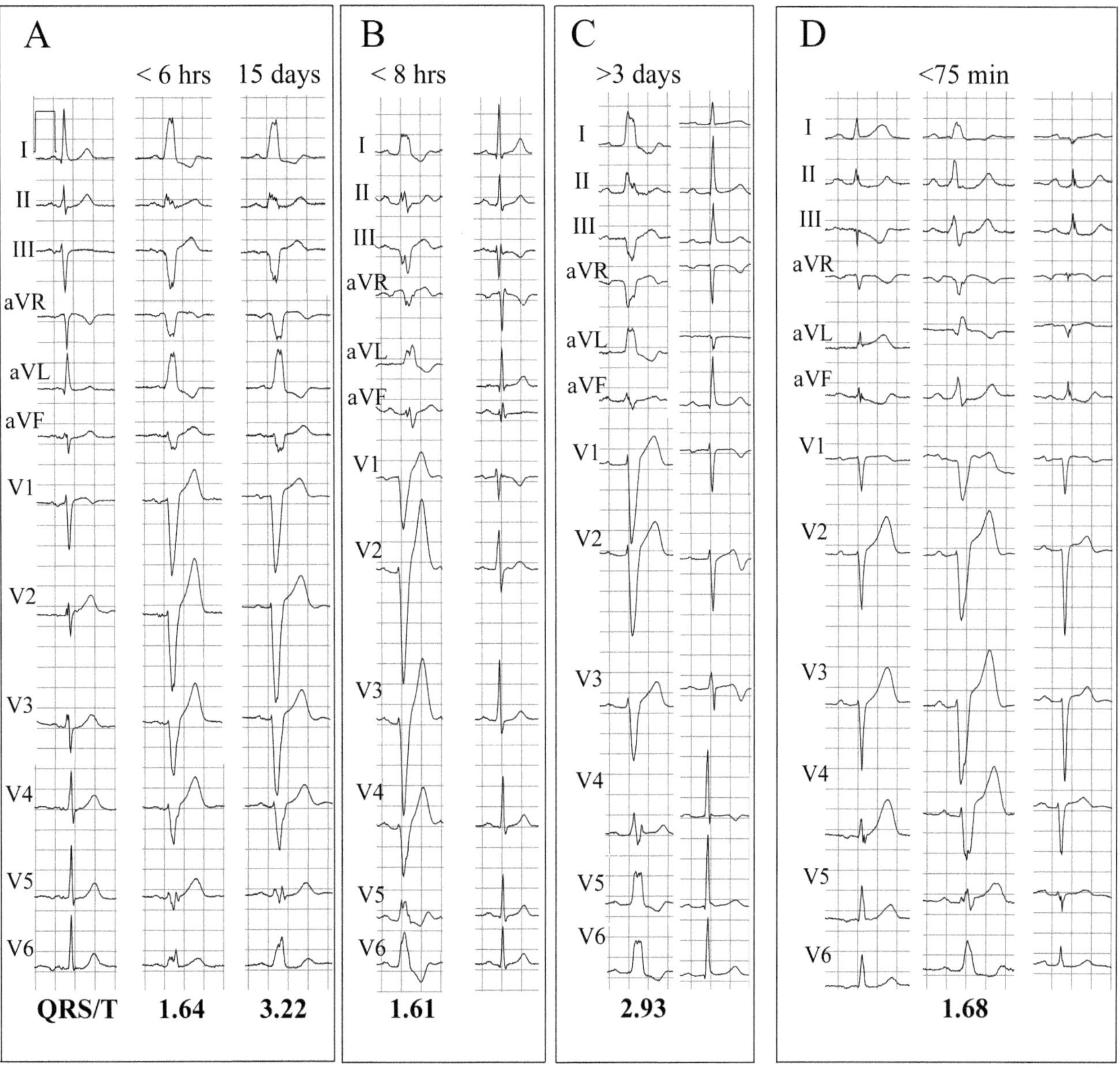

Figure 14.8. Utility of the S/T ratio in LBBB age determination. **A.** As duration of LBBB increases the S/T ratio increases from 1.64 (= new) to 3.22 (= old). **B.** A typical example of resolution of a "new" LBBB (< 8 hours duration). S/T ratio is 1.61. Resolution of LBBB results in no apparent T wave abnormalities in narrow QRS. **C.** A typical example of resolution of an "old" LBBB (< 3 days duration). S/T ratio is 2.93. Typical changes of CM with precordial TWI are evident in narrow QRS. **D.** A new onset LBBB (< 75 minute) in a setting of acute LAD thrombosis. S/T ratio is 1.68 consistent with new LBBB. Note ST segment changes in baseline tracing consistent with ischemia and loss of R waves after resolution of LBBB. (From Shvilkin et al.[42] Reproduced with permission from Elsevier.)

as well as clinical significance of these changes is the subject of further research.

CONCLUSIONS

1. CM is a normal universal property of the heart resulting from the adaptation of repolarization to the new activation sequence manifesting by T-wave changes.
2. Signs of CM can be detected during both narrow and wide QRS rhythms.
3. CM is frequently encountered in clinical practice and the knowledge of its features can help improve ECG diagnosis.

REFERENCES

1. White P. Alteration of the pulse: A common clinical condition. *Am J Med Sci.* 1915;150:82–96.
2. Currie GM. Transient inverted T waves after paroxysmal tachycardia. *Br Heart J.* 1942;4:149–152.
3. Scherf D. Alterations in the form of the T waves with changes in heart rate. *Am Heart J.* 1944;28:332–347.

4. Campbell M. Inversion of T waves after long paroxysms of tachycardia. *Br Heart J.* 1942;4:49–56.
5. Nicolai P, Medvedowsky JL, Delaage M, et al. Wolff-Parkinson-White syndrome: T wave abnormalities during normal pathway conduction. *J Electrocardiol.* 1981;14:295–300.
6. Sawada K, Hirai M, Hayashi H, et al. Spatial ventricular gradient in patients with Wolff-Parkinson-White syndrome in comparison with normal subjects: Vectorcardiographic evidence for significant repolarization changes due to preexcitation. *Intern Med.* 1995;34:738–743.
7. Nirei T, Kasanuki H, Ohnishi S, et al. Cardiac memory in patients with intermittent Wolff-Parkinson-White syndrome. *J Electrocardiol.* 1997;30:323–329.
8. Geller JC, Carlson MD, Goette A, et al. Persistent T-wave changes after radiofrequency catheter ablation of an accessory connection (Wolff-Parkinson-White syndrome) are caused by "cardiac memory". *Am Heart J.* 1999;138:987–993.
9. Herweg B, Fisher JD, Ilercil A, et al. Cardiac memory after radiofrequency ablation of accessory pathways: The post-ablation T wave does not forget the pre-excited QRS. *J Interv Card Electrophysiol.* 1999;3:263–272.
10. Poole JE, Bardy GH. Further evidence supporting the concept of T-wave memory: Observation in patients having undergone high-energy direct current catheter ablation of the Wolff-Parkinson-White syndrome. *Eur Heart J.* 1992;13:801–807.
11. Chatterjee K, Harris A, Davies G, Leatham A. Electrocardiographic changes subsequent to artificial ventricular depolarization. *Br Heart J.* 1969;31:770–779.
12. Gould L, Venkataraman K, Goswami MK, Gomprecht RF. Pacemaker-induced electrocardiographic changes simulating myocardial infarction. *Chest.* 1973;63:829–832.
13. Engel TR, Shah R, DePodesta LA, Frankl WS, Krause RL. T-wave abnormalities of intermittent left bundle-branch block. *Ann Intern Med.* 1978;89:204–206.
14. Gould L, Reddy CV, Singh B, Zen B. T-wave changes with intermittent left bundle branch block. *Angiology.* 1980;31:66–68.
15. Denes P, Pick A, Miller RH, Pietras RJ, Rosen KM. A characteristic precordial repolarization abnormality with intermittent left bundle-branch block. *Ann Intern Med.* 1978;89:55–57.
16. Bauer GE. Transient bundle-branch block. *Circulation.* 1964;29:730–738.
17. Wylie JV, Jr., Zimetbaum P, Josephson ME, Shvilkin A. Cardiac memory induced by QRS widening due to propafenone toxicity. *Pacing Clin Electrophysiol.* 2007;30:1161–1164.
18. Rosenbaum MB, Blanco HH, Elizari MV, Lazzari JO, Davidenko JM. Electrotonic modulation of the T wave and cardiac memory. *Am J Cardiol.* 1982;50:213–222.
19. Costard-Jackle A, Goetsch B, Antz M, Franz MR. Slow and long-lasting modulation of myocardial repolarization produced by ectopic activation in isolated rabbit hearts. Evidence for cardiac "memory". *Circulation.* 1989;80:1412–1420.
20. Shvilkin A, Bojovic B, Vajdic B, et al. Vectorcardiographic determinants of cardiac memory during normal ventricular activation and continuous ventricular pacing. *Heart Rhythm.* 2009;6:943–948.
21. Plotnikov AN, Shvilkin A, Xiong W, et al. Interactions between antiarrhythmic drugs and cardiac memory. *Cardiovasc Res.* 2001;50:335–344.
22. Janse MJ, Sosunov EA, Coronel R, et al. Repolarization gradients in the canine left ventricle before and after induction of short-term cardiac memory. *Circulation.* 2005;112:1711–1718.
23. Obreztchikova MN, Patberg KW, Plotnikov AN, et al. I(kr) contributes to the altered ventricular repolarization that determines long-term cardiac memory. *Cardiovasc Res.* 2006;71:88–96.
24. del Balzo U, Rosen MR. T wave changes persisting after ventricular pacing in canine heart are altered by 4-aminopyridine but not by lidocaine. Implications with respect to phenomenon of cardiac "memory". *Circulation.* 1992;85:1464–1472.
25. Yu H, McKinnon D, Dixon JE, et al. Transient outward current, Ito1, is altered in cardiac memory. *Circulation.* 1999;99:1898–1905.
26. Plotnikov AN, Yu H, Geller JC, et al. Role of l-type calcium channels in pacing-induced short-term and long-term cardiac memory in canine heart. *Circulation.* 2003;107:2844–2849.
27. Doronin SV, Potapova IA, Lu Z, Cohen IS. Angiotensin receptor type 1 forms a complex with the transient outward potassium channel Kv4.3 and regulates its gating properties and intracellular localization. *J Biol Chem.* 2004;279:48231–48237.
28. Kooshkabadi M, Whalen P, Yoo D, Langberg J. Stretch-activated receptors mediate cardiac memory. *Pacing Clin Electrophysiol.* 2009;32:330–335.
29. Patel PM, Plotnikov A, Kanagaratnam P, et al. Altering ventricular activation remodels gap junction distribution in canine heart. *J Cardiovasc Electrophysiol.* 2001;12:570–577.
30. Rosen MR, Cohen IS. Cardiac memory ... New insights into molecular mechanisms. *J Physiol.* 2006;570:209–218.
31. Wecke L, Gadler F, Linde C, et al. Temporal characteristics of cardiac memory in humans: Vectorcardiographic quantification in a model of cardiac pacing. *Heart Rhythm.* 2005;2:28–34.
32. Wecke L, Rubulis A, Lundahl G, Rosen MR, Bergfeldt L. Right ventricular pacing-induced electrophysiological remodeling in the human heart and its relationship to cardiac memory. *Heart Rhythm.* 2007;4:1477–1486.
33. Shvilkin A, Danilo P, Jr., Wang J, et al. Evolution and resolution of long-term cardiac memory. *Circulation.* 1998;97:1810–1817.
34. Ozgen N, Rosen MR. Cardiac memory: A work in progress. *Heart Rhythm.* 2009;6:564–570.
35. de Zwaan C, Bar FW, Wellens HJ. Characteristic electrocardiographic pattern indicating a critical stenosis high in left anterior descending coronary artery in patients admitted because of impending myocardial infarction. *Am Heart J.* 1982;103:730–736.
36. de Zwaan C, Bar FW, Janssen JH, et al. Angiographic and clinical characteristics of patients with unstable angina showing an ECG pattern indicating critical narrowing of the proximal LAD coronary artery. *Am Heart J.* 1989;117:657–665.

37. Shvilkin A, Ho KKL, Rosen MRR, Josephson ME. T vector direction differentiates post-pacing from ischemic T wave inversion in the precordial leads. *Circulation.* 2005,111:969-974.
38. Chen-Scarabelli C, Scarabelli TM. T-wave inversion: Cardiac memory or myocardial ischemia? *Am J Emerg Med.* 2009;27:898.e1- 898.e4
39. Byrne R, Filippone L. Benign persistent T-wave inversion mimicking ischemia after left bundle-branch block – cardiac memory. *Am J Emerg Med.* 2010;28:747.e5–747.e6
40. Antman EM, Anbe DT, Armstrong PW, et al. ACC/AHA guidelines for the management of patients with ST-elevation myocardial infarction; a report of the American College of Cardiology/American Heart Association task force on practice guidelines (committee to revise the 1999 guidelines for the management of patients with acute myocardial infarction). *J Am Coll Cardiol.* 2004;44:671-719.
41. Ellis E, Gervino EV, Litvak AD, Josephson ME, Shvilkin A. The painful LBBB syndrome review of the literature and proposed diagnostic criteria. 2014 submitted for publication.
42. Shvilkin A, Bojovic B, Vajdic B, et al. Vectorcardiographic discrimination between acute and chronic left bundle branch block. *Heart Rhythm.* 2010,7:1085-1092.
43. Wecke L, van Deursen CJ, Bergfeldt L, Prinzen FW. Repolarization changes in patients with heart failure receiving cardiac resynchronization therapy-signs of cardiac memory. *J Electrocardiol.* 2011;44:590–598.
44. Yu H, McKinnon D, Dixon JE, et al. Transient outward current, Ito1, is altered in cardiac memory. *Circulation.* 1999;99:1898–1905.

CHAPTER

15

Electrocardiographic Markers of Progressive Cardiac Conduction Disease

Vincent Probst, MD, PhD and Hervé Le Marec, MD, PhD

INTRODUCTION

Progressive cardiac conduction defect (PCCD), also called as Lenègre or Lev disease, is a common disease of adults aged more than 50 years old, which remains the main cause for pacemaker (PM) implantation.[1–3] PCCD is characterized by an age-related alteration in the conduction of the cardiac impulse through the His-Purkinje system. Until recently, PCCD was considered as a degenerative process affecting the His-Purkinje pathway in relation with aging, in which hereditary and genetic factors play only a limited role. However, during the past few years, several publications have reported pedigrees in which PCCD was transmitted as an autosomal dominant trait.[4,5]

PCCD may progress to complete atrioventricular (AV) block. The first manifestation of the disease is characterized by minor conduction defects (long PR interval, presence of hemiblock on the ECG, or minor enlargement of the QRS). The age of the first ECG manifestation as well as the rapidity of the conduction defect is variable depending on the etiology of the pathology and the patient himself.

The disease is either asymptomatic or manifests as dyspnea, dizziness, syncope, abdominal pain, heart failure, or sudden death. Syncope during exertion has been reported, and the disease can progress from a normal ECG to right bundle branch block (RBBB) and from the latter to complete heart block.

The disease can be isolated or in relation to neuromuscular dystrophy or in the context of laminopathy. During the last years, the genetic basis of the disease has been explored, and several gene defects have been identified in an isolated form of the disease.

ISOLATED PCCD

There is relatively a little information on the frequency of familial and then genetic forms of the disease. Greenspahn reported an age-related familial tendency to conduction disease among relatives of patients affected by PCCD. They observed conduction defect more frequently in relatives of patients than in controls (24/95 vs. 10/95).[6]

Recently, we used a previously described approach called genetic epidemiology, in which a geographical heterogeneity of the disease frequency is evaluated from the determination of the patient's city of birth.[7] This approach is based on the hypothesis that in an area where the population is geographically stable,

The ECG Handbook of Contemporary Challenges © 2015 Mohammad Shenasa, Mark E. Josephson, N.A. Mark Estes III
Cardiotext Publishing, ISBN: 978-1-935395-88-1

the descendents of an ancestor affected by a genetic form of a disease remain in the same area during several generations, and a major difference on the disease distribution could appear within one country or region. Using this approach, we identified a major heterogeneity of the spatial distribution of the patients implanted with a PM for PCCD (Figure 15.1). Interestingly, using this approach, we were able to identify several families affected by PCCD.

The fact that the familial factor is strong enough to induce a modification of the disease distribution in this area is clearly in favor that a major genetic factor exists for the disease.[7]

Transmission is autosomal-dominant with incomplete penetrance and variable expressivity. Recessive or sporadic forms are rare.

Mutations in 3 genes have been identified as disease causing: *SCN5A*, *SCN1B*, and *TRPM4*.[8–10] A

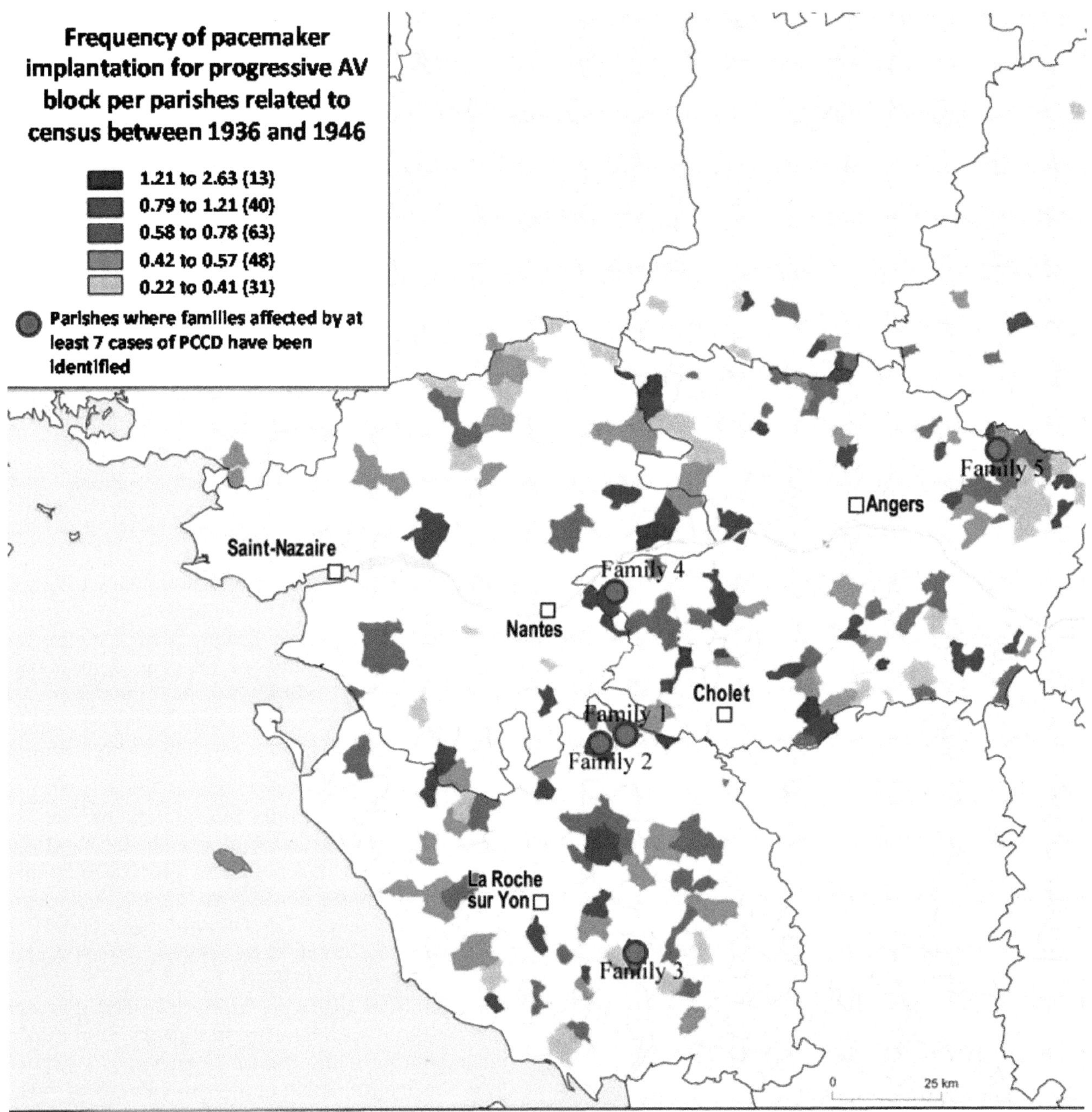

Figure 15.1. Map of the repartition of PM implantation for PCCD in the western part of France. White squares represent the main cities of Loire-Atlantique, Vendée, and Maine et Loire. Disease frequency was calculated for each Parish by comparing the number of native cases with PM implantation for PCCD to the population living in the Parish. Population was estimated with the data of the census performed in 1936 and 1946, corresponding to the average period of birth of the patients. AV, atrioventricular. (Reproduced with permission from BMJ Publishing Group Ltd.[7])

candidate gene, *GJA5*, has been associated with severe, early onset PCCD and has been described in 2 blood relatives.[11]

The type of conduction defects identified is variable depending on the gene involved. In case of *SCN5A* mutation, all types of conduction defects were observed with a homogeneous repartition between RBBB, left bundle branch block (LBBB), hemiblock, and parietal blocks (Figure 15.2). This is usually described in the Lenègre disease that is characterized by a diffuse fibrotic degeneration of the conductive system, mainly affecting the distal part of both branches.[7]

In this example, there is a typical aspect of parietal block that represents probably the more frequent aspect found in *SCN5A* mutation carriers in the first 2 patients. The third one had a RBBB associated with a long PR interval. The last one had a LBBB and a first degree AV block.

The penetrance of the conduction defect in patients carrier of *SCN5A* mutation is high (around 80%) and increases over time.[12]

The conduction defect can progress over time. As an illustration, in the patient of the Figure 15.3, there

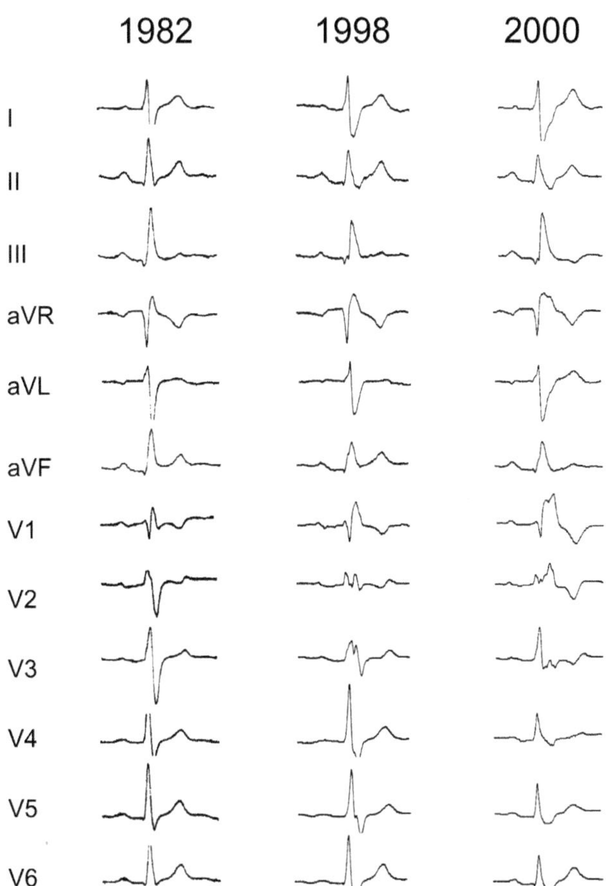

Figure 15.2. ECG aspect of *SCN5A* mutation carriers. See text for explanation.

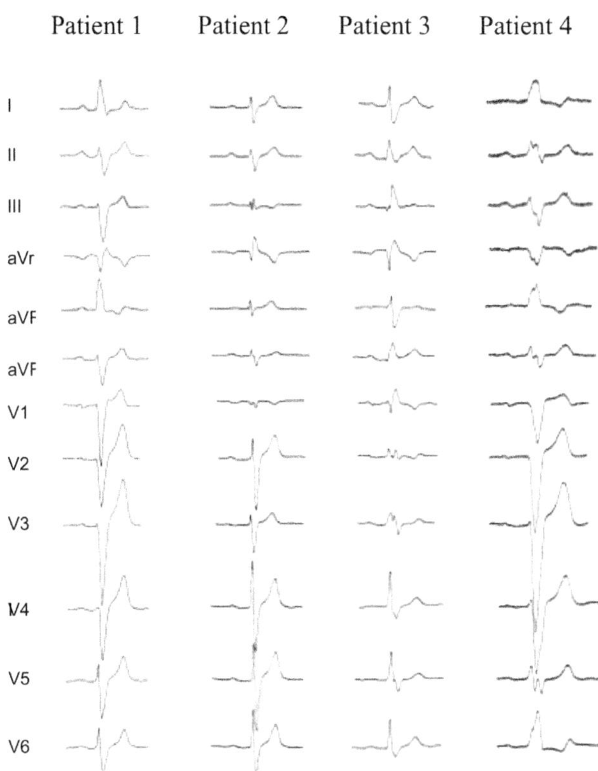

Figure 15.3. Progression of the conduction defect over time. See text for discussion.

is a clear progression of the conduction defect over time with a progressive lengthening of the QRS duration and an evolution from incomplete to complete RBBB. There is also a progressive lengthening of the PR interval with the occurrence of a first-degree AV block.

This evolution of the conduction defect over time is usual in patients carrier of an *SCN5A* mutation, but the progression is extremely variable from one patient to another and thus the presence of the mutation could not be useful at this stage to decide PM implantation in patient with only minor conduction defects.

Some cases of congenital conduction defects have also been reported in relation to *SCN5A* mutations.[8,13]

Mutations in the transient receptor potential cation channel, subfamily M, member 4 (*TRPM4*) gene have also been described.[10,14] In patients carriers of this gene mutation, the most frequent form of cardiac conduction are RBBB, followed by bifascicular block and finally complete heart block, while LBBB is infrequent (Figure 15.4). The frequency of the mutation in the patients affected by this type of conduction block remains unknown.

We also identified a third pattern of familial conduction block with a more pronounced phenotypic variability. Two-third of affected patients presented mainly with hemiblocks and parietal blocks without RBBB.

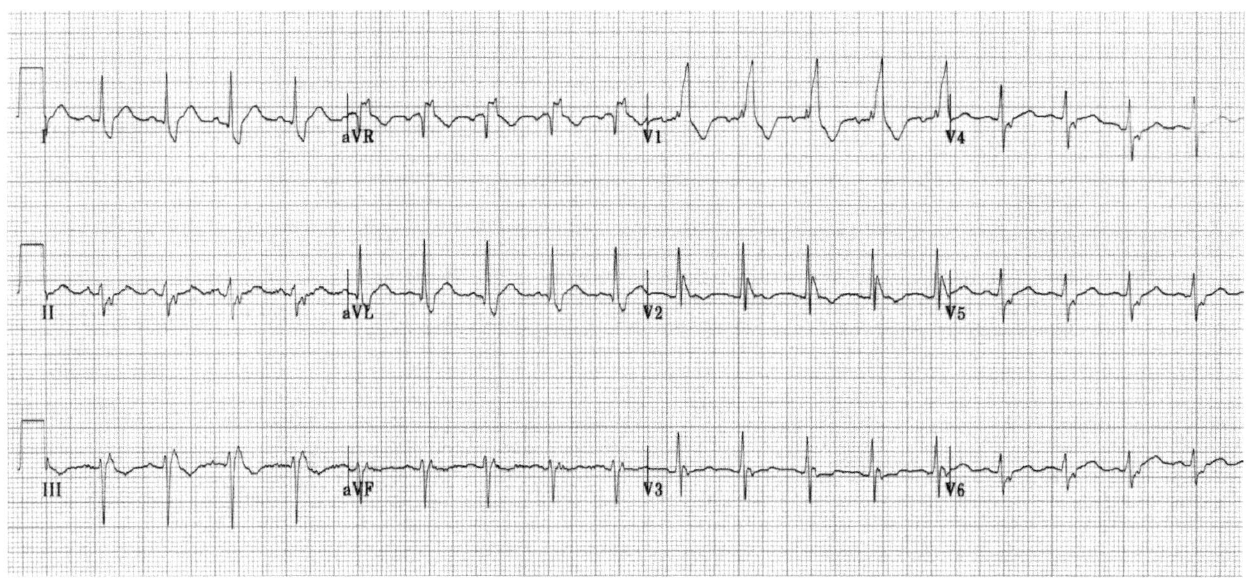

Figure 15.4. Typical aspect of bifascicular block identified in a patient carrier of a *TRPM4* mutation. See text for discussion.

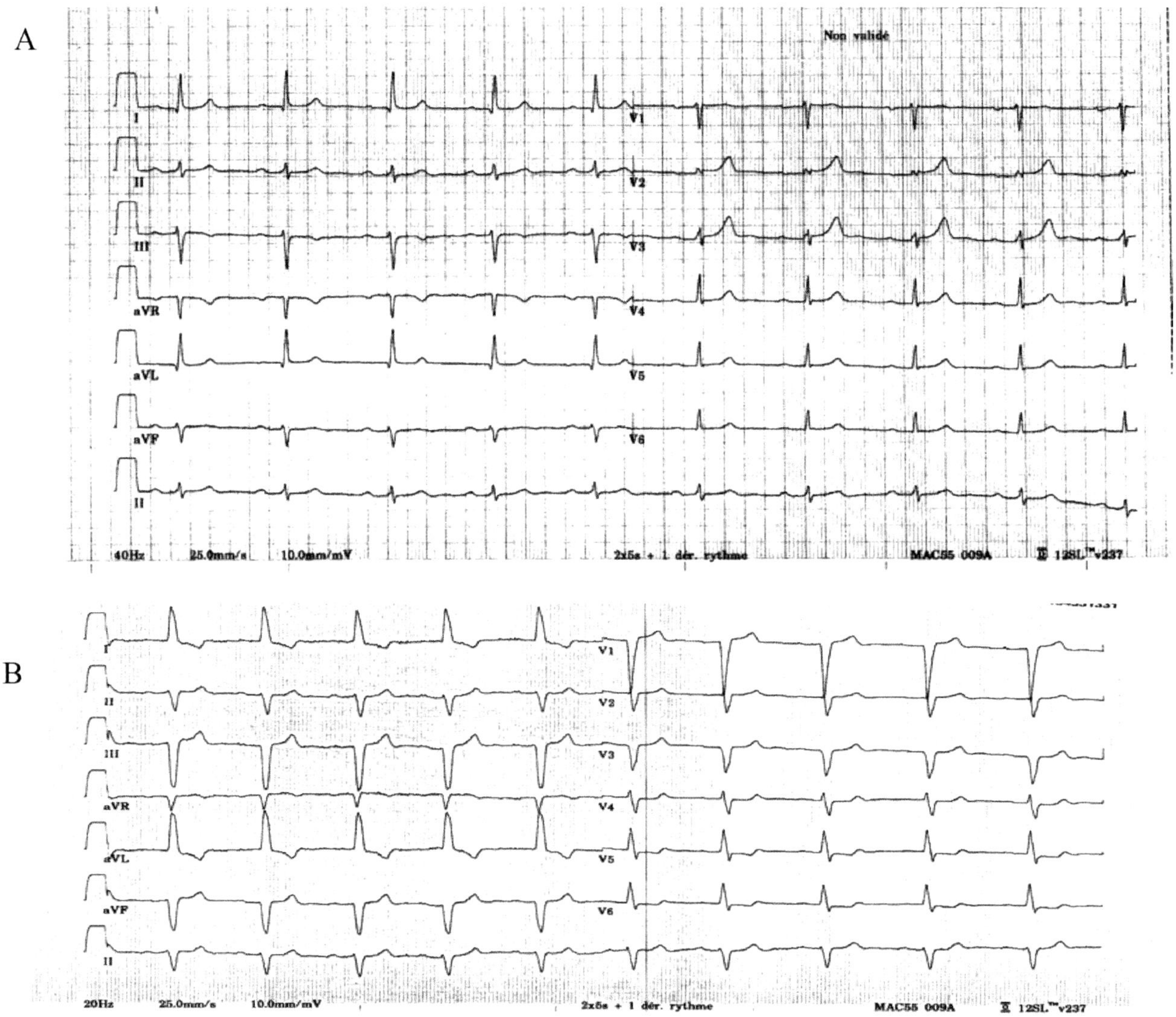

A

B

Figure 15.5. **A.** Typical aspect found at the initial phase of the disease in patients carriers of a *LMNA* mutation with a long PR interval and a left axis deviation. **B.** Later, the disease frequently progresses to complete LBBB with left axis deviation.

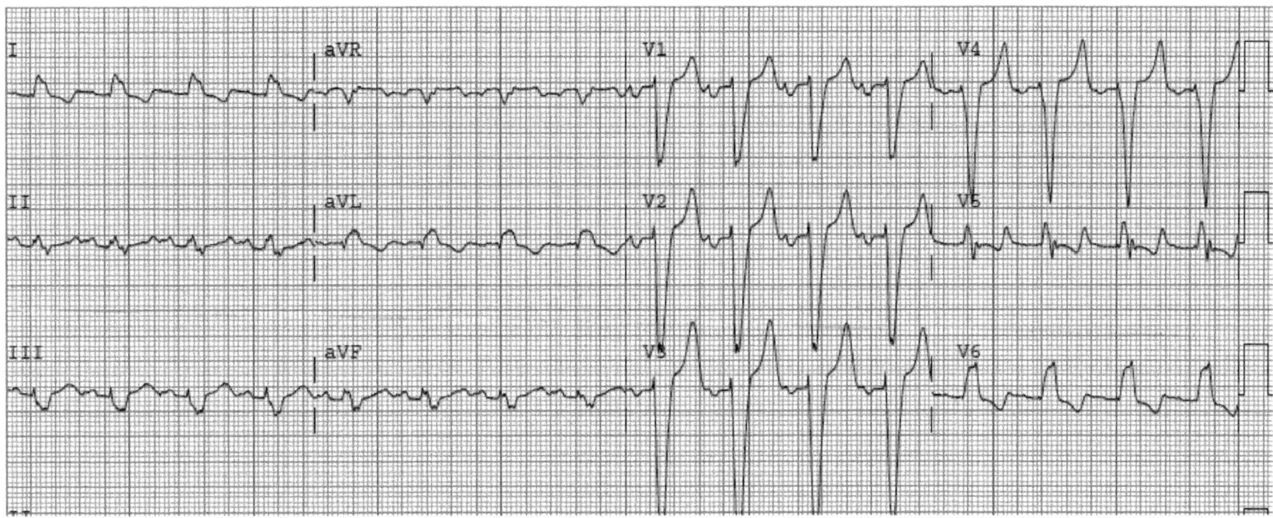

Figure 15.6. LBBB identified in a patient affected by DM1.

NONISOLATED FORMS OF PCCD

Mutations in the genes *NKX2.5*, *TBX5*, *PRKAG2*, and *LMNA* have been identified when PCCD is accompanied by congenital heart disease. Isolated PCCD has also been described in specific families, carrier of a mutation in one of these genes.

Cardiac conduction defects are particularly frequent in patients carrier of a *LMNA* mutation (Figure 15.5). While the initial cardiac descriptions were focused on left ventricular dysfunction, it is now clear that in some cases, cardiac conduction defects should be the only abnormality identified. It is important to properly identify patients who carry the *LMNA* mutation, as it is now well known that these patients have a specific risk of ventricular arrhythmias and sudden cardiac death.[15] For this reason, it is now recommended in case of cardiac conduction defects to implant an implantable cardioverter defibrillator rather than a PM.[16] Different type of conduction defect should be identified in these patients but the more frequent aspect remains a prolonged PR interval (that is the first conduction abnormalities to occur) frequently associated with a LBBB frequently incomplete initially.

TYPE 1 MYOTONIC DYSTROPHY (MD1) OR STEINERT DISEASE

MD1—also called Steinert disease—is the most common inherited neuromuscular disease in adults, with an incidence of 1:8000. MD1 is an autosomal dominant disorder involving the peripheral and cardiac muscles, leading to a multisystemic disease. The underlying genetic abnormality in MD1 is represented by the expansion of CTG triplet repeat in the 3' untranslated region of the dystrophia myotonica protein kinase gene at chromosome 19.[17]

Severe abnormalities on the ECG with prolonged PR and QRS duration prolongation or second or third-degree AV block are frequently identified in these patients and are a risk factor for sudden cardiac death (Figure 15.6).[18] Even in patients with a normal resting ECG, cardiac conduction defect can occur and invasive evaluation of the conduction should be mandatory.[19] There is no relation between the severity of the conduction defect and the severity of myotony.

CONCLUSION

Even if most of the patients affected by cardiac conduction defects are idiopathic and occur in older patients, in cases of manifestation at relatively young age (before age 60 years), a genetic origin of the disease should be suspected. In any case, in all patients affected by cardiac conduction defect a careful examination to identify other associated diseases potentially at risk of sudden cardiac death is warranted. A careful interview with a particular attention for other familial cases of the disease is also recommended.

REFERENCES

1. Lenegre J. The pathology of complete atrio-ventricular block. *Prog Cardiovas Dis.* 1964;6:317–323.
2. Lev M. Anatomic basis for atrioventricular block. *Am J Med.* 1964;37:742–748.
3. Davies MJ. Pathology of chronic AV block. *Acta Cardiol.* 1976;21:19–30.

4. Brink PA, Ferreira A, Moolman JC, et al. Gene for progressive familial heart block type I maps to chromosome 19q13. *Circulation.* 1995;91:1633–1640.
5. Stephan E, de Meeus A, Bouvagnet P. Hereditary bundle branch defect: right bundle branch blocks of different causes have different morphologic characteristics. *Am Heart J.* 1997;133:249–256.
6. Greenspahn BR, Denes P, Daniel W, Rosen KM. Chronic bifascicular block: evaluation of familial factors. *Ann Intern Med.* 1976;84:521–525.
7. Gourraud JB, Kyndt F, Fouchard S, et al. Identification of a strong genetic background for progressive cardiac conduction defect by epidemiological approach. *Heart Br Card Soc.* 2012;98:1305–1310.
8. Schott JJ, Alshinawi C, Kyndt F, et al. Cardiac conduction defects associate with mutations in SCN5A. *Nat Genet.* 1999;23:20–21.
9. Hu D, Barajas-Martínez H, Medeiros-Domingo A, et al. A novel rare variant in SCN1Bb linked to Brugada syndrome and SIDS by combined modulation of Na(v)1.5 and K(v)4.3 channel currents. *Heart Rhythm.* 2012;9:760–769.
10. Kruse M, Schulze-Bahr E, Corfield V, et al. Impaired endocytosis of the ion channel TRPM4 is associated with human progressive familial heart block type I. *J Clin Invest.* 2009;119:2737–2744.
11. Makita N, Seki A, Sumitomo N, et al. A connexin40 mutation associated with a malignant variant of progressive familial heart block type I. *Circ Arrhythm Electrophysiol.* 2012;5:163–172.
12. Probst V, Wilde AA, Barc J, et al. SCN5A mutations and the role of genetic background in the pathophysiology of Brugada syndrome. *Circ Cardiovasc Genet.* 2009;2:552–557.
13. Bezzina CR, Rook MB, Groenewegen WA, et al. Compound heterozygosity for mutations (W156X and R225W) in SCN5A associated with severe cardiac conduction disturbances and degenerative changes in the conduction system. *Circ Res.* 2003;92:159–168.
14. Liu H, El Zein L, Kruse M, et al. Gain-of-function mutations in TRPM4 cause autosomal dominant isolated cardiac conduction disease. *Circ Cardiovasc Genet.* 2010;3:374–385.
15. van Rijsingen IA, Arbustini E, Elliott PM, et al. Risk factors for malignant ventricular arrhythmias in lamin a/c mutation carriers a European cohort study. *J Am Coll Cardiol.* 2012;59:493–500.
16. Anselme F, Moubarak G, Savouré A, et al. Implantable cardioverter-defibrillators in lamin A/C mutation carriers with cardiac conduction disorders. *Heart Rhythm.* 2013;10:1492–1498.
17. Brook JD, McCurrach ME, Harley HG, et al. Molecular basis of myotonic dystrophy: Expansion of a trinucleotide (CTG) repeat at the 3' end of a transcript encoding a protein kinase family member. *Cell.* 1992;68:799–808.
18. Groh WJ, Groh MR, Saha C, et al. Electrocardiographic abnormalities and sudden death in myotonic dystrophy type 1. *N Engl J Med.* 2008;358:2688–2697.
19. Wahbi K, Meune C, Porcher R, et al. Electrophysiological study with prophylactic pacing and survival in adults with myotonic dystrophy and conduction system disease. *JAMA.* 2012;307:1292–1301.

CHAPTER

16

Sex- and Ethnicity-Related Differences in Electrocardiography

Anne B. Curtis, MD and Hiroko Beck, MD

CHAPTER SUMMARY

Electrocardiography (ECG) is one of the most commonly used diagnostic tools in medicine, due to its ease, cost effectiveness, and versatility in the diagnosis and treatment of patients. Although many factors that affect the ECG are well documented,[1] sex- and ethnicity-related differences have been less well appreciated. In this chapter, we will review physiological variability reflected in electrocardiographic measurements in relation to differences in sex and ethnicity. In addition, current data regarding sex-specific electrocardiographic markers for various pathological conditions will be reviewed.

SEX AND ETHNIC DIFFERENCES IN PR DURATION AND P-WAVE MORPHOLOGY

PR duration and P-wave morphology have been studied as prognostic markers for the prediction of cardiovascular disease outcomes, including atrial fibrillation, stroke, and all-cause mortality.[2–5] Sex- and ethnic-specific definitions of normal PR duration and P-wave morphology may assist in the utilization of such prognostic markers. Sex differences in PR duration have been reported in several studies. In 1960, Simonson et al studied 566 healthy individuals (424 men and 142 women), using a supine, resting 12-lead ECG recorded on standard direct-writing instruments. Manual measurements were made in duplicate by 2 investigators. Statistical analysis of their data revealed significantly shorter PR durations in women (155 ms vs. 167 ms, $P \leq 0.0001$). The average relative body weight of men was approximately 5% higher than that of women. Both women and men had similar distributions of weight groups (underweight, normal weight, and overweight). This was the first study that revealed significant sex differences in the ECG, taking relative weight into consideration.[6] This observation of shorter PR intervals in women has been reported in multiple subsequent studies. Mansi et al evaluated ethnic differences in PR intervals and found no significant variation in mean PR interval among Saudi, Indian, Jordanian, Filipino, and Caucasian subjects; however, PR intervals were shorter in women in all ethnic groups.[7] Most recently, PR duration and P-wave indices in 1252 individuals (59% women) free of cardiovascular disease and its risk factors were studied. Standard 12-lead ECGs were digitally acquired at 10 mm/mV calibration and a speed of 25 mm/s. P-wave durations and PR intervals were automatically measured. PR intervals (9.6 ms difference, $P < 0.001$), heart rate-adjusted PR intervals

The ECG Handbook of Contemporary Challenges © 2015 Mohammad Shenasa, Mark E. Josephson, N.A. Mark Estes III
Cardiotext Publishing, ISBN: 978-1-935395-88-1

Table 16.1. Sex, age, and ethnicity-related differences in PR duration from the MESA cohorts. Adapted with permission.[8]

PR Duration (ms)	Age Group	Caucasians		African Americans		Hispanics		Chinese	
		Women	Men	Women	Men	Women	Men	Women	Men
Mean (SD)	45 to 64 years	155 (23)	167 (25)	165 (22)	174 (24)	155 (21)	159 (19)	154 (18)	162 (19)
	65 years and older	162 (22)	176 (32)	160 (19)	178 (31)	163 (18)	162 (17)	158 (19)	160 (24)

SD, standard deviation.

(8.6 ms difference, $P < 0.001$), and P-wave durations (6.1 ms difference, $P < 0.001$) were significantly shorter in women in this study as well. This study also found significant ethnic differences in PR intervals as well, with longer PR intervals in African Americans compared to Caucasians. PR intervals in Caucasians were significantly longer than in Chinese or Hispanic subjects (Table 16.1).[8]

The physiological basis for these sex differences in P-wave duration and PR intervals are not well understood, but the smaller size of women's hearts, both absolute and in relation to body weight, may be a contributing factor.[6] Baseline differences in vagal tone may also play a role in the sex difference in PR intervals. A recent study which reported PR interval as one of the predictors for risk of atrial fibrillation used PR interval definitions stratified by sex due to the shorter PR intervals in women.[9] With the increasing use of P-wave duration and PR intervals as diagnostic tools, it is critical to revisit the definitions of normal ranges, as present standards were derived from groups of men.

SEX DIFFERENCES IN QRS DURATION

Representing the time of ventricular activation, QRS duration is clinically relevant in multiple ways, such as indications for cardiac resynchronization therapy (CRT) and evaluation for conduction system disease. Similar to PR intervals and P-wave duration, QRS duration has also been reported to vary based on sex. In addition to shorter PR intervals in women, Simonson et al reported shorter QRS durations in women (67 ms vs. 90 ms in men, $P \leq 0.0001$).[6] Mansi's study revealed no significant differences in QRS duration among ethnic groups, but QRS durations were shorter in women in each ethnic group.[7] The etiology of this sex difference in QRS duration is unknown, but the smaller anatomical size of women's hearts may be a key factor.[6] The importance of defining QRS duration by sex, particularly in left bundle branch block (LBBB), has been advocated by Strauss et al, as women have been reported to show response to CRT with QRS durations starting at 130 ms, whereas men do not exhibit responses when the QRS duration is <140 ms.[10] A corollary to this observation is that women in general respond better to CRT, which may reflect more "dyssynchrony" for any particular QRS value compared to men, given that their normal range is shorter than that of men.

SEX DIFFERENCES IN THE QT INTERVAL

Sex differences in ventricular repolarization patterns between women and men have been studied extensively. They are important as they have direct implications for susceptibility to ventricular arrhythmias. It has been shown that a longer QT interval and a lower T-wave amplitude, which reflect a longer duration of repolarization, are present on the surface ECGs of women as compared to men (Figure 16.1).[11–13] Bidoggia et al measured repolarization in 27 castrated men, 26 women with virilization syndromes, and 53 control subjects pair-matched for age and sex. The study reported delayed repolarization in

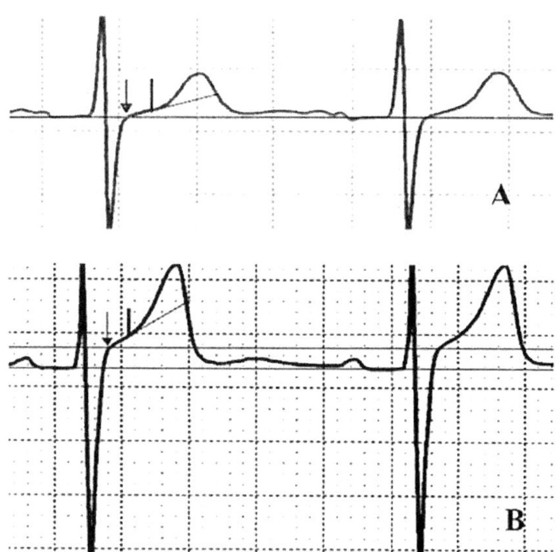

Figure 16.1. Female and male pattern in lead V_3. The 2 horizontal lines represent the Q-Q line and the line parallel to the Q-Q line at the level of the J point, respectively. The arrow marks the J point; the short vertical line marks the point 60 ms after the J point; the oblique line connects the J point with the above point. **A.** Female pattern: the J point is at the level of the Q-Q line, and the ST angle is 19 degrees. **B.** Male pattern: the J point is > 0.1 mV above the Q-Q line, and the ST angle is 36 degrees. Modified with permission.[16]

castrated men compared to normal men and shorter and faster repolarization in women with virilization compared to normal women and castrated men.[11] Sex differences in QT duration become apparent from the time of puberty[14–16] and subside after the age of 50 (Table 16.2, Figure 16.2).[14,16] The QT interval shortens during puberty in boys, and this difference persists through early adulthood. This age-related change, along with Bidoggia's findings, suggests that testosterone may contribute to sex differences in QT duration. At the receptor level, androgen receptors have been identified in the ventricles, and androgen receptor mRNA has been identified in infant male and female human right ventricles, suggesting its involvement in repolarization.[17–19]

The effect of female hormones on QT duration has been investigated as well. One such study involved the relationship of the menstrual cycle and the QT interval. Nakagawa et al reported shorter QT intervals during the luteal phase of the menstrual cycle by approximately 10 ms and suggested that estrogen-induced QT prolongation may be counteracted by sympathetic tone and serum progesterone.[20] However, other studies showed no significant changes in QT interval duration during the menstrual cycle.[21–23] One study reported QTc reduction in the luteal phase only after autonomic blockade.[22,24] These conflicting findings suggest a complex interaction of multiple factors affecting QT intervals, including sex hormones and sympathetic tone.

Despite dramatic changes in autonomic balance and hormonal changes during pregnancy, a study of long QT syndrome (LQTS) found that there was not a higher risk of cardiac events during pregnancy in women with LQTS, although there was an increased risk during the 9-month postpartum period. The authors postulated that relative tachycardia during pregnancy may have a protective effect on women by shortening QT duration, while during the postpartum period, the reduction in resting heart rate in combination with increased physical and emotional stress may induce arrhythmia triggers.[24,25]

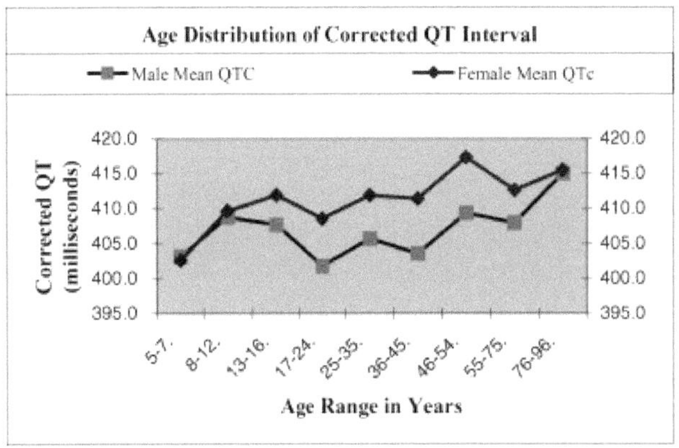

Figure 16.2. Average QTc in 9 age groups of women and men. Modified with permission.[50]

Estrogen replacement therapy has been shown to prolong the QT interval in multiple studies conducted in postmenopausal women.[26–28] It has been reported that long-term hormone replacement therapy with estrogen alone increases the QT interval and heart rate variability, whereas progestin-estrogen replacement therapy does not change QT duration, suggesting that progestin may counteract the effect of estrogen on QT prolongation.[26,29] The Heart and Estrogen/Progestin Replacement Study reported

Table 16.2. Distribution of heart rate, QTc duration, and T-wave amplitude. Adapted with permission.[16]

Age Group in Years	Male Mean HR (SD)	Female Mean HR (SD)	*P* Value	Male Mean QTc (SD)	Female Mean QTc (SD)	*P* Value	Male Mean T (SD)	Female Mean T (SD)	*P* Value
5-7	89.6 (11.7)	87.2 (12.9)	0.334	403.2 (16.4)	402.6 (10.0)	0.84	5.3 (2.1)	4.9 (2.3)	0.297
8-12	77.5 (11.9)	82.6 (11.1)	0.023	408.8 (11.9)	409.7 (14.9)	0.725	5.2 (2.2)	4.2 (1.6)	0.005
13-16	71.8 (13.6)	75.8 (14.7)	0.134	407.7 (13.6)	411.9 (14.9)	0.118	4.5 (2.3)	3.7 (1.5)	0.037
17-24	70.3 (11.2)	73.0 (10.4)	0.23	401.8 (14.6)	408.6 (15.5)	0.033	5.3 (2.1)	3.0 (1.2)	<0.001
25-35	70.3 (12.0)	74.5 (9.3)	0.046	405.7 (15.8)	411.9 (14.6)	0.042	3.7 (1.8)	3.0 (1.4)	0.024
36-45	70.1 (10.8)	73.5 (9.6)	0.11	403.6 (11.3)	411.4 (13.1)	0.003	4.2 (1.6)	2.5 (1.3)	<0.001
46-54	70.1 (13.9)	74.3 (11.8)	0.061	409.4 (14.4)	417.3 (14.5)	0.002	4.0 (1.9)	2.8 (1.3)	<0.001
55-75	64.1 (10.4)	70.5 (12.4)	0.001	408.0 (11.8)	412.6 (10.2)	0.004	4.3 (1.7)	2.6 (1.1)	<0.001
76-98	67.5 (14.8)	72.2 (11.7)	0.032	415.1 (15.6)	415.5 (14.4)	0.98	4.2 (2.1)	3.4 (1.4)	0.007

HR, heart rate; QTc, corrected QT interval; mean T, mean T-wave voltage (X0.1 mV).

that estrogen-progestin replacement therapy did not reduce the risk of arrhythmias in a population of post-menopausal women with coronary heart disease.[24,30] These observations suggest a QT-prolonging effect of estrogen and a potential protective effect of progestin against QT prolongation and arrhythmia.

For patients with congenital LQTS, an international registry reported that women had a higher risk of a first cardiac event between ages 1 and 40 years.[24,31] Sex differences in acquired QT prolongation due to medications have been described in several studies (Table 16.3), although it is not clear if all QT-prolonging medications are associated with sex-related differences in the degree of QT prolongation. For acquired LQTS from drugs such as antidepressants, antiarrhythmic drugs, and antibiotics, female sex has been recognized as an independent risk factor for ventricular arrhythmias.[32–34] More than 68% of drug-induced torsades de pointes (TdP) occurs in women.[24,35–37] TdP due to antiarrhythmic drugs occurs more often in women, well out of proportion to the number of women who are prescribed these medications.

There are several antiarrhythmic drugs that prolong the QT interval that have been reported to have a greater effect on QT-interval prolongation in women, including sotalol and quinidine. The effect of d,l-sotalol on ventricular repolarization measured by the JTc interval was found to be significantly more pronounced in women compared to men.[38] Somberg et al reported marked QTc prolongation in women with sotalol as well.[39] Quinidine has also been reported to have a greater effect on QTc prolongation in women compared to men.[40] Although a higher incidence of TdP in women with ibutilide has been reported,[41,42] QT prolongation by ibutilide does not differ between men and women.[43] Thus, not all QT-prolonging medications have a more pronounced effect on the QT interval in women. Even a medication that affects QT intervals more in women may not result in increased arrhythmic events. Further investigations are warranted to elucidate the mechanisms behind sex differences in QT-prolonging medications. In the meantime, these medications should be used with particular caution in women, given the effect of these drugs on QT intervals in women.

ETHNIC DIFFERENCES IN QT INTERVALS

There have been a few studies that compare QT intervals between different ethnic groups. In a large-scale population-based, prospective cohort study of 15,792 participants, QTc intervals were longer in women than in men as described earlier. With respect to ethnicity, QTc intervals were longer in Caucasians than in African Americans. This racial difference persisted after adjustment for multiple factors including body mass index, systolic blood pressure, and chest size, reaching statistical significance ($P < 0.01$) in both men and women.[44] In another study, QTc was found to be greater in Chinese subjects than in Caucasians.[45] Mansi et al found no significant differences in QTc among Saudi, Indian, Jordanian, Filipino, and Srilankan women when compared to Caucasians.[7] The lack of available data comparing ethnicity limits our understanding of variability in QT duration as a reflection of ventricular repolarization and its effect on clinical outcomes.

PROGNOSTIC VALUE OF THE ECG BY SEX AND ETHNICITY

The ECG is a simple diagnostic tool whose value is enhanced if sex- and ethnicity-related differences are understood. Rautaharju et al proposed the use of several repolarization variables in post-menopausal women as predictors of the risk of congestive heart failure (CHF) and all-cause mortality, based on a large scale Cox regression analysis of 38,283 participants in the Women's Health Initiative during 9 years of follow-up. These variables included a wide QRS/T angle, which was associated with a 3-fold increased risk of CHF, and myocardial infarction by ECG with over a 2-fold increase in the risk of incident CHF.[46] This same

Table 16.3. Sex differences in response to drugs.

Publications	*n* = Sample Size	Medication	Method of Measurement	Sex Differences in Ventricular Repolarization		
				Women	Men	*P*-value
Lehmann, 1999	*n* = 1897 (26% women)	d,l-Sotalol	JTc ≥ 390 ms	16.20%	10.30%	0.003
Somberg, 2012	*n* = 15 (60% women)	Sotalol	Change in QTc	34 ± 8ms	21 ± 12ms	<0.05
Kannankeril, 2011	*n* = 253 (60% women)	Ibutilide	Change in QTc	39 ± 27ms	39 ± 29ms	NS
El-Eraky, 2003	*n* = 48 (44% women)	Quinidine	Change in QTc	33 ± 16ms	24 ± 17ms	<0.05

NS, not statistically significant.

group also reported that ventricular repolarization abnormalities in post-menopausal women were important predictors of coronary heart disease. Using the same cohorts of post-menopausal women, they found several ECG abnormalities as dominant mortality risk predictors of coronary heart disease, including wide QRS/T angle, ECG evidence of myocardial infarction, reduced heart rate variability, and QT prolongation.[47]

Sex differences in the clinical manifestation of Brugada syndrome (BrS) have been described as well. Benito et al found that among 384 patients, men experienced syncope more frequently (18% vs. 14% in women, $P < 0.05$) and more often had aborted sudden cardiac death (6% vs. 1% in women, $P < 0.05$). More sudden cardiac death or ventricular fibrillation occurred in men compared to women (11.6% vs. 2.8% in women, $P = 0.003$). With these findings, they concluded that men with BrS present a greater risk profile and worse prognosis than women.[48]

The diagnostic and prognostic value of the ECG in left ventricular hypertrophy (LVH) has been reported by ethnicity. When LVH was defined by MRI, Jain et al found Romhilt–Estes score, Framingham score, Cornell voltage, Cornell duration product, and Framingham-adjusted Cornell voltage predicted increased cardiovascular disease risk, and these parameters had particularly high sensitivity among African-American patients.[49] As more information become available on the diagnostic and prognostic value of the ECG by sex and ethnicity, its utility may be expected to increase.

SUMMARY

- Sex differences exist in certain elements of the ECG.
- PR and QRS durations are shorter in women, possibly due to anatomical differences in heart size. Differences in vagal tone may also be responsible for differences in the PR interval.
- QTc interval durations are longer in women from puberty to about 50 years of age.
- QTc intervals may be shortened by testosterone and prolonged by estrogen.
- Some QT prolonging drugs are reported to affect ventricular repolarization more in women compared to men.
- The ECG may have prognostic value by gender and ethnicity in various disease processes, including coronary artery disease, CHF, and BrS.

REFERENCES

1. Surawicz B, Knilans TK. *Chou's Electrocardiography in Clinical Practice.* 6th ed. Philadelphia, PA: Saunders Elsevier;2008.
2. Soliman EZ, Prineas RJ, Case LD, Zhang ZM, Goff Jr, DC. Ethnic distribution of electrocardiographic predictors of atrial fibrillation and its impact on understanding the ethnic distribution of ischemic stroke in the Atherosclerosis Risk in Communities Study (ARIC). *Stroke.* 2009;40:1204–1211.
3. Schnabel RB, Sullivan LM, Levy D, et al. Development of a risk score for atrial fibrillation (Framingham Heart Study): A community-based cohort study. *Lancet.* 2009;373:739–745.
4. Cheng S, Keyes MJ, Larson MG, et al. Long-term outcomes in individuals with prolonged PR interval or first-degree atrioventricular block. *JAMA.* 2009;301:2571–2577.
5. Magnani JW, Johnson VM, Sullivan LM, et al. P wave duration and risk of longitudinal atrial fibrillation in persons ≥ 60 years old (from the Framingham Heart Study). *Am J Cardiol.* 2011;107:917–921.
6. Simonson E, Blackburn H, Puchner TC, et al. Sex differences in the electrocardiogram. *Circulation.* 1960;22:598–601.
7. Mansi IA, Nash IS. Ethnic differences in electrocardiographic intervals and axes. *J Electrocardiol.* 2001;34:303–307.
8. Soliman EZ, Alonso A, Misialek JR, et al. Reference range of PR duration and P-wave indices in individuals free of cardiovascular disease: the Multi-Ethnic Study of Atherosclerosis (MESA). *J Electrocardiol.* 2013;46:702–706.
9. Nielsen JB, Pietersen A, Graff C, et al. Risk of atrial fibrillation as a function of the electrocardiographic PR interval: results from the Copenhagen ECG study. *Heart Rhythm.* 2013;10:1249–1256.
10. Strauss DG, Selvester RH, Wagner GS. Defining left bundle branch block in the era of cardiac resynchronization therapy. *Am J Cardiol.* 2011;107:927–934.
11. Bidoggia H, Maciel JP, Norberto C, et al. Sex differences on the electrocardiographic pattern of cardiac repolarization: Possible role of testosterone. *Am Heart J.* 2000;140:678–683.
12. Merri M, Benhorin J, Alberti M, Locati E, Moss AJ. Electrocardiographic quantitation of ventricular repolarization. *Circulation.* 1989;80:1301–1308.
13. Gambil CL, Wilkins ML, Haisty WK, et al. T wave amplitudes in normal populations. Variation with ECG lead, sex and age. *J Electrocardiol.* 1995;28:191–197.
14. Rautaharju PM, Zhou SH, Wong S, et al. Sex differences in the evaluation of the electrocardiographic QT interval with age. *Can J Cardiol.* 1992;8:690–695.
15. Stramba-Badiale M, Spagnolol D, Bosi G, Bosi G, Schwartz PJ. Are gender differences in QTc present at birth? MISNES Investigators. Multicenter Italian Study on Neonatal Electrocardiography and Sudden Infant Death Syndrome. *Am J Cardiol.* 1995;75:1277–1278.
16. Surawicz B, Parikh SR. Prevalence of male and female patterns of early ventricular repolarization in the normal ECG of males and females from childhood to old age. *J Am Coll Cardiol.* 2002;40:1870–1876.
17. Krieg M, Smith K, Bartsch W. Demonstration of a specific androgen receptor in heart muscle. Relationship between binding, metabolism and tissue levels of androgens. *Endocrinology.* 1978;103:1686–1694.

18. McGill HC, Anselmo VC, Buchanan JM, Sheridan PJ. The heart is a target organ for androgen. *Science.* 1977;196:319–321.
19. Marsh JD, Lehmann MH, Ritchie RH, et al. Androgen receptors mediate hypertrophy in cardiac myocytes. *Circulation.* 1998;98:256–261.
20. Nakagawa M, Ooie T, Takahashi N, et al. Influence of menstrual cycle on QT interval dynamics. *Pacing Clin Electrophysiol.* 2006;29:607–613.
21. Rodriguez I, Kilborn MJ, Liu JT, Pezzullo JC, Woosley RL. Drug-induced QT prolongation in women during the menstrual cycle. *JAMA.* 2001;285:1322–1326.
22. Burke JH, Ehlert FA, Kruse JT, et al. Gender-specific differences in the QT interval and the effect of autonomic tone and menstrual cycle in healthy adults. *Am J Cardiol.* 1997;79:178–181.
23. Hulot JS, Demolis JL, Riviere R, et al. Influence of endogenous estrogens on QT interval duration. *Eur Heart J.* 2003;24:1663–1667.
24. Yang P, Clancy CE. Effects of sex hormones on cardiac repolarization. *J Cardiovasc Pharmacol.* 2010;56:123–129.
25. Seth R1, Moss AJ, McNitt S, et al. Long QT syndrome and pregnancy. *J Am Coll Cardiol.* 2007;49:1092–1098.
26. Haseroth K, Seyffart K, Wehling M, Christ M. Effects of progestin-estrogen replacement therapy on QT-dispersion in postmenopausal women. *Int J Cardiol.* 2000;75:161–165.
27. Kadish AH, Greenland P, Limacher MC, et al. Estrogen and progestin use and the QT interval in postmenopausal women. *Ann Noninvasive Electrocardiol.* 2004;9:366–374.
28. Carnethon MR, Anthony MS, Cascio WE, et al. A prospective evaluation of the risk of QT prolongation with hormone replacement therapy: The atherosclerosis risk in communities study. *Ann Epidemiol.* 2003;13:530–536.
29. Gokce M, Karahan B, Yilmaz R, et al. Long term effects of hormone replacement therapy on heart rate variability, QT interval, T dispersion and frequencies of arrhythmia. *Int J Cardiol.* 2005;99:373–379.
30. Grady D, Herrington D, Bittner V. Cardiovascular disease outcomes during 6.8 years of hormone therapy: Heart and Estrogen/progestin Replacement Study follow-up (HERS II). *JAMA.* 2002;288:49–57.
31. Locati EH, Zareba W, Moss AJ, et al. Age- and sex-related differences in clinical manifestations in patients with congenital long-QT syndrome: findings from the International LQTS Registry. *Circulation.* 1998;97:2237–2244.
32. Abi-Gerges N, Philp K, Pollard C, et al. Sex differences in ventricular repolarization: from cardiac electrophysiology to torsade de pointes. *Fundam Clin Pharmacol.* 2004;17:139–151.
33. Pham TV, Rosen MR. Sex, hormones, and repolarization. *Cardiovasc Res.* 2002;53:740–751.
34. James AF, Choisy SC, Hancox JC. Recent advances in understanding sex differences in cardiac repolarization. *Prog Biophys Mol Biol.* 2007;94:265–319.
35. Drici MD, Knollmann BC, Wang WX, Woosley RL. Cardiac actions of erythromycin: influence of female sex. *JAMA.* 1998;280:1774–1776.
36. Makkar RR, Fromm BS, Steinman RT, Meissner MD, Lehmann MH. Female gender as a risk factor for torsades de pointes associated with cardiovascular drugs. *JAMA.* 1993;270:2590–2597.
37. Lehmann MH, Hardy S, Archibald D, quart B, MacNeil DJ. Sex difference in risk of torsade de pointes with d,l-sotalol. *Circulation.* 1996;94:2535–2541.
38. Lehmann MH, Sterling H, Archibald D, MacNeil DJ. JTc prolongation with d,l-sotalol in women versus men. *Am J Cardiol.* 1999;83:354–359.
39. Somberg JC, Preston RA, Ranada V, Cvetanovic I, Molnar J. Gender differences in cardiac repolarization following intravenous sotalol administration. *J Cardiovasc Pharmacol Ther.* 2012;17:86–92.
40. El-Eraky H, Thomas SH. Effects of sex on the pharmacokinetic and pharmacodynamics properties of quinidine. *Br J Clin Pharmacol.* 2003;56:198–204.
41. Gowda RM1, Khan IA, Punukollu G, et al. Female preponderance in ibutilide-induced torsade de pointes. *Int J Cardiol.* 2004;95:219–222.
42. Hreiche R, Morissette P, Turgeon J. Drug-induced long QT syndrome in women: review of current evidence and remaining gaps. *Gend Med.* 2008;5:124–135.
43. Kannankeril PJ, Norris KJ, Carter S, Roden DM. Factors affecting the degree of QT prolongation with drug challenge in a large cohort of normal volunteers. *Heart Rhythm.* 2011;8:1530–1534.
44. Vitelli LL, Crow RS, Shahar E, et al. Electrocardiographic findings in a healthy biracial population. *Am J Cardiol.* 1998;81:453–459.
45. Fei L, Statters DJ, Camm J. QT-interval dispersion on 12-lead electrocardiogram in normal subjects: its reproducibility and relation to the T wave. *Am Heart J.* 1994;127:1654–1655.
46. Rautaharju PM, Kooperberg C, Larson JC, LaCroix A. Electrocardiographic predictors of incident congestive heart failure and all-cause mortality in postmenopausal women. *Circulation.* 2006;113:481–489.
47. Rautaharju PM, Kooperberg C, Larson JC, LaCroix A. Electrocardiographic abnormalities that predict coronary heart disease events and mortality in postmenopausal women. *Circulation.* 2006;113:473–480.
48. Benito B, Sarkozy A, Mont L, et al. Gender differences in clinical manifestations of Brugada syndrome. *J Am Coll Cardiol.* 2008;52:1567–1573.
49. Jain A, Tandri H, Dalal D, et al. Diagnostic and prognostic utility of electrocardiography for left ventricular hypertrophy defined by magnetic resonance imaging in relationship to ethnicity: The Multi-Ethnic Study of Atherosclerosis (MESA). *Am Heart J.* 2010;159(4):652–658.
50. Surawicz B, Parikh SR. Differences between ventricular repolarization in men and women: description, mechanisms, and implications. *Ann Noninvasive Electrocardiol.* 2003;8:333–340.

CHAPTER

17

Electrocardiograms in Biventricular Pacing

John Rickard, MD, MPH, Victor Nauffal, MD, and Alan Cheng, MD

INTRODUCTION

The simple 12-lead ECG is an integral component to select appropriate candidates for cardiac resynchronization therapy (CRT) as well as assessing the adequacy of biventricular pacing in those who have undergone implantation of a CRT-capable device. The ECG provides important information about left and right ventricular (LV/RV) lead position, as well as suggesting possible pacing problems, such as anodal stimulation and loss of LV capture. In addition, QRS duration and morphology have been shown to be important determinants of favorable outcomes in CRT recipients. Thus, an ECG should be part of any pre-CRT workup and post-CRT patient assessment.

QRS PATTERNS DURING RV PACING

In patients pacing from the RV, the QRS vector takes on a different direction from native conduction and can provide clues on lead location (e.g., RV apex vs. outflow tract). When placed in the apex, the QRS vector typically takes on a left superior frontal axis, although a right superior axis vector is seen uncommonly.[1] As the RV lead is placed further into the right ventricular outflow tract (RVOT), the vector changes from a superior to an inferior axis, maintaining a leftward direction. Eventually, as the RV lead progresses from the RVOT and closer towards the pulmonary valve, a transition from a right inferior to a left inferior axis occurs.[2]

RV pacing most commonly generates a dominant negative deflection or left bundle branch block (LBBB)-like pattern in lead V_1. In 8% to 10% of patients, however, a dominant R wave or right bundle branch block (RBBB)-like pattern is observed.[3,4] The cause of a RBBB-like pattern in RV pacing may be due to inappropriately positioned recording electrodes or fusion with the intrinsic rhythm. A dominant R wave can also be seen with RV pacing when V_1 is recorded from the third intercostal space.[1] Lowering the V_1 recording electrode to the fifth intercostal space should eliminate the dominant R wave with standard RV pacing.[4] This situation has been termed as "pseudo-RBBB" by Klein et al.[3] When a dominant R wave is present in V_1 with RV pacing, the transition between positive and negative should occur by V_3.[4] When a dominant R wave persists at V_4, LV pacing should be strongly suspected. Pacing leads intended

The ECG Handbook of Contemporary Challenges © 2015 Mohammad Shenasa, Mark E. Josephson, N.A. Mark Estes III
Cardiotext Publishing, ISBN: 978-1-935395-88-1

for the RV may be placed inadvertently into the LV via a patent foramen ovale or atrial septal defect, inadvertent cannulation of the subclavian artery with passage of the lead across the aortic valve, perforation of the ventricular septum or through a ventricular septal defect (VSD), perforation of the right ventricular free wall with epicardial migration of the electrode, or placement in a coronary vein.[5–8]

QRS PATTERNS DURING LV PACING FROM THE CORONARY SINUS (CS)

Pacing from a ventricular branch of the CS should produce a RBBB-like pattern in V_1, although a LBBB-like pattern can sometimes occur.[1] Basilar pacing locations typically produce dominant R waves in leads V_4 to V_6 while more apical sites demonstrate dominant negative deflections in V_4 to V_6.[1] The CSos, sometimes covered by the Thebesian valve, is located at the base of the Triangle of Koch and gives rise to the CS that runs along the atrial side of the mitral valve annulus. The initial portion of the CS is supported by extensions of myocardial tissue until it reaches the Valve of Vieussens (also the location of the Ligament of Marshall/Vein) where it becomes the great cardiac vein (GCV). The GCV continues to track along the mitral valve annulus, where it tapers off and becomes the anterior interventricular vein that courses anteriorly along the left side of the left anterior descending artery. Throughout the CS and GCV, venous branches can be seen, and their locations are often described based on right anterior oblique (RAO) and left anterior oblique (LAO) radiographic viewpoints. When viewed from an LAO perspective, these tributaries can roughly be divided into 3 main regions: (1) the posterior segment branches; (2) lateral segment branches, and (3) the anterior segment branches. When viewed from an RAO angle, these branches are further segmented into a basal portion, mid portion, and an apical portion (Figure 17.1).[9] Traditionally, veins in the posterolateral region are most commonly targeted for LV lead placement. Anteriorly placed leads are thought to elicit inferior response rates from CRT and hence are less commonly seen.[10] A computed tomography analysis of coronary veins in 121 cadaveric hearts by Spencer et al found that 11% did not have a coronary vein branch overlaying the posterolateral area of the heart. An additional 18% had posterolateral veins that were too small to place a 5F lead and therefore prohibited lead implantation.[11] This may explain some of the reported nonresponse rates and emphasizes the variability of the coronary venous anatomy. A careful assessment of periprocedural images is necessary for optimization of lead placement and response to therapy.

Pacing from posterior or lateral veins typically manifests a RBBB-like pattern with a right inferior axis although a right superior axis is less commonly seen (Figure 17.2).[1] For unclear reasons, rarely, a left axis deviation with either a superior or inferior axis can also be noted.[1] Pacing in a lateral branch of the middle cardiac vein typically produces a RBBB pattern,

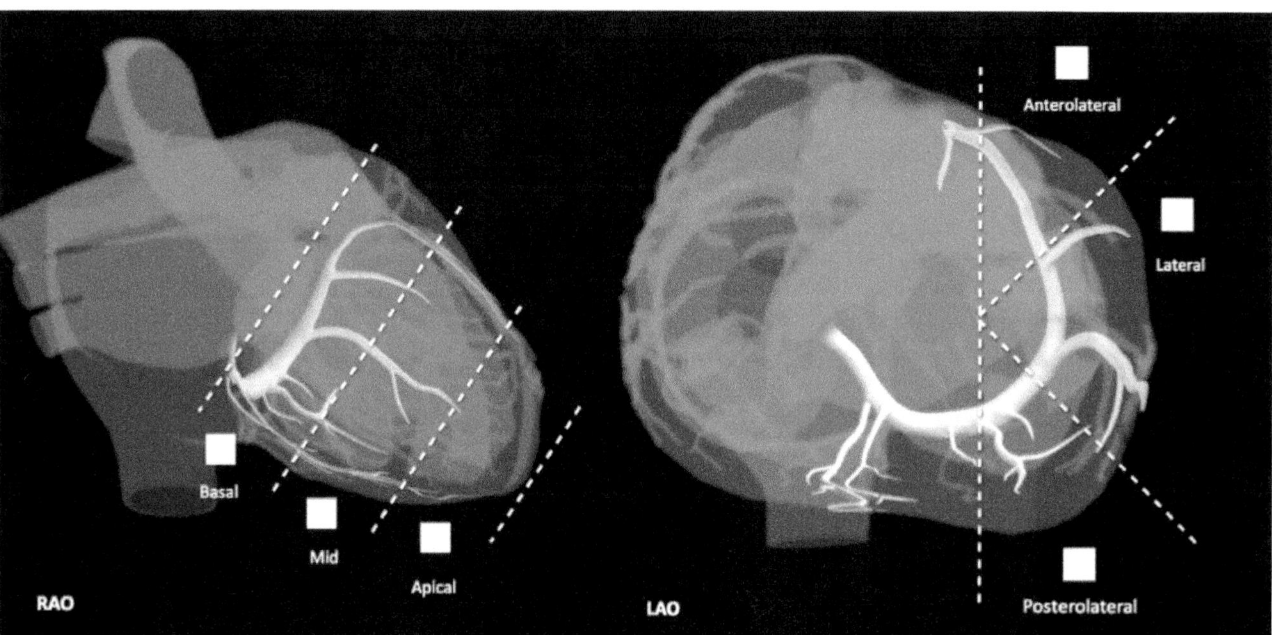

Figure 17.1. Cartoon renditions of coronary sinus anatomy in the right and left anterior oblique angles. RAO view demonstrating basal, mid, and apical segmentation of coronary veins. LAO view demonstrating coronary venous branching into 3 major posterolateral, lateral, and anterolateral regions. (Reproduced with permission from Boston Scientific.)

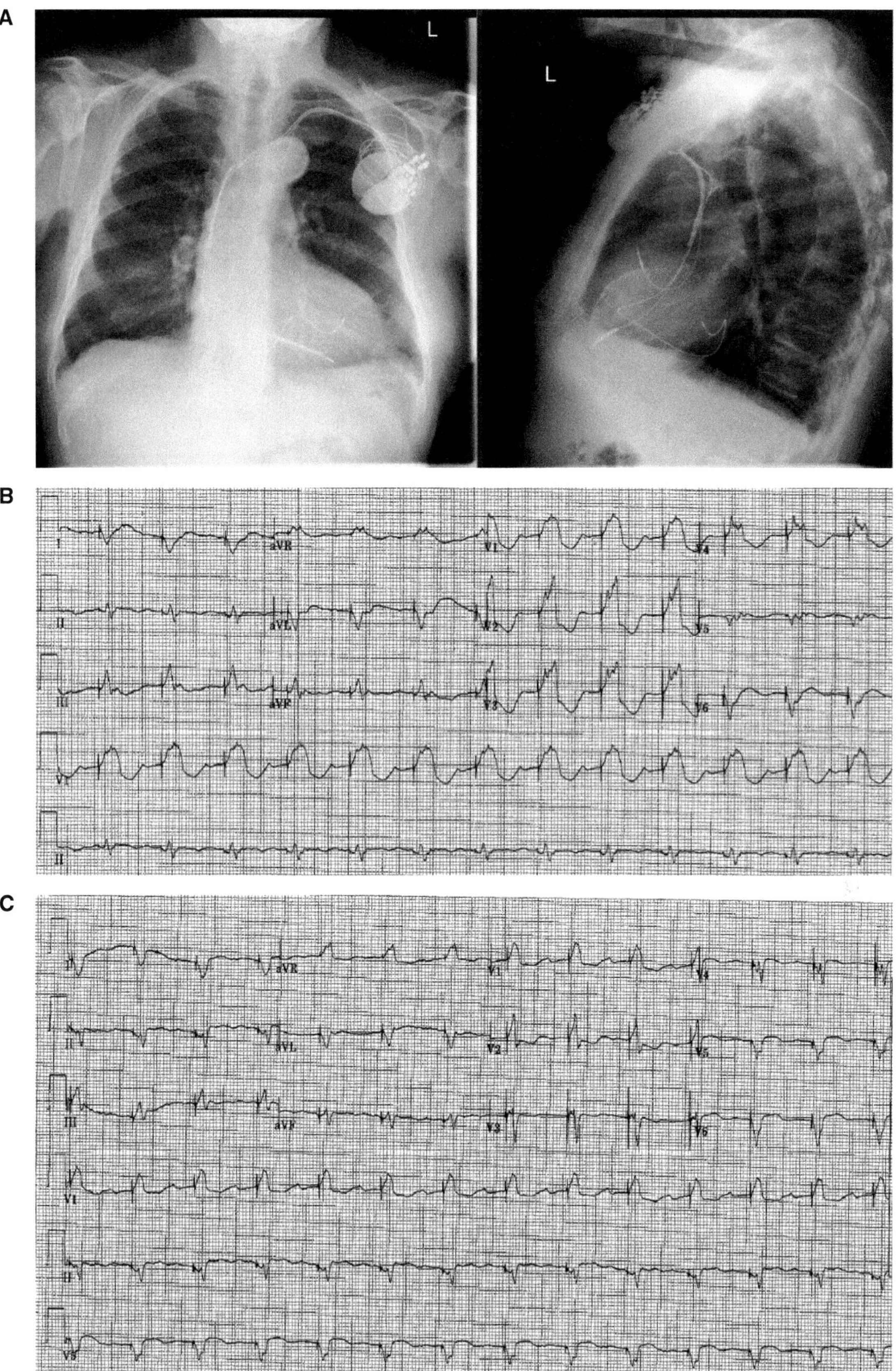

Figure 17.2. LV single-chamber and BiV pacing with LV lead in mid-posterior coronary sinus branch. **A.** CXR demonstrating a mid-posterior lead position for the LV lead. The right ventricular lead is apically placed. **B.** ECG showing LV alone pacing from the above position, demonstrating a wide RBBB-like complex in V_1 and a right inferior axis. **C.** ECG showing biventricular pacing from the above position demonstrating a RBBB-like complex in V_1 and a right superior axis.

although a LBBB morphology can also be noted.[1,12] A LBBB pattern is more commonly noted from a branch of the middle cardiac vein than from other CS branches.[12] Typically, pacing from the middle cardiac vein or its branches yields a superior axis, usually directed leftwards.[1] Pacing from the anterolateral veins typically produces a RBBB pattern.[1,12,13] LBBB may also be seen during pacing from the anterior interventricular vein.[12]

QRS PATTERNS DURING BIVENTRICULAR PACING

The vector of biventricular paced QRS waveforms changes depending on the location of the RV lead, the degree of anisotropic conduction between the RV and LV, and programmed differences in the V-V paced timing. Assuming simultaneous RV and LV pacing, the biventricular-paced waveform typically takes on a right superior axis when the RV lead is placed in the apex and a right inferior axis when placed in the outflow tract.[2] A vector from any of the other 3 quadrants is less common but does not necessarily signify a pacing problem (see Figure 17.2C).[2] In addition, lead V_1 also commonly demonstrates a dominant positive deflection during biventricular pacing, although a LBBB-like pattern also may occur particularly when the RV lead is placed in the outflow tract. A RBBB-like pattern in V_1, however, does not guarantee biventricular pacing, as a minority of patients with RV-only pacing can manifest this finding.

If a LBBB-like pattern is found in V_1 in a patient assumed to be biventricular pacing, troubleshooting should commence to ensure no pacing issues are present (Figure 17.3). Causes of a LBBB-like pattern with biventricular pacing include: incorrect placement of lead V_1 too high on the chest, latency with left LV pacing, placement of the LV lead in a middle cardiac or anterior interventricular vein, ventricular fusion with the native complex, and loss of LV capture (Figure 17.4).[2,14,15] In a study of 54 patients with biventricular pacing, 7% had a LBBB morphology all of whom had an LV lead positioned in a middle cardiac vein.[16] Of note, a LBBB-like pattern does not necessarily imply that biventricular pacing is inadequate. Local scar, ischemia, and varying participation of the His-Purkinje system may contribute to this finding.[2]

ANODAL STIMULATION

During cathodal capture, a single wavefront is initiated which paces cardiac tissue, representing the desired mechanism of cardiac pacing. In certain circumstances, however, hyperpolarization of local tissue may occur resulting in capture at the anode.[17] This can occur when the surface area of the cathode and anode dipoles are similar in size. In the case of biventricular pacing, this may undermine the ability to generate a V-V offset especially when the LV lead cathode is pacing to an RV anode. In patients who require a V-V offset (typically LV first) for proper resynchronized ventricular pacing, anodal capture will prevent this from occurring since both the LV and RV are being stimulated simultaneously. This could result in CRT nonresponse and clinical deterioration.[18] This situation is most commonly seen in CRT pacemakers (when LV pacing is programmed to occur between an LV electrode and the RV ring electrode) but has been observed in CRT defibrillators as well.[19] Anodal capture is far more common with dedicated rather than integrated bipolar RV defibrillator leads and at high-pacing outputs.[17] Since anodal capture biventricular pacing results from stimulating the RV and LV simultaneously, the QRS morphology generated is often similar to that seen with simultaneous biventricular pacing without anodal stimulation (Figure 17.5).[18,19]

QRS CHANGES AND RESPONSE TO CRT

Whether changes in the axis or duration of the paced complex following CRT have prognostic value is an area of ongoing study. In terms of axis changes, Sweeney et al performed a detailed analysis of ECGs in 202 patients undergoing CRT.[20] The authors found that increased LV activation times and a lower QRS score, a marker of LV scar burden, were associated with improved response, defined as a reduction in LV end-systolic volume (LVESV) ≥ 10% from baseline. In addition, increasing R-wave amplitudes in V_1 and V_2 as well as left-to-right frontal axis shifting was positively associated with response.[19]

Multiple papers have reported on the association between QRS duration changes and reverse ventricular remodeling with mixed results. On one hand, widening of the QRS duration following CRT is not thought to represent areas of slow ventricular activation. In addition, the QRS complex following CRT may remain unchanged or actually lengthen despite improvements in mechanical dyssynchrony.[21] A few clinical studies support this lack of association. Reuter et al found no correlation between QRS changes and response to CRT in a cohort of 47 patients.[22] Gold et al found no association between QRS narrowing and improved outcomes from the REVERSE study.[23]

Conversely, multiple studies have demonstrated a positive correlation between QRS narrowing and improved outcomes. Alonso et al were among the first to report a positive association between

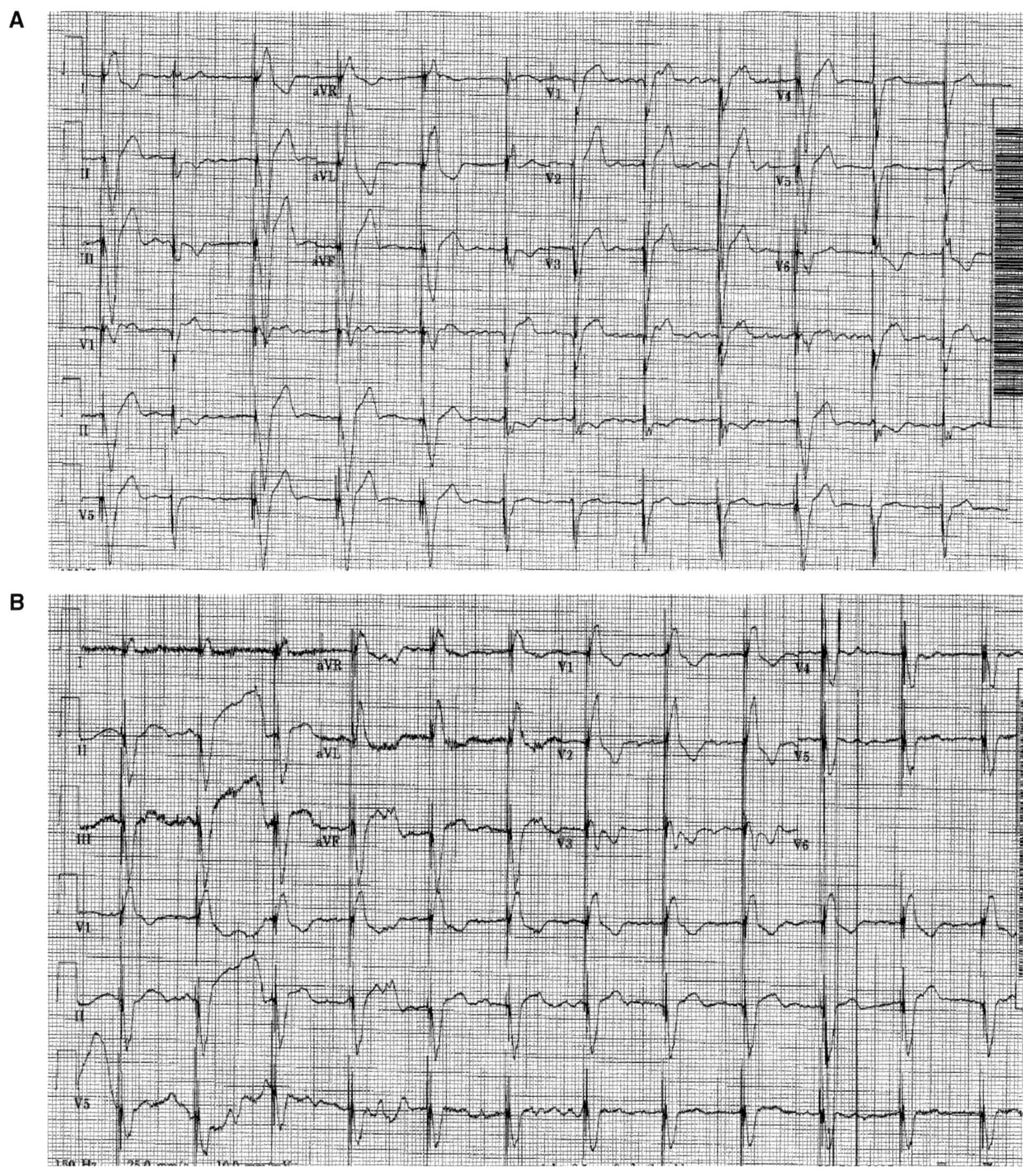

Figure 17.3. ECG of a 72-year-old female with clinical deterioration following CRT implant placed 12 months prior to this ECG. On CXR lead is in a posterolateral coronary branch. **A.** Note the LBBB pattern. LV lead from patient was found to be programmed at sub-threshold pacing outputs; hence, the patient was RV pacing 100% of the time. **B.** ECG after adjustment of LV pacing output. Note the left superior axis during biventricular pacing.

clinical response and QRS narrowing in a cohort of 26 patients undergoing CRT, in which response was defined as survival with improved symptoms and exercise tolerance.[24] Responders were found to have significantly greater QRS narrowing than nonresponders.[24] Lecoq et al looked at a cohort of 139 patients undergoing CRT, in which response was defined as freedom from death or hospitalization and improvement in New York Heart Association class, peak VO_2, or 6-minute hall walk at 6 months.[25] There was a significantly greater QRS narrowing in responders than nonresponders.[25] Iler et al looked at the association between all-cause mortality and QRS narrowing following CRT.[26] In this study, QRS widening was noted to be an independent predictor of death or heart transplant.[26] Rickard et al showed an association

A

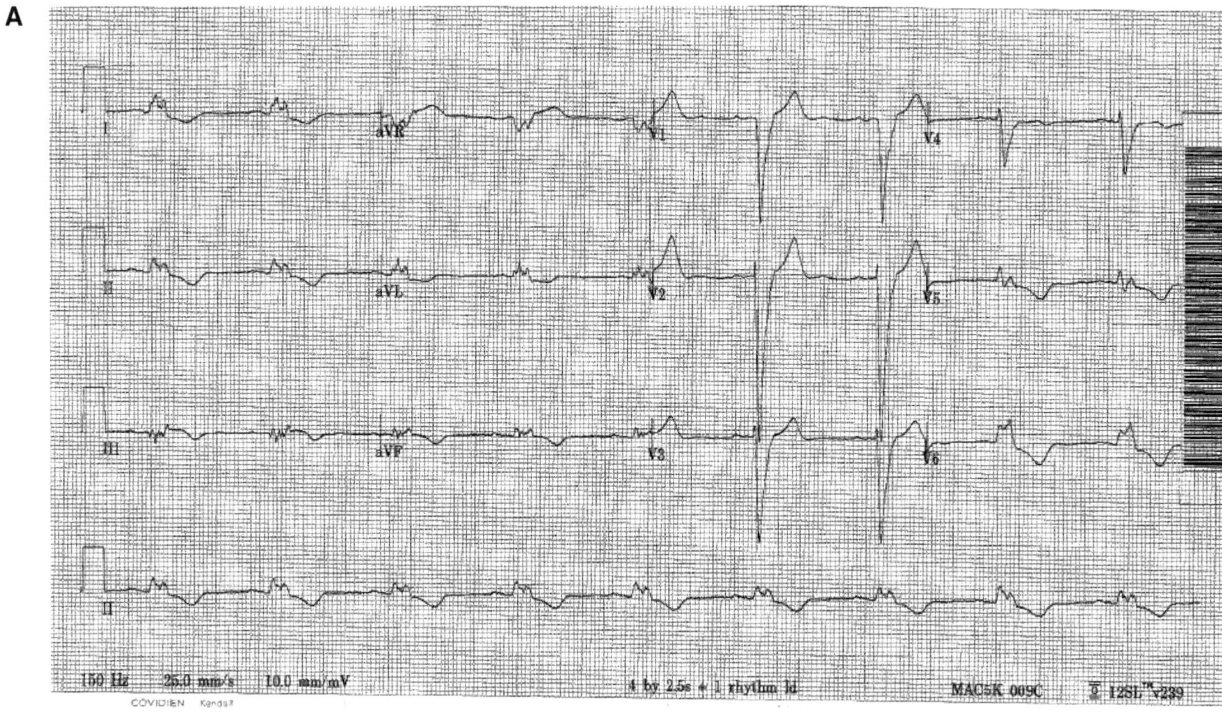

B

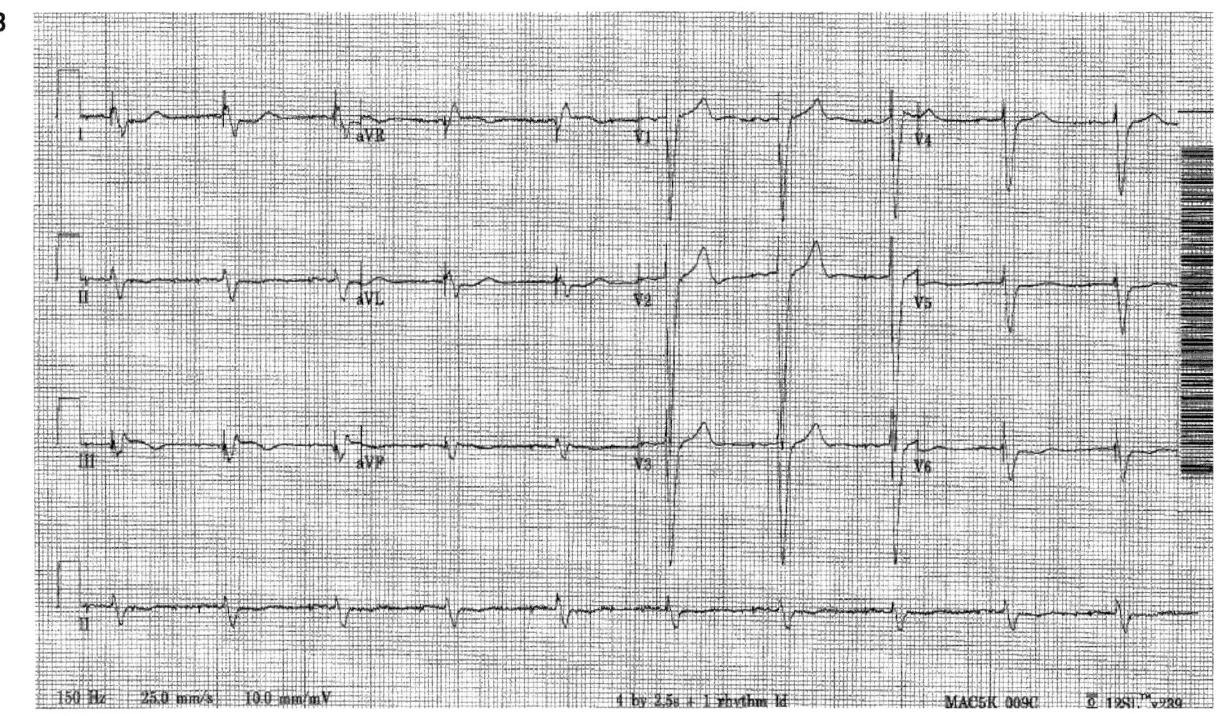

Figure 17.4. A 56-year-old male with nonresponse to CRT. On presentation, paced AV delay was set at 260 to 300 ms and sensed AV delay at 180 to 210 ms. **A.** Underlying nonpaced 12-lead ECG. AV delay is approximately 170 ms. **B.** 12-lead ECG presenting paced QRS complex. QRS morphology demonstrates a fused complex rather than a true biventricular paced waveform due to long programmed AV delays.

(Continued)

with reverse ventricular remodeling defined as a reduction in LVESV ≥ 10% using the change in QRS duration indexed to the baseline QRS duration.[27] The applicability of this index was independently verified in a separate, small Italian cohort.[28] Hsing et al documented a positive correlation between QRS narrowing and response from the large PROSPECT-ECG substudy.[29] In addition, the converse association, QRS widening, and LVEF deterioration has also been demonstrated.[30]

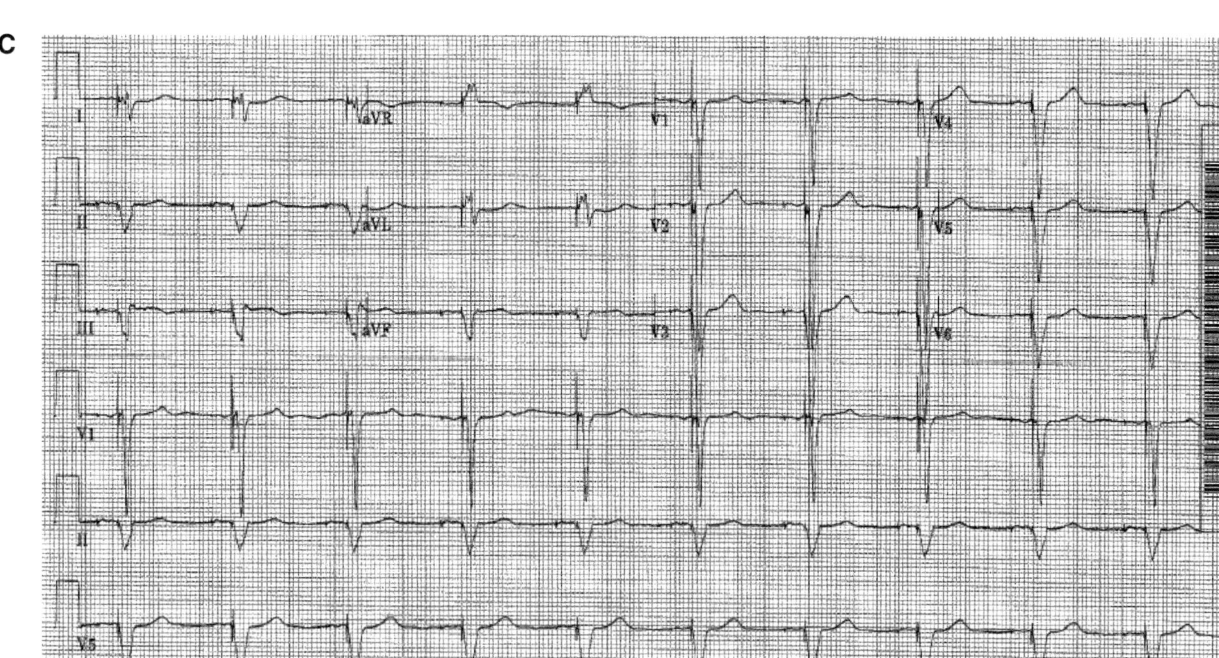

Figure 17.4. (*Continued*) C. 12-lead ECG when AV delays are shortened to promote nonfused biventricular pacing.

Looking at the totality of literature data, it appears QRS narrowing does have an association with improved response to CRT. There does exist, however, significant overlap between responders and nonresponders who experience QRS narrowing. One subgroup in which QRS narrowing may have the best predictive value is patients who are upgraded from near 100% right ventricular pacing.[31] In this subgroup, narrowing of the QRS complex appeared to be a strong predictor of response.[31]

THE IMPORTANCE OF THE QRS COMPLEX AND PREDICTING RESPONSE TO CRT

QRS DURATION

It has long been noted that patients with wider baseline QRS durations derive greater benefit from CRT than those with narrower QRS durations. In patients with both a LBBB and nonLBBB, the wider the QRS duration the greater the LV electrical activation delay.[32] Subgroup analyses from many of the clinical

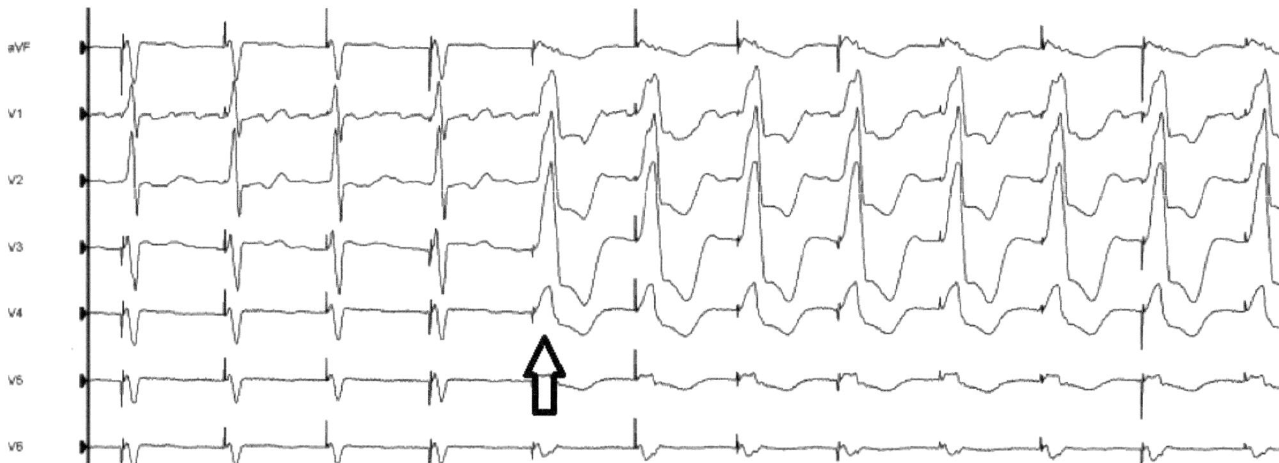

Figure 17.5. Testing LV single-chamber pacing in a patient with a biventricular pacing device. Note the initial narrow QRS pattern due to anodal stimulation at high pacing threshold that changes to a wide RBBB-like pattern (arrow) as pacing output is reduced.

trials of CRT have demonstrated superior benefit of CRT at wider QRS durations.[33–37] In a meta-analysis of 5 large, randomized controlled trials of CRT, benefit was noted above a QRS duration of 150 ms but was not realized at narrower durations.[38] With the results of 3 large clinical trials, CRT has been shown to be ineffective in patients with a QRS duration <120 ms and without a need for frequent ventricular pacing.[39–41] The ECHO-CRT trial actually suggested that CRT may result in harm in this population.[41] Whether there is a degree of QRS widening after which benefit from CRT declines is an area of ongoing study. In a prospective, longitudinal observational study of 3319 patient undergoing CRT, patients with a baseline QRS <200 ms had greater survival benefit from CRT compared to patients with a QRS >200 ms.[42]

QRS Morphology

In addition to QRS duration, QRS morphology has also been shown to be an important determinant of response to CRT. LBBB results in significant delay between LV septal and lateral wall activation. In patients undergoing CRT, the presence of a LBBB prior to CRT has consistently been shown to be a strong marker of a favorable response.[43–47] How LBBB is defined has increasingly been shown to be an important determinant of CRT responsiveness. Strauss et al proposed a stricter definition of LBBB defined as the following: QS or rS in V_1, QRS duration ≥140 ms in men or ≥130 ms in women, and midQRS notching/slurring in at least 2 of the leads I, aVL, V_1, V_2, V_5, or V_6 with the midQRS notching/slurring beginning after the first 40 ms of the QRS onset but before 50% of the QRS duration.[48] Patients meeting this stricter definition have been noted to have greater mechanical dyssynchrony than those with a looser, traditional definition of LBBB.[49]

The response to CRT in patients with a nonLBBB morphology (a RBBB or a nonspecific interventricular conduction delay) is more controversial. Patients with a nonLBBB can have left-sided electrical activation delay but often times to a much lesser extent than patients with a LBBB.[32,50] The term "RBBB masking LBBB" has been used to refer to patients with an atypical RBBB with a wide QRS duration.[50] Compared to patients with a LBBB, patients with nonLBBB morphologies derive less benefit from CRT.[43,44] In subgroup analyses from the MADIT-CRT trial, no clinical benefit was observed in patients with nonLBBB morphologies.[51] In patients with a nonLBBB, the QRS duration may be an important determinant of response such that patients with a greater QRS duration may derive benefit. Patients with a nonLBBB and a QRS duration <150 ms are unlikely to benefit from CRT, especially if they are minimally symptomatic.[52]

Interplay Between QRS Duration and Morphology

While both QRS duration and morphology are important predictors of response to CRT, the 2 are intimately linked raising the question of which is of more importance. Patients with a LBBB more commonly have a wider QRS duration than patients with a nonLBBB.[53] The relative importance of QRS duration versus morphology is a question of ongoing investigation. In a single center cohort of 496 patients, QRS morphology was found to be a more important determinant of benefit from CRT compared to QRS duration.[53] Contrary to this, in a larger cohort of 3782 patients from 5 randomized controlled trials, QRS duration, but not QRS morphology, was found to be a potent predictor of outcome.[54]

CONCLUSIONS

The ECG plays a pivotal role in any patient either being considered for or implanted with a CRT-capable device. The ECG can provide a simple, noninvasive means of troubleshooting potential CRT problems and assessing adequacy of biventricular pacing. Anodal capture is likely under-recognized and should be looked for whenever a CRT patient is assessed especially patients with a CRT-P device with elevated LV pacing thresholds. The association between QRS narrowing and response to CRT is controversial although the totality of evidence supports a link. The ECG is a pivotal tool in assessing candidates for CRT as both QRS morphology and duration have been shown to be potent predictors of outcome following CRT. Whether QRS duration or QRS morphology is a more potent predictor of response is an area of ongoing investigation.

SUMMARY

- The ECG is an instrumental noninvasive tool that should be used in the assessment of CRT candidates and their follow-up.
- Routine ECG can reliably troubleshoot pacing problems and assess adequacy of biventricular pacing.
- Anodal capture is an overlooked complication of CRT and should especially be suspected in the setting of a CRT-P device with elevated LV pacing thresholds.
- Whether QRS narrowing is a determinant of response to CRT is still controversial with a trend in the literature towards a positive association.
- QRS duration and morphology remain potent predictors of response to CRT with the relative contribution of each currently unknown.

REFERENCES

1. Barold SS, Herweg B, Giudici M. Electrocardiographic follow up of biventricular pacemakers. *Ann Non Invasive Electrocardiol.* 2005;10:231–255.
2. Barold SS, Herweg B. Usefulness of the 12-lead electrocardiogram in the follow-up of patients with cardiac resynchronization devices. Part 1. *Cardiol J.* 2011;18:476–486.
3. Klein HO, Becker B, Sareli P, et al. Unusual QRS morphology associated with transvenous pacemakers. The pseudo RBBB pattern. *Chest.* 1985;87:517–521.
4. Coman JA, Trohman RG. Incidence and electrocardiographic localization of safe right bundle branch block configuration during permanent ventricular pacing. *Am J Cardiol.* 1995;76:781–784.
5. Wynn GJ, Weston C, Cooper RJ, Somauroo JD. Inadvertant left ventricular pacing through a patent foramen ovale: identification, management, and implications for postpacemaker implantation checks. *BMJ Case Rep.* 2013;27:2103.
6. Van Gelder BM, Bracke FA, Oto A, et al. Diagnosis and management of inadvertently placed pacing and ICD leads in the left ventricle: a multicenter experience and review of the literature. *Pacing Clin Electrophysiol.* 2000;23(5):877–883.
7. Sharifi M, Sorkin R, Sharifi V, Lakier JB. Inadvertent malposition of a transvenous-inserted pacing lead in the left ventricular chamber. *Am J Cardiol.* 1995;76(1):92–95.
8. Shettigar UR, Loungani RR, Smith CA. Inadvertent permanent ventricular pacing from the coronary vein. An electrocardiographic, roentgenographic, and echocardiographic assessment. *Clin Cardiol.* 1989;12:267–274.
9. Spencer JH, Anderson SE, Iaizzo PA. Human coronary venous anatomy: Implications for interventions. *J Cardiovasc Transl Res.* 2013;2:208–217.
10. Wilton SB. Shibata MA, Sondergaard R, et al. Relationship between left ventricular lead position using a simple radiographic classification scheme and long term outcome with resynchronization therapy. *J Interv Card Electrophysiol.* 2008;23:219–227.
11. Spencer JH, Larson AA, Drake R, Iaizzo PA. A detailed assessment of the human coronary venous system using contrast computed tomography of perfusion-fixed specimens. *Heart Rhythm.* 2014;11(2):282–288.
12. Giudici MC, Tigrett DW, Carlson JI, et al. Electrocardiographic patterns during: pacing the great cardiac and middle cardiac veins. *Pacing Clin Electrophysiol.* 2007;30:1376–1380.
13. Altmikas R, Nathan AW. Left ventricular pacing via the great cardiac vein in a patient with tricuspid and pulmonary valve replacement. *Heart.* 2001;85:91.
14. Grimley SR, Suffoletto MS, Gorcsan J III, Schwartzman D. Electrocardiographically concealed variation in left ventricular capture: A case with implications for resynchronization therapy in ischemic cardiomyopathy. *Heart Rhythm.* 2006;3:739–742.
15. Herweg B, Ilercil A, Madramootoo C, et al. Latency during left ventricular pacing from the lateral cardiac veins. A cause of ineffective biventricular pacing. *Pacing Clin Electrophysiol.* 2006;29:574–581.
16. Refaat M, Mansour M, Singh JP, Ruskin J, Heist EK. Electrocardiographic characteristics in right ventricular vs biventricular pacing in patients with paced right-bundle branch block QRS pattern. *J Electrocardiol.* 2011;44:289–295.
17. Ranjan R, Chiamvimon N, Thakor N, Tomaselli G, Marban E. Mechanism of anode stimulation in the heart. *Biophys J.* 1998;74:1850–1863.
18. Dendy KF, Poweel BD, Cha YM, et al. Anodal stimulation: An underrecognized cause of nonresponders to cardiac resynchronization therapy. *Indian Pacing Electrophysiol.* 2011;11(3):64–72
19. Tamborero D, Mont L, Alanis R, et al. Anodal capture in cardiac resynchronization therapy implications for device programming. *Pacing Clin Electrophysiol.* 2006;29:940–945.
20. Sweeney MO, van Bommel RJ, et al. Analysis of ventricular activation using surface electrocardiography to predict left ventricular reverse volumetric remodeling during cardiac resynchronization therapy. *Circulation* 2010;121:626–634.
21. Leclercq C, Faris O, Tunin R, et al. Systolic improvement and mechanical resynchronization does not require electrical synchrony in the dilated failing heart with left-bundle branch block. *Circulation.* 2002;106:1760–1763.
22. Reuter S, Garrigue S, Bordachar P, et al. Intermediate results of biventricular pacing in heart failure: Correlation between clinical and hemodynamic data. *Pacing Clin Electrophysiol.* 2000;23:1713–1717.
23. Gold MR, Thébault C, Linde C, et al. Effect of QRS duration and morphology on cardiac resynchronization therapy outcomes in mild heart failure: Results from the Resynchronization Reverses Remodeling in Systolic Left Ventricular Dysfunction (REVERSE) study. *Circulation.* 2012;126:822–829.
24. Alonso C, Leclerq C, Victor F, et al. Electrocardiographic predictive factors of long-term clinical improvement with multivariate biventricular pacing in advanced heart failure. *Am J Cardiol.* 1999;84:1417–1421.
25. Lecoq G, Leclerq C, Leray E, et al. Clinical and electrocardiographic predictors of a positive response to cardiac resynchronization therapy in advanced heart failure. *Eur Heart J.* 2005;26:1094–1100.
26. Iler MA, Hu T, Ayyagari S, et al. Prognostic value of electrocardiographic measurements before and after cardiac resynchronization device implantation in patients with heart failure due to ischemic or non-ischemic cardiomyopathy. *Am J Cardiol.* 2008;101:359–363.
27. Rickard J, Popovic Z, Verhaert D, et al. The QRS narrowing index predicts reverse left ventricular remodeling following cardiac resynchronization therapy. *Pacing Clin Electrophysiol.* 2011;34:604–611.
28. Copploa G, Bonaccorso P, Corrado E, et al. The QRS narrowing index for easy and early identification of responders to cardiac resynchronization therapy. *Int J Cardiol.* 2014;170:440–441.
29. Hsing JM, Selzman KA, Leclercq C, et al. Paced left ventricular QRS width and ECG parameters predict outcomes after cardiac resynchronization therapy:

PROSPECT-ECG substudy. *Circ Arrhythm Electrophysiol.* 2011;4:851–857.
30. Rickard J, Jackson G, Spragg DD, et al. QRS prolongation induced by cardiac resynchronization therapy correlates with deterioration in left ventricular function. *Heart Rhythm.* 2012;10:1674–1678.
31. Rickard J, Cheng A, Spragg D, et al. QRS narrowing is associated with reverse remodeling in patients with chronic right ventricular pacing upgraded to cardiac resynchronization therapy. *Heart Rhythm.* 2013;10:55–60.
32. Varma N. Left ventricular conduction delays and relation to QRS configuration in patients with left ventricular dysfunction. *Am J Cardiol.* 2009;103:1578–1585.
33. Bristow MR, Saxon LA, Boehmer J, et al. Cardiac resynchronization therapy with or without an implantable defibrillator in advanced chronic heart failure. *N Engl J Med.* 2004;350:2140–2150.
34. Cleland JG, Daubert JC, Erdmann E, et al. The effect of cardiac resynchronization on morbidity and mortality in heart failure. *N Engl J Med.* 2005;352:1539–1549.
35. St. John Sutton M, Ghio S, Plappert T, et al. On behalf of the resynchronization reverses remodeling in systolic left ventricular dysfunction (REVERSE) study group. *Circulation.* 2009;120:1858–1865.
36. Moss AJ, Hall WJ, Cannom DS, et al. Cardiac-resynchronization therapy for the prevention of heart-failure events. *N Engl J Med.* 2009;361:1329–1338.
37. Tang AS, Wells GA, Talajic M, et al. Resynchronization-defibrillation for ambulatory heart failure trial investigators. *N Engl J Med.* 2010;363:2385–2395.
38. Sipahi I, Carrigan TP, Rowland DY, Stambler BS, Fang JC. Impact of QRS duration on clinical event reduction with cardiac resynchronization therapy: Meta-analysis of randomized controlled trials. *Arch Intern Med.* 2011;171:1454–1462.
39. Thibault B, Harel F, Ducharme A, et al. Cardiac resynchronization therapy in patients with heart failure and a QRS complex <120 milliseconds: the Evaluation of Resynchronization Therapy for Heart Failure (LESSER-EARTH) trial. *Circulation.* 2013;127:873–881.
40. Beshai JF, Grimm RA, Nagueh SF, et al. Cardiac-resynchronization therapy in heart failure with narrow QRS complexes. *N Engl J Med.* 2007;357:2461–2471.
41. Ruschitzka F, Abraham WT, Singh JP, et al. Cardiac-resynchronization therapy in heart failure with a narrow QRS complex. *N Engl J Med.* 2013;369:1395–1405.
42. Gasparini M, Leclercq C, Yu CK, et al. Absolute survival after cardiac resynchronization therapy according to baseline QRS duration: a multinational 10-year experience: Data from the Multicenter International CRT Study. *Am Heart J.* 2014;167:203–209.
43. Adelstein EC, Saba S. Usefulness of baseline electrocardiographic QRS complex pattern to predict response to cardiac resynchronization therapy. *Am J Cardiol.* 2009;103:238–242.
44. Rickard J, Kumbhani DJ, Gorodeski EZ, et al. Cardiac resynchronization therapy in non-left bundle branch block morphologies. *Pacing Clin Electrophysiol.* 2010;33:590–595.
45. Wokhlu A, Rea RF, Asirvatham SJ, et al. Upgrade of *de novo* cardiac resynchronization therapy: Impact of paced or intrinsic QRS morphology on outcomes and survival. *Heart Rhythm.* 2009;6:1439–1447.
46. Bilchick KC, Kamath S, DiMarco JP, Stukenborg GJ. Bundle-branch block morphology and other predictors of outcome after cardiac resynchronization therapy in Medicare patients. *Circulation.* 2010;122:2022–2030.
47. Rickard J, Kumbhani DJ, Popovic Z, et al. Characterization of super-response to cardiac resynchronization therapy. *Heart Rhythm.* 2010;7:885–889.
48. Strauss DG, Selvester RH, Wagner GS. Defining left bundle branch block in the era of cardiac resynchronization therapy. *Am J Cardiol.* 2011;107(6):927–934.
49. Anderson LG, Wu KC, Wiselander B, et al. Left ventricular mechanical dyssynchrony by cardiac magnetic resonance is greater in patients with strict vs nonstrict electrocardiogram criteria for left bundle-branch block. *Am Heart J.* 2013;165: 956–963.
50. Fantoni C, Kawabata M, Massaro R, et al. Right and left ventricular activation sequence in patient with heart failure and right bundle branch block: a detailed analysis using three-dimensional non-fluoroscopic electroanatomic mapping system. *J Cardiovasc Electrophysiol.* 2005;16:112–119.
51. Zareba W, Klein H, Cygankiewicz I, et al. Effectiveness of cardiac resynchronization therapy by QRS morphology in the multicenter automatic defibrillator implantation trial-cardiac resynchronization therapy (MADIT-CRT). *Circulation.* 2011;123:1061–1072.
52. Epstein AE, DiMarco JP, Ellenbogen KA, et al. 2012 ACCF/AHA/HRS focused update incorporated into the ACCF/AHA/HRS 2008 guidelines for device-based therapy of cardiac rhythm abnormalities: a report of the American College of Cardiology Foundation/ American Heart Association Task Force on Practice Guidelines and the Heart Rhythm Society. *J Am Coll Cardiol.* 2013;61:e6–e75.
53. Dupont M, Rickard J, Baranowski B, et al. Differential response to cardiac resynchronization therapy and clinical outcomes according to QRS morphology and QRS duration. *J Am Coll Cardiol.* 2012; 60:592–598.
54. Cleland JG, Abraham WT, Linde C, et al. An individual patient meta-analysis of five randomized trials assessing the effects of cardiac resynchronization therapy on morbidity and mortality in patients with symptomatic heart failure. *Eur Heart J.* 2013;46:3547–3456.

CHAPTER

18

Effect of Cardiac and Noncardiac Drugs on Electrocardiograms: Electrocardiographic Markers of Drug-Induced Proarrhythmias (QT Prolongation, TdP, and Ventricular Arrhythmias)

Chinmay Patel, MD, Eyad Kanawati, MD, and Peter Kowey, MD

INTRODUCTION

The ECG is an indispensable tool in evaluating the effects of drugs on the cardiac electrical system. Various cardiac and noncardiac drugs affect a variety of cardiac ion channels, either therapeutically or as an untoward effect. In this chapter, the basic electrophysiologic effects of antiarrhythmic drugs on cardiac ion channels, action potential, and their correlation with the ECG will be discussed to provide a framework for evaluating drug efficacy and proarrhythmia.

CARDIAC ACTION POTENTIAL

The cardiac action potential has 5 phases (Figure 18.1).[1] In nonpacemaker cells, during the resting *phase 4*, the myocardial membrane potential is maintained at a steady level of approximately –85 to –90 mV by the Na^+-K^+ ATPase pump. *Phase 0* defines the opening of voltage-gated Na channels and rapid influx of Na^+ ions (I_{Na}) that changes the membrane potential to about +40 mV, followed by rapid inactivation of the majority of the Na channels. However, a small fraction of sodium channels remains open and continues to carry inward sodium current. This is called late sodium current ($I_{Na\text{-}L}$). Brief, transient outward potassium current (I_{to}) then follows, which leads to the characteristic spike and dome appearance (*phase 1*). The L-type calcium channel drives the inward calcium current ($I_{Ca\text{-}L}$) that defines the beginning of *phase 2* of action potential. *Phase 2* represents a delicate balance between inward currents ($I_{Ca\text{-}L}$, $I_{Na\text{-}L}$) and outward

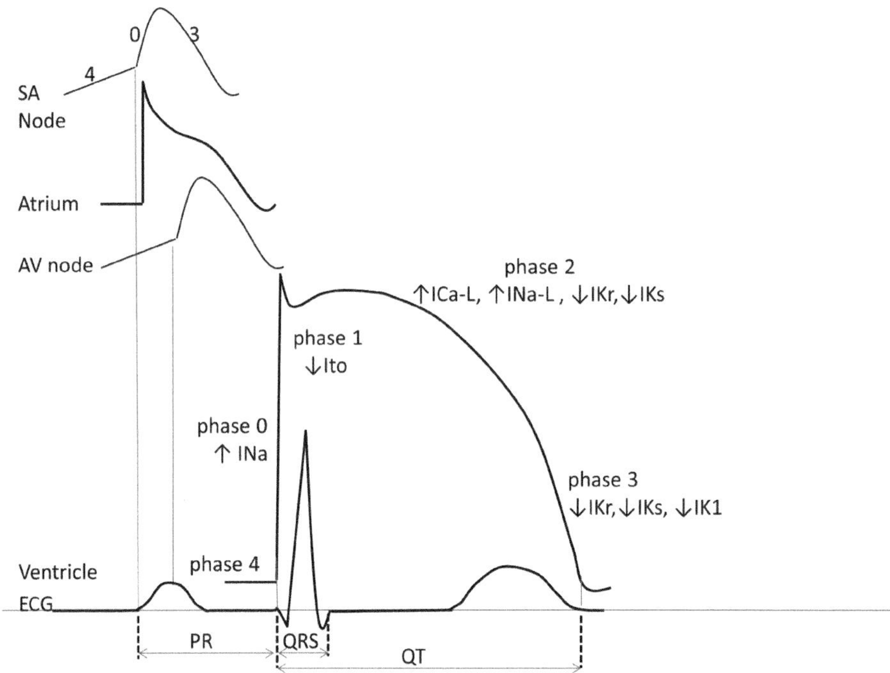

Figure 18.1. Schematic presentation of action potential of various cardiac cell types and their relationship to the surface ECG.

potassium currents (slow activating (I_{Ks}) and rapidly activating (I_{Kr}) delayed rectifier potassium current). During *phase 3*, there is a gradual decay of the inward $I_{Ca\text{-}L}$, and outward potassium current (I_{Kr}, I_{Ks}, and I_{K1}) predominates. This brings the membrane potential back to baseline (*phase 4*) with the recovery of fast Na^+ channels in preparation for ventricular reexcitation.

For practical purposes, the cardiac cellular action potential can be divided into 2 subtypes: the slow, calcium-mediated action potential and the fast, sodium channel-mediated action potential (see Figure 18.1).[1] Myocytes in the SA and AV nodes exhibit automaticity due to spontaneous phase 4 depolarization, rendering them as pacemaker cells. Compared to other cardiac cell types, their resting membrane potential is less negative (−60 mV) during the early part of phase 4.[2] Spontaneous phase 4 depolarization results from pacemaker current (I_F) that largely carries Na^+ into the cell. This brings the membrane potential close to threshold potential, resulting in phase 0 depolarization, that is, mediated by $I_{Ca\text{-}L}$. This particular action potential is characterized by a slowly rising upstroke. In contrast, atrial, ventricular, and His-Purkinje system myocytes do not have pacemaker current, and phase 0 is mediated by fast I_{Na} with rapid upstroke of the action potential.[1]

CARDIAC ACTION POTENTIAL AND THE ECG

As stated previously, the SA node has the highest rate of spontaneous phase 4 diastolic depolarization and hence serves as the primary pacemaker of the heart.[2] Pacemaker cell action potential acts as a current source that propagates to neighboring atrial cells via gap junctions that leads to activation of fast Na^+ channels and conduction of the electrical impulse to the entire atrial myocardium, leading to inscription of the P wave.[1] Conduction delay in the AV node manifests at the PR interval. This is followed by rapid propagation via fast sodium current in the His-Purkinje system that leads to sequential activation of the entire ventricular myocardium that produces the QRS complex on the surface ECG.[1] The QT interval corresponds to the duration of ventricular cell action potential. Dispersion in duration and sequence of ventricular myocyte repolarization leads to inscription of the T wave.[3]

DRUGS AND ECG: BASIC PRINCIPLES

Cardio-active drugs influence the cardiac electrical cycle either by direct effects on membrane ion channels or by indirectly altering the autonomic input to the heart.

Heart Rate

Drugs can affect the heart rate by altering the automaticity of the sinus node. The intrinsic heart rate or rate of spontaneous depolarization of pacemaker cells is determined by the interplay between baseline membrane potential, threshold potential, and the slope of

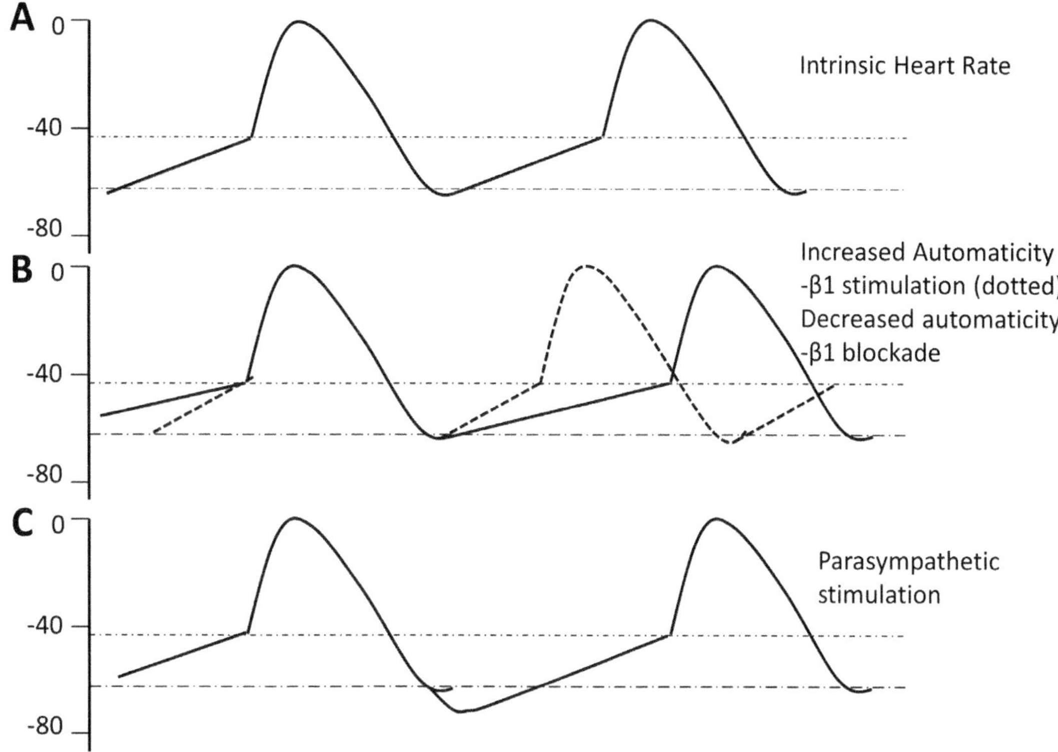

Figure 18.2. Electrophysiologic and autonomic effects of drugs that affect heart rate. See the text for detailed explanation.

spontaneous phase 4 depolarization (Figure 18.2A).[2] Changes in any of these factors affect the rate of impulse formation—*automaticity*—and hence heart rate.

Both the SA and the AV node are richly innervated with muscarinic cholinergic receptors and β1 adrenergic receptors. Sympathetic stimulation via activation of β1-adrenergic receptors enhances I_{Ca-L} and inward I_F thus augmenting the slope of phase 4, thereby increasing automaticity (see Figure 18.2B).[4] Sympathomimetic drugs like dobutamine, dopamine, norepinephrine, epinephrine, and isoproterenol cause tachycardia by this mechanism. Cocaine increases the level of circulating catecholamines that leads to sinus tachycardia by a similar mechanism. On the other hand, β-blockers and drugs with antiadrenergic properties decrease the slope of phase 4 depolarization and decrease the heart rate (see Figure 18.2B).[4] Ivabradine, a selective I_F blocker, leads to bradycardia by a similar mechanism.[5]

In contrast, parasympathetic stimulation via acetylcholine activates the outward potassium current (I_{K-Ach}) and inhibits the inward I_{Ca-L}.[6] An increase in outward potassium current drives the membrane potential to a more negative resting potential, and a decrease in calcium current slows the rate of diastolic depolarization, resulting in a slower rate of impulse formation (see Figure 18.2C). The effects of digoxin on heart rate and the PR interval are mediated via increased parasympathetic tone.

PR Interval

In a similar fashion, autonomic input affects the rate of impulse conduction through the AV node and is reflected as changes in the PR interval. Sympathetic stimulation shortens the PR interval, and parasympathetic stimulation prolongs the PR interval.

P Wave and QRS Complex

The duration of the P wave and the QRS complex is a reflection of conduction velocity, or total depolarization time, of atrial and ventricular muscle mass respectively, via fast I_{Na}. Slowing of conduction velocity leads directly to prolongation of the P wave and QRS duration (Figure 18.3A).

QT Interval

The QT interval/ventricular cell action potential duration (APD) is a fine balance between inward currents (I_{Na}, I_{Ca-L}, I_{Na-L}) and outward currents (I_{Ks}, I_{Kr}, I_{K1}).[3,7] Drugs that increase the net inward current increase the duration of ventricular cell action potential, and the drugs that decrease the net inward

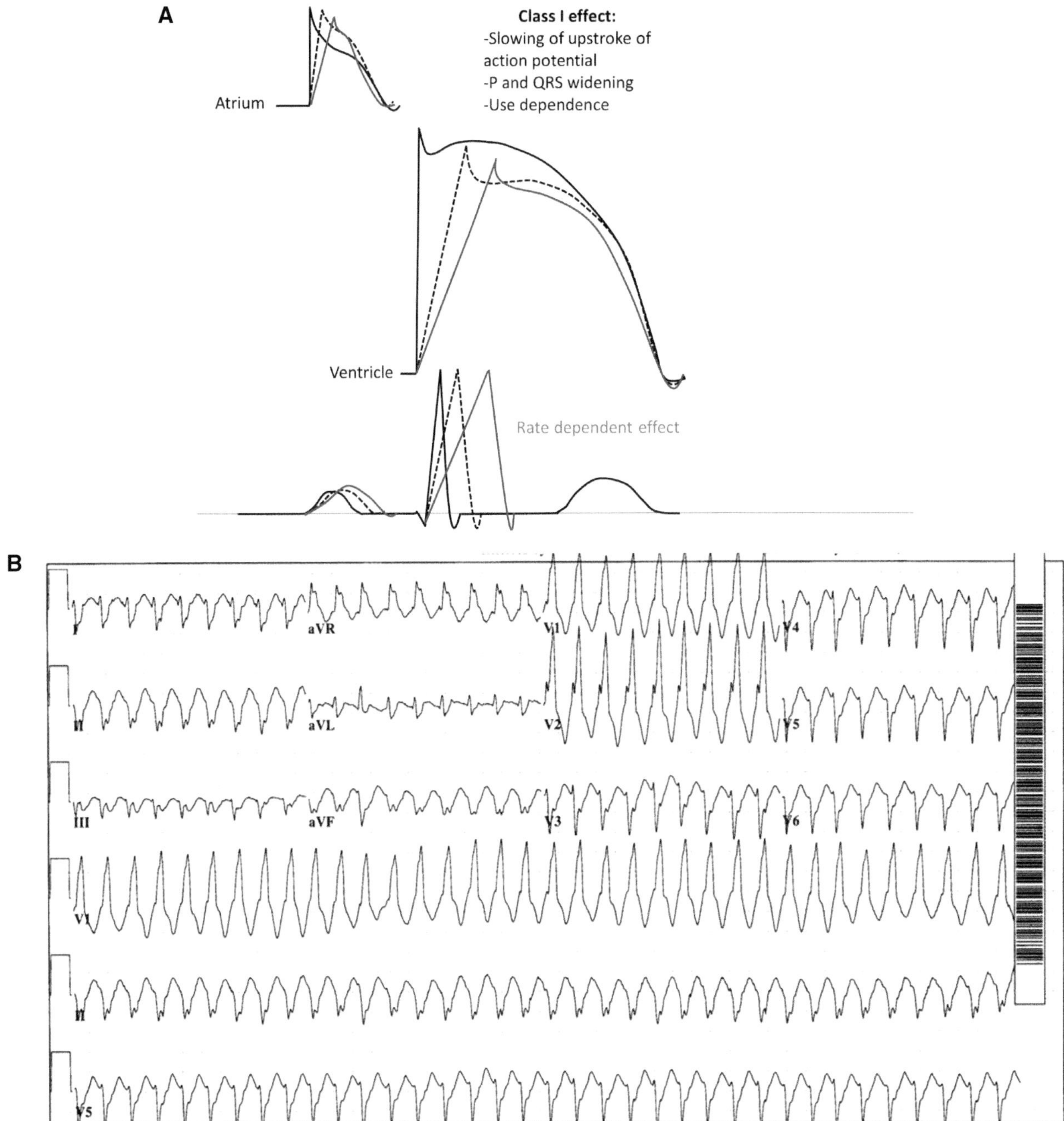

Figure 18.3. Class I ECG effects. **A.** Schematic presentation of use dependency and ECG correlates. **B.** ECG of a patient who presented with atrial flutter with 1:1 AV conduction in the setting of flecainide therapy. Slowing of conduction decreased the rate of atrial flutter, thus promoting 1:1 AV nodal conduction. Use dependent I_{Na} block caused prolongation of QRS during mimicking VT. *Source:* Used with permission from Dr. Gan-Xin Yan, Lankenau Medical Center, Wynnewood, PA, USA.

current decrease the duration of ventricular action potential, and the QT interval.[7]

MECHANISMS OF DRUG-INDUCED ARRHYTHMIA

Mechanistically, any arrhythmia can be caused by automaticity, reentry, or triggered activity.[8] Triggered activity is mediated by *early after-depolarization (EAD)* or *delayed after-depolarization (DAD)*. Drugs that prolong the QT interval lead to EAD-mediated proarrhythmia, and drugs that cause calcium overload lead to DAD-mediated proarrhythmia.

Enhanced automaticity is the mechanism of arrhythmia for sympathomimetic drugs.[8,9] Adrenergic stimulation can also promote intracellular calcium overload and may cause arrhythmia mediated by *triggered activity*. *Reentry* is a prominent mechanism of drug-induced arrhythmia caused by sodium channel-blocking drugs.[8,9] Drug-induced slowing of conduction within diseased myocardium can cause wavelength shortening and increases the likelihood of sustained reentry.

VAUGHAN WILLIAMS CLASSIFICATION

The effects of drugs on the ECG have been described by Vaughan Williams based on the predominant ion current or receptor. The Vaughan Williams classification is presented below. Noncardiac drugs are also included based on their predominant ion channel effects.

Class I ECG Effects

Class I effects are caused by slowing of the upstroke of phase 0 of the I_{Na}-mediated action potential of atrial and ventricular myocytes (see Figure 18.3A). This leads to decreased conduction velocity.[10] Pure *class I ECG changes* are prolongation of the P wave and QRS durations. If there is a significant prolongation of P wave and QRS complex duration, it may result in mild prolongation of the PR and QT intervals; however, the JT interval remains unchanged.[10]

Use-dependence is a specific class I effect that describes more pronounced sodium channel blockade at faster rates (see Figure 18.3A).[11] In general, drug binding to sodium channels occurs during phases 0 and 2, and dissociation occurs during phase 4. During tachycardia, phase 4 is abbreviated, not allowing adequate time for dissociation of the drug from its receptor. A higher degree of sodium channel blockade is seen at higher heart rates and is concentration-dependent. Thus, higher doses of these drugs result in further slowing of conduction velocity, leading to prolongation of the QRS duration.

The extent of sodium channel blockade with class I antiarrhythmic drugs depends on heart rate, membrane potential, and the rate of onset/recovery of the block.[10] Pure class IC drugs such as flecainide and propafenone have the most pronounced sodium channel blocking effects even at normal heart rates, and can cause significant conduction slowing.

Class IA drugs such as quinidine, procainamide, and disopyramide have moderate sodium channel effects and generally cause slowing of conduction only at rapid heart rates. They also have class III effects, discussed below. Class IB drugs such as lidocaine and mexiletine have no effects on normal inward sodium current but cause significant slowing of conduction in partially depolarized tissue like ischemic myocardium. For all practical purposes, class IB drugs have no discernible effects on the ECG.

Class I Proarrhythmia

Class IC drugs are frequently used in patients with atrial fibrillation (AF).[12] The slowing of conduction in AF can result in development of atrial flutter with a very slow flutter cycle length. This may result in rare cases in 1:1 atrioventricular conduction with fast ventricular rates at 150 to 200 bpm (see Figure 18.3B). In many cases, fast ventricular rate may be associated with marked QRS prolongation due to use-dependent enhanced blockade of fast sodium channels and further conduction slowing.[10] Wide QRS tachycardia thus can mimic ventricular tachycardia (VT). Similarly, enhanced slowing of conduction during sinus tachycardia in patients receiving flecainide has been shown to be associated with development of monomorphic VT.[13] This kind of proarrhythmia is much more common in patients with ischemic cardiomyopathy, since sodium channels in ischemic myocytes are more sensitive to sodium channel blockade.

Since conduction in the His-Purkinje system is sodium channel-dependent, any drug with class I effects can precipitate higher degrees of AV block in patients with preexisting conduction system disease. Several psychotropic drugs, including tricyclic antidepressants, neuroleptics like thioridazine, and antipsychotics like loxapine, also block I_{Na} and have been shown to cause ventricular proarrhythmia.[14] Although its clinical significance is unknown, sodium channel blocker can induce the ECG pattern of the Brugada syndrome and in some cases provoke ventricular fibrillation in susceptible patients.[15]

Class II and IV ECG Effects

Class II and IV ECG effects are decrease in heart rate and prolongation of the PR interval. β-adrenergic blocking agents and nondihydropyridine calcium channel blockers (CCB) decrease the slope of spontaneous phase 4 depolarization, resulting in decreased SA node automaticity and prolonged AV nodal conduction[10] (see Figure 18.2). Large doses of any of these agents can cause profound sinus bradycardia, a variable degree of AV nodal block, and the suppression of automaticity of escape pacemaker cells. The dihydropyridine CCBs such as nifedipine are predominantly peripheral vasodilators and may cause reflex tachycardia.

Class III ECG Effects

Class III effects are caused by prolongation of phase 3 of the cardiac action potential (Figure 18.4A). Drugs that block one of the outward potassium currents such as I_{Kr}, I_{Ks}, or increase the late inward sodium current

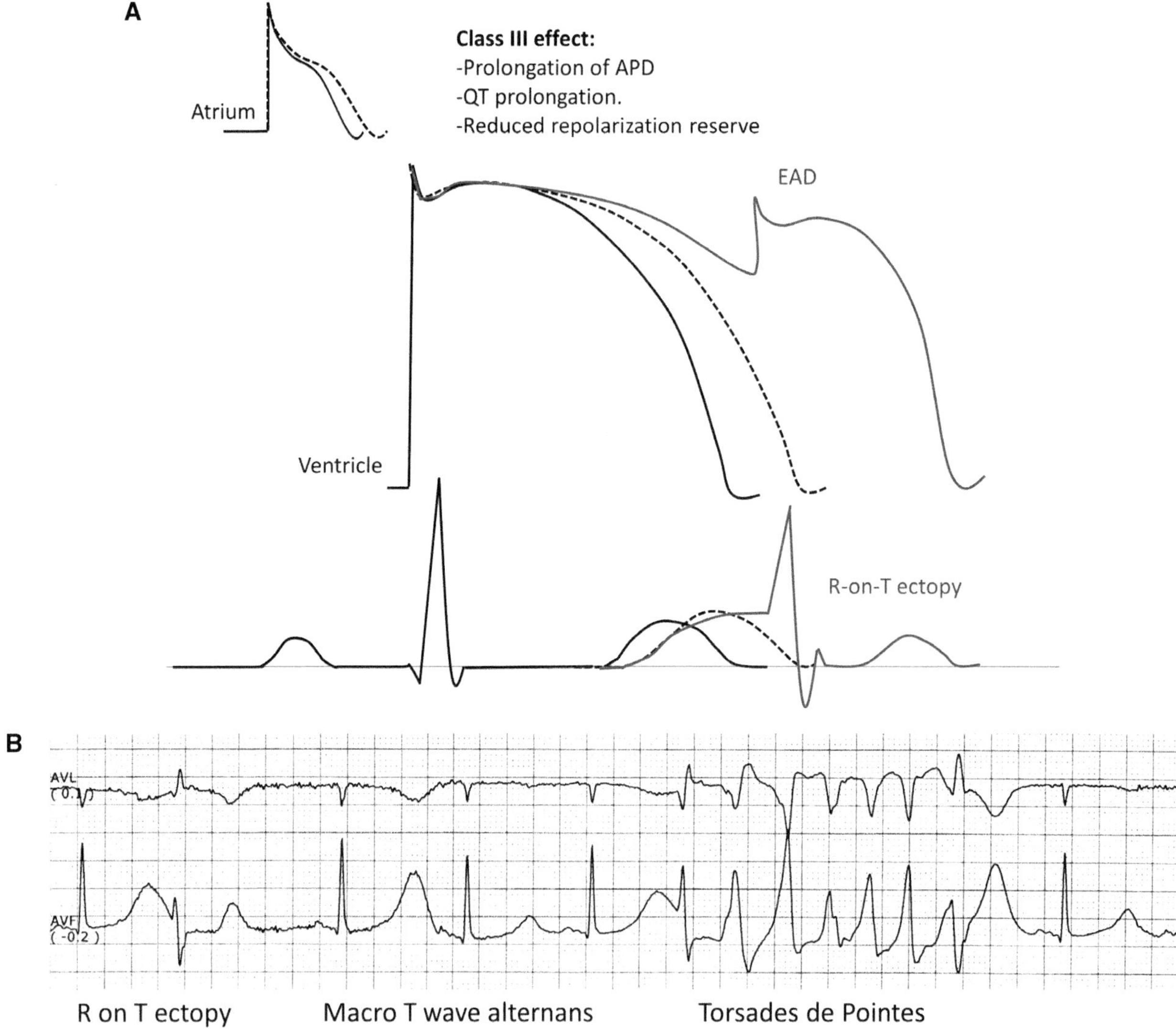

Figure 18.4. Class III ECG effects. **A.** Schematic presentation of Class III effects on action potential, EAD, and their ECG correlates. **B.** Rhythm strip of a patient who presented with sotalol-induced TdP, showing macro-T wave alternans, an R-on-T ectopic beat, and torsades de pointes.

prolong the duration of ventricular cell action potential reflected as JT/QT interval prolongation on the ECG.[10] Pure class III agents do not have any effects on I_{Na} or $I_{Ca\text{-}L}$, so they do not generally affect heart rate or QRS duration.

Reverse use-dependence is a specific property of class III antiarrhythmic drugs (dofetilide, sotalol) that block I_{Kr} current.[16] A greater degree of prolongation of repolarization is observed during bradycardia than during tachycardia. This results in limited drug effects during tachycardia and pronounced drug effects during bradycardia. APD and QT interval can prolong significantly at slower heart rates, which facilitates torsade de pointes (TdP). Drugs that block I_{Ks} current in addition to I_{Kr} (amiodarone, azimilide) do not exhibit reverse use-dependence and have a lower incidence of TdP.[17]

Antiarrhythmic drugs such as dofetilide, ibutilide, and azimilide are pure class III agents. A complete list of cardiac and noncardiac drugs that have been shown to block outward potassium, especially I_{Kr}, and prolong the QT interval (and thus have a potential to harm) can be found at www.QTdrugs.org.[18]

Dofetilide is a commonly used drug in treatment of AF that is a selective I_{Kr} blocker. It prolongs repolarization in atrial and ventricular myocytes.[10,12] Its sole ECG effect is prolongation of the JT/QT interval. Due to its potential to cause TdP, dofetilide should not be used in patients with a baseline QTc greater than 440 ms, and dose reduction is recommended if the QTc interval increases to more than 500 ms (or 15% from baseline).

Sotalol is a class III antiarrhythmic drug with noncardioselective β-adrenergic/class II effects.[10] The

ECG effects of sotalol include slowing of heart rate and prolongation of PR and QTc interval.

Ibutilide, a drug approved for chemical cardioversion of AF, has ECG effects similar to those of dofetilide.[10] Azimilide (I_{Kr} and I_{Ks} blocker) leads to about a 25% increase in QT interval with less of a potential to cause TdP due to lack of reverse use-dependent properties.

Class III Proarrhythmia—TdP

TdP is a polymorphic VT seen in the setting of QT interval prolongation. The QT interval is the ECG correlate of ventricular cell APD.[7,19] A balance between depolarizing inward currents (I_{Na}, $I_{Ca\text{-}L}$, and $I_{Na\text{-}L}$), repolarizing outward currents (I_{Kr}, I_{Ks}, I_{K1}, I_{to}, and $I_{K\text{-}ATP}$), and their time/voltage-dependent properties determines ventricular cell APD and hence QT interval (see Figure 18.4A). Any drug that decreases net repolarizing forces (increases the depolarizing current and/or decreases repolarizing current) leads to QT prolongation.[20] A reduced repolarization reserve/decreased net repolarizing force is the principal abnormality in drug-induced QT prolongation irrespective of the ionic currents involved.[20] Reduction of repolarization reserve leads to prolongation of ventricular APD and amplifies the intrinsic heterogeneity of ventricular myocardium due to preferential prolongation of cells with baseline poor repolarization forces like midmyocardial M cells.[21] The resultant increase in dispersion of repolarization creates a vulnerable window across the ventricular wall.

Activation of inward current (reactivation of $I_{Ca\text{-}L}$ or sodium-calcium exchange current) leads to EADs (see Figure 18.4A). EADs that do not reach threshold potential cause abnormal T-wave morphology and further QT prolongation. It is suggested that sub-threshold EAD alternans is the cellular mechanism for macro-T-wave alternans. EADs that reach the threshold for reexcitation of sodium channels lead to R-on-T extrasystoles. Such extrasystoles may capture the vulnerable window, resulting in TdP.[21] Abnormal reverse use-dependent prolongation of the QT interval under such conditions further promotes arrhythmogenesis.

Studies of congenital long QT syndrome have shown that the longer the QT interval, the higher the risk of TdP. However, QT prolongation is not the sole determinant of the development of TdP. Drugs like amiodarone and ranolazine consistently prolong the QT interval but rarely lead to TdP.[21] On the other hand, many patients with congenital long QT syndrome have near-normal QT intervals when they develop TdP. Dispersion of repolarization is another important determinant of TdP.[21] Studies using arterially perfused left ventricular wedge preparations show that QT-prolonging drugs do not cause TdP unless dispersion of repolarization reaches a critical threshold value. Drugs such as sotalol, dofetilide, and erythromycin produce dose-dependent prolongation of the QT interval that is associated with increased dispersion of repolarization.

ECG Index of Dispersion of Repolarization—$T_{peak\text{-}end}$ Interval

Although the QT interval on the surface ECG is a surrogate for APD of ventricular myocytes, there is no well-defined ECG marker that reflects dispersion of repolarization. It is agreed that the T wave reflects repolarization of ventricular myocardium, but the exact cellular basis of the T wave is a matter of controversy.[3] Studies have suggested electrophysiologic heterogeneity in the cells spanning the ventricular wall.

There are at least 3 different populations of cells across the ventricular wall: (1) epicardial; (2) endocardial; and (3) midmyocardial (M) cells.[22] Cardiac ion channels are expressed differentially in these subgroups of cells and respond differently when subjected to changes in heart rate and drugs. M cells are characterized by poor baseline repolarization forces due to smaller I_{Ks}, larger $I_{Na\text{-}L}$, and larger Na-Ca exchange currents, and have a longer APD than epicardial and endocardial myocytes.[22] The APD of M cells prolongs much more than that of other cell types in response to slowing of the heart rate, or in the presence of APD-prolonging agents.

Studies using arterially perfused canine left ventricular wedge preparations have shown that the differential time course of repolarization of the 3 myocardial cell types leads to the inscription of the electrocardiographic T wave.[7,19] The end of repolarization of epicardial myocytes coincides with the peak of the T wave, and the end of repolarization of M cells coincides with the end of the T wave.[7,19] The interval from the peak of the T wave to the end of the T wave ($T_{peak\text{-}end}$) closely correlates with transmural dispersion of repolarization (TDR). It has been suggested that $T_{peak\text{-}end}$ interval is an important noninvasive index of spatial dispersion of repolarization, importantly TDR.[23] Many studies have shown that $T_{peak\text{-}end}$ interval and importantly $T_{peak\text{-}end}$/QT ratio is increased in arrhythmogenic conditions like acute myocardial infarction, Brugada syndrome, long QT syndrome, and short QT syndrome, and can be used as an ECG surrogate of dispersion of repolarization.[24–26] Temporal changes in $T_{peak\text{-}end}$ interval and their QT interval relationship may be particularly valuable for the prediction of ventricular proarrhythmia.

Irrespective of offending drug and ion current involved, when a "torsadogenic" milieu is present,

12-lead ECGs (see Figure 18.4B) show a constellation of findings that may include the following:

- Significant QT interval prolongation (>500 ms).
- Abnormal T-wave morphology.
- Increase in $T_{peak-end}$ interval and $T_{peak-end}$/QT ratio from baseline.
- Beat-to-beat change in QT interval.
- Macro-T-wave alternans.
- R-on-T extra-systole.
- TdP that may or may not be pause-dependent.

MULTI-ION CHANNEL BLOCKING DRUGS

Quinidine and Class IA drugs

Although quinidine is a class IA agent, in addition to $I_{Na,}$ it blocks I_{Kr}, I_{Ks}, and I_{to}. *In vitro*, even at lower concentrations, quinidine predominantly blocks I_{Kr} and prolongs APD. At higher concentration, quinidine additionally blocks I_{Na} and blunts APD prolongation. It also has vagolytic effects. Expected ECG changes are *class I and class III effects*, including prolongation of P and QRS duration, and QT interval prolongation. In toxic concentrations, sinus bradycardia or sinus arrest, sinus tachycardia, notching and prolongation of the P wave and QRS complex, organization of AF to atrial flutter, and 1:1 AV conduction of flutter can occur. By slowing conduction, quinidine can promote monomorphic VT in patients with a substrate for VT. Quinidine syncope represents TdP in the setting of significant QT interval prolongation.

The ECG effects of procainamide and disopyramide are similar to those of quinidine but are less pronounced.[10] Disopyramide has strong anticholinergic effects that cause sinus bradycardia. Procainamide is acetylated in the liver to an active metabolite N-acetylprocainamide, which blocks I_{Kr} and leads to QT prolongation.[10]

Amiodarone, Dronedarone, and Ranolazine

Amiodarone, although a class III drug, exhibits electrophysiologic properties of all 4 Vaughan Williams classes.[10] In addition to block I_{Kr} and I_{Ks}, it blocks inward I_{Na}, I_{Ca-L}, and has β-blocking properties. Intravenous administration of amiodarone has prominent antiadrenergic and I_{Ca-L} blocking effects; hence it slows heart rate and prolongs AV nodal conduction. Chronic therapy leads to blockade of I_{Kr} and I_{Ks} in addition to I_{Na} and I_{Ca-L}.[10] Sinus bradycardia, PR interval prolongation, and QRS and QT interval prolongation are common after chronic therapy. Occasionally, sino-atrial exit block, sinus arrest, and AV block can occur. Because of use-dependent I_{Na} blockade, amiodarone therapy slows conduction of reentry circuits in patients with reentrant VT resulting in slow VT with a wide QRS complex. Although the QT interval is prolonged, because of preferential prolongation of the APD of epicardial and endocardial myocytes as compared to M cells, TDR is minimal.[27] With I_{Ks} blockade, amiodarone does not exhibit significant reverse use-dependent QT prolongation. As a result of all of these unique electrophysiologic effects, amiodarone has a remarkably low incidence of TdP.[28]

Dronedarone is an amiodarone congener with electrophysiologic properties similar to but generally not as marked as amiodarone.[29] With clinical doses, the ECGs show mild QT-interval prolongation.

Ranolazine is an antianginal drug that also blocks I_{Kr} and is a potent blocker of I_{Na-L}.[30] Mild QT-interval prolongation is observed in patients on ranolazine therapy. Because of I_{Na-L} blockade, ranolazine does not cause TdP.

NA⁺ K⁺ ATPASE BLOCKER: DIGOXIN

Digoxin is a cardiac glycoside currently used for heart failure.[31] It inhibits Na^+ K^+ ATPase leading to intracellular sodium accumulation, resulting in intracellular calcium overload via the Na^+-Ca^{2+} exchanger. The rise of intracellular calcium levels causes the positive inotropic effect associated with digoxin, but it also contributes to abnormal automaticity/triggered activity via DADs. Digoxin also increases vagal tone, causing direct inhibition of the SA and AV nodes.

Digoxin's earliest ECG effects are a decrease in T-wave amplitude and shortening of QT interval.[31] "Digitalis effect" refers to mild ST-segment depression with upward concavity, depression of the first part of the T wave, and prominent U waves. Digoxin-induced arrhythmias are a result of increased vagal tone, increased automaticity/trigger activity in atrial, ventricular, or His-Purkinje system myocytes, and combination thereof. The earliest manifestation of digoxin toxicity is premature ventricular complexes. Less-common but well-described arrhythmias with digoxin toxicity are paroxysmal atrial tachycardia with variable degrees of AV block and bi-directional VT.

Increased vagal tone can manifest as variable degrees of AV block, sinus bradycardia, or sino-atrial exit block or arrest. Shortening of the atrial refractory period can result in AF. In patients with chronic AF on digoxin therapy, regularization of ventricular rate often is an indication of digoxin toxicity. Increased automaticity/trigger activity can result in atrial tachycardia, junctional tachycardia, or fascicular tachycardia. When triggered activity originates in the His-Purkinje system, the ECG shows right bundle branch block with either left axis deviation (suggestive of origin in the left posterior fascicle) or right axis deviation (suggestive of origin in the left anterior fascicle). Sometimes, the site of triggered activity alternates between the 2 fascicles, resulting in classically described bi-directional VT.

COCAINE AND OTHER RECREATIONAL DRUGS

Cocaine, a recreational drug, blocks I_{Kr}, I_{Na}, and the reuptake of catecholamines at adrenergic nerve endings.[32] Sinus tachycardia and ST-T changes suggestive of ischemia are frequently seen in patients with cocaine intoxication. It can cause monomorphic VT due to I_{Na} blockade and TdP due to I_{Kr} blockade. A hyperadrenergic state induced by cocaine can promote calcium overload and resultant triggered atrial and ventricular arrhythmia. Cocaine intoxication has also been shown to induce a type-1 Brugada-like pattern in predisposed individuals.[15,32] Additionally, recreational drugs such as ecstasy, ice, crystal, the love pill, Eve, Death, ma-huang, khat, bath salts, LSD, PCP, and cannabis result in hyperadrenergic states with expected sympathomimetic effects.

CONCLUSION

- Knowledge of the cardiac action potential, electrophysiologic properties of drugs, and mechanisms of arrhythmia is integral to understanding the effects of various drugs on the ECG
- Categorization of drug effects by Vaughan Williams class helps to understand these principles, even though drugs may have effects that cut across several of the defined classes, and can have effects that the nosology does not take into account.
- Relating drug-induced arrhythmia to arrhythmia mechanism promotes understanding and facilitates the treatment of these remarkably common but dangerous clinical entities.

REFERENCES

1. Grant AO, Carboni M. In: Podrid PJ, Kowey PR, eds. *Cardiac Arrhythmia: Mechanisms, Diagnosis and Management.* 2nd ed. Philadelphia, PA: Lippincott Williams and Wilkins; 2001:37–51. Brown HF. Electrophysiology of the sinoatrial node. *Physiol Rev.* 1982;62:505–530.
2. Patel C, Burke JF, Patel H, et al. Is there a significant transmural gradient in repolarization time in the intact heart? Cellular basis of the T wave: a century of controversy. *Circ Arrhythm Electrophysiol.* 2009;2:80–88.
3. Zhang H, Vassalle M. Mechanisms of adrenergic control of sino-atrial node discharge. *J Biomed Sci.* 2003;10:179–192.
4. Roubille F, Tardif JC. New therapeutic targets in cardiology: Heart failure and arrhythmia: HCN channels. *Circulation.* 2013;127:1986–1996.
5. Vassalle M, Zhang H. On the mechanisms of cholinergic control of the sinoatrial node discharge. *J Cardiovasc Pharmacol.* 2001;37:173–186.
6. Antzelevitch C. Cellular basis for the repolarization waves of the ECG. *Ann N Y Acad Sci.* 2006;1080:268–281.
7. Wit AL, Rosen MR. Pathophysiologic mechanisms of cardiac arrhythmias. *Am Heart J.* 1983;106:798–811.
8. Zipes DP. Mechanisms of clinical arrhythmias. *J Cardiovasc Electrophysiol.* 2003;14:902–912.
9. Kowey PR, Yan G-X, Crijns H. Antiarrhythmic drugs. In: Fuster V, O'Rouke R, Walsh R, Poole-Wilson P, eds: *Hurst's The Heart.* 12th ed, Columbus, OH: McGraw-Hill; 2008:1077–1095.
10. Ranger S, Talajic M, Lemery R, et al. Kinetics of use-dependent ventricular conduction slowing by antiarrhythmic drugs in humans. *Circulation.* 1991;83:1987–1994.
11. Patel C, Salahuddin M, Jones A, et al. Atrial fibrillation: pharmacological therapy. *Curr Probl Cardiol.* 2011;36:87–120.
12. Ranger S, Talajic M, Lemery R, Roy D, Nattel S. Amplification of flecainide-induced ventricular conduction slowing by exercise. A potentially significant clinical consequence of use-dependent sodium channel blockade. *Circulation.* 1989;79:1000–1006.
13. Sala M, Coppa F, Cappucciati C, et al. Antidepressants: Their effects on cardiac channels, QT prolongation and Torsade de Pointes. *Curr Opin Investig Drugs.* 2006;7:256–263.
14. Antzelevitch C, Brugada P, Borggrefe M, et al. Brugada syndrome: Report of the second consensus conference. *Heart Rhythm.* 2005;2:429–440.
15. Hondeghem LM, Snyders DJ. Class III antiarrhythmic agents have a lot of potential but a long way to go. Reduced effectiveness and dangers of reverse use dependence. *Circulation.* 1990;81:686–690.
16. Groh WJ, Gibson KJ, Maylie JG. Comparison of the rate-dependent properties of the class III antiarrhythmic agents azimilide (NE-10064) and E-4031: Considerations on the mechanism of reverse rate-dependent action potential prolongation. *J Cardiovasc Electrophysiol.* 1997;8:529–536.
17. Fenichel RR, Malik M, Antzelevitch C, et al. Drug-induced torsades de pointes and implications for drug development. *J Cardiovasc Electrophysiol.* 2004;15:475–495.
18. Yan GX, Lankipalli RS, Burke JF, Musco S, Kowey PR. Ventricular repolarization components on the electrocardiogram: Cellular basis and clinical significance. *J Am Coll Cardiol.* 2003;42:401–409.
19. Roden DM. Taking the "idio" out of "idiosyncratic": Predicting torsades de pointes. *Pacing Clin Electrophysiol.* 1998;21:1029–1034.
20. Antzelevitch C. Role of transmural dispersion of repolarization in the genesis of drug-induced torsades de pointes. *Heart Rhythm.* 2005;2:S9–S15.
21. Antzelevitch C, Sicouri S, Litovsky SH, et al. Heterogeneity within the ventricular wall. Electrophysiology and

pharmacology of epicardial, endocardial, and M cells. *Circ Res.* 1991;69:1427–1449.

22. Antzelevitch C, Sicouri S, Di Diego JM, et al. Does Tpeak-Tend provide an index of transmural dispersion of repolarization? *Heart Rhythm.* 2007;4:1114–1116.
23. Barbhaiya C, Po JR, Hanon S, Schweitzer P. Tpeak - Tend and Tpeak - Tend /QT ratio as markers of ventricular arrhythmia risk in cardiac resynchronization therapy patients. *Pacing Clin Electrophysiol.* 2013;36:103–108.
24. Gupta P, Patel C, Patel H, et al. T(p-e)/QT ratio as an index of arrhythmogenesis. *J Electrocardiol.* 2008;41:567–574.
25. Panikkath R, Reinier K, Uy-Evanado A, et al. Prolonged Tpeak-to-Tend interval on the resting ECG is associated with increased risk of sudden cardiac death. *Circ Arrhythm Electrophysiol.* 2011;4:441–447.
26. Sicouri S, Moro S, Litovsky S, Elizari MV, Antzelevitch C. Chronic amiodarone reduces transmural dispersion of repolarization in the canine heart. *J Cardiovasc Electrophysiol.* 1997;8:1269–1279.
27. Hohnloser SH, Klingenheben T, Singh BN. Amiodarone-associated proarrhythmic effects. A review with special reference to torsade de pointes tachycardia. *Ann Intern Med.* 1994;121:529–535.
28. Patel C, Yan GX, Kowey PR. Dronedarone. *Circulation.* 2009;120:636–644.
29. Antzelevitch C, Burashnikov A, Sicouri S, Belardinelli L. Electrophysiologic basis for the antiarrhythmic actions of ranolazine. *Heart Rhythm.* 2011;8:1281–1290.
30. Hauptman PJ, Kelly RA. Digitalis. *Circulation.* 1999;99:1265–1270.
31. Ramirez FD, Femenia F, Simpson CS, et al. Electrocardiographic findings associated with cocaine use in humans: Asystematic review. *Expert Rev Cardiovasc Ther.* 2012;10:105–127.

INDEX